Non Invasive Brain Stimulation
in Psychiatry and Clinical Neurosciences

Bernardo Dell'Osso • Giorgio Di Lorenzo
Editors

Non Invasive Brain Stimulation in Psychiatry and Clinical Neurosciences

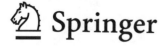

Editors
Bernardo Dell'Osso
ASST Fatebenefratelli Sacco
University of Milan
Milano
Italy

Giorgio Di Lorenzo
University of Rome Tor Vergata
Roma
Italy

ISBN 978-3-030-43358-1   ISBN 978-3-030-43356-7   (eBook)
https://doi.org/10.1007/978-3-030-43356-7

This Springer imprint is published by the registered company Springer Nature Switzerland AG
The registered company address is: Gewerbestrasse 11, 6330 Cham, Switzerland

Foreword

Non Invasive Brain Stimulation in Psychiatry and Clinical Neurosciences, edited by Bernardo Dell'Osso and Giorgio Di Lorenzo, and published by Springer, is a timely and authoritative text and a rare combination of a cutting-edge and user-friendly guide to TMS and tDCS. It includes seminal contributions from world renowned experts in this emerging field. Building on a foundational understanding of the mechanism of action of brain stimulation techniques, the book then translates these insights into clinical applications across a fascinating range of neuropsychiatric conditions. It carefully weighs the efficacy and safety of these approaches. These new treatments may be especially promising for depression and anxiety disorders, OCD, ADHD, addiction, as well as developmental disorders and dementia. This work spearheads the development of novel clinical neuroscience treatments based on the emerging understanding of underlying neural circuits and human behavior.

Eric Hollander
Albert Einstein College of Medicine,
Psychiatric Research Institute at Montefiore-Einstein
The Bronx, NY, USA

Foreword

This volume provides updated, cutting-edge information about the different brain stimulation technologies and lays out the neuroscience beyond NIBS. It brings essential guidance to clinicians on how to use NIBS in different diagnoses, including depression, psychosis, OCD, ADHD, Tourette, addictions, dementia, and anxiety. The Editors and the Contributors summarize in a clear, yet scientifically accurate and clinically useful, manner the state of the art of this exciting development in psychiatry in recent years. The Reader will come up with both an understanding of the neuroscience basis and how to clinically use those important tools that are currently available. This volume is an important addition to the bookshelves of every professional who is interested in understanding and treating disorders of the brain.

Joseph Zohar
Chaim Sheba Medical Center
Tel HaShomer, Israel

Acknowledgements

The Editors acknowledge the valuable contribution of Doctors Eleonora Piccoli, Federica Giorgetti, Laura Molteni, Rita Cafaro and Monica Macellaro of the University of Milan (Sacco Hospital) and Doctors Tommaso B. Jannini, Lucia Longo and Rodolfo Rossi of the University of Rome Tor Vergata in relation to proofs revision.

In recognition of the ongoing collaborations and contributions to the present volume, Editors acknowledge the following organizations:

- "Aldo Ravelli" Center for Neurotechnology and Brain Therapeutic, University of Milan, Milan, Italy;
- Associazione Italiana per le Terapie Somatiche in Psichiatria (AITESP);
- BrainTrends Ltd, IRCCS Fondazione Santa Lucia, Rome, Italy;
- European College of Neuropsychopharmacology (ECNP) Thematic Working Group on Neuromodulation;
- European Conference on Brain Stimulation in Psychiatry;
- Società Italiana di Psichiatria (SIP), Gruppo di Brain Stimulation in Psichiatria.

Contents

NIBS 2020: How TMS and tDCS Acquisitions Have Set New Standards in Clinical Neuroscience

1

Bernardo Dell'Osso and Giorgio Di Lorenzo

At the beginning of the millenium, not many neuroscientists and even less patient treating doctors could have predicted such a massive development in the field of non-invasive brain stimulation—otherwise known as "NIBS"—which became an innovative tool for neurophysiologic research, psychological and cognitive investigation, and, ultimately, clinical treatment of a wide spectrum of neuropsychiatric conditions. Indeed, transcranial magnetic stimulation (TMS) and transcranial direct current stimulation (tDCS) the main NIBS techniques—have become the mainstay of translational neuroscience as research tools for understanding cognitive and behavioral states. In addition, their efficacy has been acknowledged within guideline-recommended algorithms for the treatment of different neurological conditions and psychiatric disorders [1–3].

There are many reasons regarding the unprecedented growth of preclinical and clinical investigation with NIBS techniques. One of these is represented by their accessibility and possibility to be associated with other research methodologies and clinical devices, including structural and functional neuroimaging, electroencephalography, genetics, and epigenetics investigation. This has permitted our increased understanding of the network activity underlying both healthy human brain

B. Dell'Osso (✉)
Department of Biomedical and Clinical Sciences 'Luigi Sacco', University of Milan, ASST Fatebenefratelli-Sacco, Milan, Italy

'Aldo Ravelli' Research Center for Neurotechnology and Experimental Brain Therapeutics, Department of Health Sciences, University of Milan, Milan, Italy

Department of Psychiatry and Behavioural Sciences, Stanford University, Stanford, CA, USA
e-mail: bernardo.dellosso@unimi.it

G. Di Lorenzo
Department of Systems Medicine, University of Rome Tor Vergata, Rome, Italy

Psychiatry and Clinical Psychology Unit, Fondazione Policlinico Tor Vergata, Rome, Italy

IRCCS Fondazione Santa Lucia, Rome, Italy

© Springer Nature Switzerland AG 2020
B. Dell'Osso, G. Di Lorenzo (eds.), *Non Invasive Brain Stimulation in Psychiatry and Clinical Neurosciences*,
https://doi.org/10.1007/978-3-030-43356-7_1

functions as well as connectivity changes associated with dysfunctional states characterizing neuropsychiatric disorders.

On the other hand, as the acronym "NIBS" literally indicates, TMS and tDCS are considered safe and well-tolerated interventions for the investigation of neurophysiology, cognitive, affective, and other behavioral domains in healthy controls, as well as for the treatment of patients affected by different neuropsychiatric disorders. Indeed, the use of NIBS in neuroscience research not only allows us to investigate cortical excitability, cerebral connectivity, and neuroplasticity [4, 5] but, in relation to the clinical use of NIBS as therapeutic interventions, TMS and tDCS are considered by many clinicians and patients better tolerated than many psychotropic drugs, in light of their lack of systemic side-effects, including weight gain and sexual dysfunctions, which are often responsible for poor therapy compliance and treatment withdrawal in medicated patients. The favorable safety and tolerability profile of NIBS, however, is not to be claimed at the expense of the clinical efficacy of these interventions. For instance, since 2008, the American F.D.A. approved four different TMS devices for the treatment of Major Depressive Disorder with poor response to standard antidepressants. Lastly, NIBS techniques may also serve as adjuvants to support therapeutic activities across various disciplines, including re-learning or rehabilitative approaches, with encouraging results from field studies.

On this basis, the present book was conceived as a compendium of the latest acquisitions in the evolving field of NIBS, through the valuable contributions of a series of international experts in the areas of brain stimulation and neurophysiology, clinical psychology, neurology, and psychiatry. Across three sections, respectively, focused on (1) basic mechanisms of actions and rationale for the application of NIBS techniques in clinical neuroscience; (2) efficacy and safety of TMS; and (3) tDCS for the investigation and treatment of neuropsychiatric conditions and behavioral alterations, we sought to present a comprehensive and updated state of the art for NIBS in the aforementioned fields.

Because the unprecedented development of NIBS opened new ways for neuroscience by allowing researchers to validate their correlational theories through the direct manipulation of brain function for the first time [6], and for clinicians to safely approach difficult-to-treat conditions, we firmly believe that it deserves a place of priority in the modern education and wealth of knowledge of neuropsychiatrists, neurophysiologists, clinical psychologists, and other professionals involved in the study of neural mechanisms underlying emotions, cognition, and behavioral alterations.

Whether NIBS research in clinical neuroscience will contribute to the identification of biomarkers for specific diseases in the future still represents one of the greatest challenges; however, clinicians are currently focusing their efforts in identifying the best candidates and predictors of response to TMS and tDCS, optimizing stimulation parameters and anatomical targets. Notably, we have already been noticing the use of NIBS as therapeutic interventions for conditions that have been traditionally considered poor targets for psychotropic medications like, for instance, addictive behaviors and eating disorders with remarkable results [7].

Under these premises, we hope the present book will succeed in representing the uniqueness of NIBS as a translational research tool in clinical neuroscience through the peculiar capacity of TMS and tDCS to embrace different clinical and preclinical disciplines advancing their mutual understanding of brain functioning and alterations.

References

1. Lefaucheur JP, Antal A, Ayache SS, Benninger DH, Brunelin J, Cogiamanian F, Cotelli M, De Ridder D, Ferrucci R, Langguth B, Marangolo P, Mylius V, Nitsche MA, Padberg F, Palm U, Poulet E, Priori A, Rossi S, Schecklmann M, Vanneste S, Ziemann U, Garcia-Larrea L, Paulus W. Evidence-based guidelines on the therapeutic use of transcranial direct current stimulation (tDCS). Clin Neurophysiol. 2017;128(1):56–92s.
2. Lefaucheur JP, André-Obadia N, Antal A, Ayache SS, Baeken C, Benninger DH, Cantello RM, Cincotta M, de Carvalho M, De Ridder D, Devanne H, Di Lazzaro V, Filipović SR, Hummel FC, Jääskeläinen SK, Kimiskidis VK, Koch G, Langguth B, Nyffeler T, Oliviero A, Padberg F, Poulet E, Rossi S, Rossini PM, Rothwell JC, Schönfeldt-Lecuona C, Siebner HR, Slotema CW, Stagg CJ, Valls-Sole J, Ziemann U, Paulus W, Garcia-Larrea L. Evidence-based guidelines on the therapeutic use of repetitive transcranial magnetic stimulation (rTMS). Clin Neurophysiol. 2014;125(11):2150–206.
3. Milev RV, Giacobbe P, Kennedy SH, Blumberger DM, Daskalakis ZJ, Downar J, Modirrousta M, Patry S, Vila-Rodriguez F, Lam RW, MacQueen GM, Parikh SV, Ravindran AV, CANMAT Depression Work Group. Canadian Network for Mood and Anxiety Treatments (CANMAT) 2016 clinical guidelines for the management of adults with major depressive disorder: section 4. Neurostimulation treatments. Can J Psychiatr. 2016;61(9):561–75.
4. Di Lazzaro V, Rothwell J, Capogna M. Noninvasive stimulation of the human brain: activation of multiple cortical circuits. Neuroscientist. 2018;24(3):246–60.
5. Reinhart RM, Cosman JD, Fukuda K, Woodman GF. Using transcranial direct-current stimulation (tDCS) to understand cognitive processing. Atten Percept Psychophys. 2017;79(1):3–23.
6. Farzan F, Vernet M, Shafi MM, Rotenberg A, Daskalakis ZJ, Pascual-Leone A. Characterizing and modulating brain circuitry through transcranial magnetic stimulation combined with electroencephalography. Front Neural Circuits. 2016;10:73.
7. Yavari F, Shahbabaie A, Leite J, Carvalho S, Ekhtiari H, Fregni F. Noninvasive brain stimulation for addiction medicine: from monitoring to modulation. Prog Brain Res. 2016;224:371–99.

Part I

Introducing NIBS: From Research to Clinical Practice

Neurophysiological Bases and Mechanisms of Action of Transcranial Magnetic Stimulation

2

Vincenzo Di Lazzaro and Emma Falato

2.1 Introduction

Transcranial Magnetic Stimulation (TMS) is a neurophysiological technique that allows a noninvasive, painless stimulation of the human brain through the intact scalp.

Different brain areas can be targeted by TMS, depending on the position of the coil. TMS effects on motor areas have been better characterized compared to non-motor areas since the output produced by the stimulation of the primary motor area of one side can be easily recorded from muscles of the contralateral side of the body.

The application of noninvasive TMS to the human brain for assessing central motor pathways was described for the first time in 1985, in the *Lancet* journal, by A.T. Barker, R. Jalinous and I.L. Freeston, from the University of Sheffield [1].

The new TMS technique had a unique potential and some advantages compared to noninvasive transcranial electrical stimulation (TES), which was developed in 1980 by P.A. Merton and H.B. Morton [2]. Compared to TMS, TES requires high current densities to overcome the skull and to generate action potentials, resulting in painful and low tolerable stimulation.

The interest in TMS raised during the years and a consistent number of studies on this topic have advanced our knowledge of the human brain [3], even if many limitations exist due to the artificial nature of the stimulation. So far, many protocols of TMS stimulation have been tested and described, and different cortical circuits activated by TMS have been characterized [4, 5]. TMS can be used alone or in combination with other techniques in order to test corticospinal and cortico-cortical connectivity and brain plasticity, to map brain functions, and study specific cortical functions by inducing a "virtual lesion" in a targeted area [6–8].

V. Di Lazzaro (✉) · E. Falato
Unit of Neurology, Neurophysiology and Neurobiology, Università Campus Bio-Medico, Rome, Italy
e-mail: V.DiLazzaro@unicampus.it

© Springer Nature Switzerland AG 2020
B. Dell'Osso, G. Di Lorenzo (eds.), *Non Invasive Brain Stimulation in Psychiatry and Clinical Neurosciences*,
https://doi.org/10.1007/978-3-030-43356-7_2

A milestone in TMS history has been the demonstration that protocols based on repetitive TMS (rTMS) can induce prolonged effects, which outlast the period of stimulation [9, 10]. This evidence opened exciting research and clinical scenarios in which rTMS protocols are used for neuromodulatory/therapeutic purposes.

To date, TMS has a recognized role in the clinical and research settings. Stimulation protocols have been standardized, and safety limits of TMS stimulation have been established [11, 12]. Indeed, specific rTMS protocols received Food and Drug Administration (FDA) approval for the treatment of drug-resistant unipolar major depression.

In this chapter, we will review the evidence and the hypotheses on the neurophysiological bases and on the mechanisms of action of TMS, focusing on TMS application to the primary motor cortex.

2.2   How TMS Is Delivered

TMS is based on the Faraday's principle of electromagnetic induction, according to which a time-varying magnetic field will induce an electric current [13]. In TMS, a brief electric current is delivered through a capacitor to a coil, made of loops of copper wire embedded in a plastic case. Perpendicularly to the coil plane, a focal magnetic field is induced, which penetrates the scalp and the skull without attenuation and generates an electric current. If sufficiently strong, the induced electric current will change the electrical potential of the conductive superficial neuronal membranes leading to an action potential [14, 15].

The most widespread TMS devices can provide monophasic or biphasic pulse shapes with a determined width. More recently, TMS devices with controllable pulse parameters have been introduced [16].

Different types of coil exist, for superficial and deep targets of stimulation, and their effects have been modelled [17, 18]. Among the most frequently used coils, there are the figure-of-eight coil (which induces a more focal stimulation) and the circular coil (which induces a nonfocal stimulation of the brain) [4].

Focal coils can be oriented so as to induce currents in the brain with different directions: more commonly, the coil is kept perpendicularly to the central sulcus, and a posterior-to-anterior (PA) directed current is induced in the brain.

TMS spatial resolution and corticospinal output vary depending on several factors, including the shape of the stimulating coil, its position above the scalp, coil orientation, stimulation intensity, pulse waveform, ongoing voluntary muscle contraction, and other variables [19–22].

2.3   Single-Pulse TMS

The responses that can be recorded at the muscular level after TMS are named as motor-evoked potentials (MEPs) [1, 23–25] (Fig. 2.1). The optimal scalp location to evoke MEPs in the targeted muscle is defined as "hot-spot", while the minimum

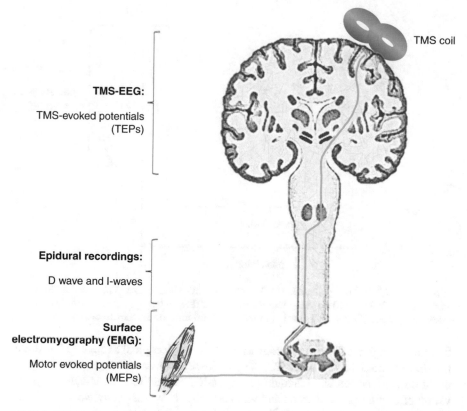

Fig. 2.1 TMS-induced responses at different recording levels

TMS stimulation intensity able to elicit consistent MEPs (with peak-to-peak amplitudes of at least 50 μV in each trial) in at least 5 out 10 consecutive TMS stimuli at rest is defined as resting motor threshold or RMT [12]. For each MEP, objective measures such as onset latency, peak latency, amplitude, and area can be obtained (Fig. 2.2). MEP amplitude, usually measured peak-to-peak, has an intrinsic variability of multifactorial origin [26, 27]. The mechanisms through which primary motor cortex TMS produces MEPs are partially understood due to the complexity of cortical circuits and the difficulty in assessing the interactions between the induced current in the brain and the neural networks, which are composed of different cell types, with different orientations and sizes. The physiological effects produced by motor cortex stimulation have been characterized first in animals, using direct electrical stimulation of the motor cortex together with the direct recording of the evoked corticospinal activity from the high cervical cord. These recordings revealed that a single electrical stimulus delivered to the motor cortex could produce a high-frequency (>600 Hz) repetitive discharge of corticospinal axons originating both from direct and indirect activation of corticospinal cells [28–30]. The earliest wave that is still recordable after cerebral cortex ablation was

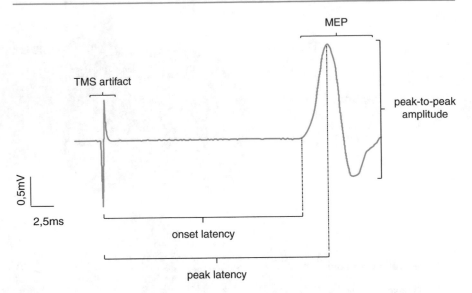

Fig. 2.2 Motor-evoked potential (MEP) elicited by single-pulse Transcranial Magnetic Stimulation (TMS) at 110% resting motor threshold (RMT) intensity, recorded from superficial electromyography (EMG) at the level of the contralateral first dorsal interosseous muscle

thought to originate from direct activation of the corticospinal axons and has therefore been termed the "D" wave [29]. The following waves that require the integrity of the cerebral cortex were thought to originate from indirect, trans-synaptic, activation of corticospinal neurons and were termed "I" waves. They were numbered in order of their appearance (I1, I2, I3, …). The interval between I-waves is about 1.5 ms, which corresponds to a discharge frequency of about 600 Hz. The same high-frequency corticospinal activity was subsequently recorded in humans after motor cortex TMS through epidural high cervical electrodes implanted for the treatment of chronic pain. This unique setting has provided relevant insight [31]. Indeed, it has been shown that also in humans the TMS-induced corticospinal descending activity is made by multiple descending high-frequency waves. Several studies showed that the composition of the corticospinal volleys in terms of D- and I-waves is influenced by the parameters of stimulation (stimulation intensity, coil type, and coil orientation) and by changes in cortical excitability (e.g., changes induced by voluntary contraction) [31, 32]. When the stimulating coil is aligned to induce a current perpendicularly to the line of the central sulcus (approximately posterior–anterior in the brain; PA), TMS evokes the earliest trans-synaptic response that, in analogy with animal recordings, is termed I1-wave. At higher intensities, this wave is followed by later waves numbered in order of their appearance (I2, I3, etc.) [31]. Only at very high stimulus intensity, a short-latency D-wave is evoked. When the induced current flows parallel to the line of the central sulcus (approximately lateral-to-medial in the brain; LM), only a D-wave is preferentially recruited. If the orientation of the induced current is kept perpendicular to the line of the central sulcus, but it is reversed (approximately anterior–posterior in the

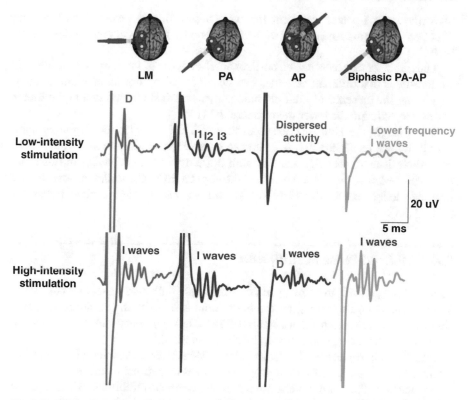

Fig. 2.3 Epidural recordings from the cervical cord of descending volleys evoked by lateromedial (LM), posterior–anterior (PA), anterior–posterior (AP), or biphasic (PA-AP) transcranial magnetic stimulation (TMS) at low and high intensity in patients with cervical epidural electrodes. At lower intensities of stimulation, the different orientations of the induced current evoke different cortico-spinal activities: LM TMS evokes D-waves; PA TMS elicits three I-waves; AP TMS evokes a dispersed activity, and no clear waves can be identified; biphasic TMS (PA followed by AP) evokes longer latency and lower frequency I-waves. At high intensity, all the directions of the induced current only evoke the high-frequency I-waves

brain; AP), the evoked activity is less synchronized, with some later peaks of latencies compared to those of the I-waves evoked by PA stimulation [31]. Similar findings have been obtained with biphasic stimulation (a PA-induced current followed by an AP-induced current): using biphasic TMS discharges, a corticospinal activity with a frequency that is half of that of the I-waves (about 330 Hz) has been recorded in some patients [4] (Fig. 2.3). These findings suggest that motor cortex TMS may activate not only the corticospinal neurons responding with a high-frequency discharge at I-wave frequency, but also different populations of corticospinal neurons responding at lower frequencies. However, these activities are usually not evident in volleys recorded at the epidural level because, as in animals, these volleys are dominated by fast conducting axons whose discharge is larger and more synchronous, particularly at high stimulation intensity. Only at lower intensities, different corticospinal outputs can be detected. Indeed, at high intensities of stimulation, the high-frequency I-waves represent the only output that is recorded with all the directions of the induced current in the brain and by both focal and nonfocal coils [4, 31] (Fig. 2.3).

Thus, the direct recording of corticospinal activity in humans and in animals demonstrates that different activities can be produced by transcranial stimulation, suggesting the presence of multiple independent cortical circuits within the motor cortex projecting to the lower motor neurons [4].

Interestingly, the simultaneous recording of TMS and electroencephalography (EEG), known as TMS-EEG, is emerging as a very useful clinical tool to assess cortico-cortical connectivity together with corticospinal connectivity. In this case, the TMS-evoked responses are recorded through the EEG electrodes as positive and negative deflections in the EEG signal and are called TMS-evoked potentials (TEPs) [33].

2.4   Paired-Pulse Stimulation

In paired-pulse TMS protocols, pairs of stimuli are delivered using two connected TMS stimulators. Depending on the interstimulus interval and stimulus intensity, the interaction between pairs of stimuli delivered to the primary motor cortex can be inhibitory or facilitatory, as assessed by MEP amplitude.

Specific paired-pulse TMS protocols have been described. Among the most frequently used in research, for their proposed role as an indirect measure of interneuronal function, there are the short-interval intracortical inhibition (SICI) and the intracortical facilitation (ICF) protocols. SICI and ICF are elicited by pairing a subthreshold conditioning stimulus and a suprathreshold test stimulus, delivered at 1–5 ms (SICI) or 8–30 ms (ICF) interstimulus interval (ISI), respectively. The result is a suppression (SICI) or a facilitation (ICF) of MEP amplitude [34, 35]. SICI has been mainly related to the activation of GABA-A receptors and to a reduction of late I-waves [36–38], while ICF has been in part attributed to glutamatergic NMDA receptor activation, even if it is less well understood [39, 40]. Other paired-pulse protocols are the short-interval intracortical facilitation (SICF) and the long-interval intracortical inhibition (LICI) (for more details see [4]).

Several other TMS protocols are used in research, being TMS a very versatile tool. These protocols include the interhemispheric inhibition (IHI), in which two TMS coils (one for each hemisphere) are used, and the very interesting protocols in which TMS is paired with peripheral electrical stimulation: short-latency afferent inhibition (SAI), long-latency afferent inhibition (LAI), and paired associative stimulation (PAS). For a more comprehensive list and description of TMS protocols, see [12]. Interestingly, epidural recordings in humans have shown that inhibitory protocols only suppress the later components of the corticospinal volley with no effect on the I1-wave [4]. This observation provides further support to the existence of independent cortical circuits producing different corticospinal activities with only some of them under a GABAergic inhibitory control.

2.5   Repetitive TMS (rTMS)

In rTMS, a repetitive stimulation, with biphasic or monophasic stimuli, is delivered over the scalp. rTMS targeting primary motor area showed to be able to induce prolonged effects on corticospinal excitability, which outlasted the stimulation from several minutes to some hours [9, 41]. The mechanisms underlying rTMS effects are still largely unknown. rTMS application on motor areas is commonly studied through the analysis of MEPs size before and after rTMS stimulation. In contrast, rTMS effects over nonmotor areas have more indirect outcome measures, including EEG and MRI connectivity measures and behavioral tests, whose interpretation requires more caution.

To date, existing evidence suggests that rTMS might induce changes in cortical and subcortical neurotransmitter release, with consequent prolonged changes in synaptic activity [42, 43].

rTMS applied to the dorsolateral prefrontal cortex (DLPFC), as in the treatment of depression, is thought to act not only on the stimulated area but also in distant regions, which are anatomically and/or functionally connected [44, 45].

rTMS classical protocols include low-frequency (LF) rTMS (≤1 Hz) and high-frequency (HF) rTMS (>1 Hz). Other popular rTMS protocols are the continuous theta-burst stimulation (cTBS) and the intermittent theta-burst stimulation (iTBS) (Fig. 2.4). Classically, LF rTMS and cTBS were considered inhibitory protocols,

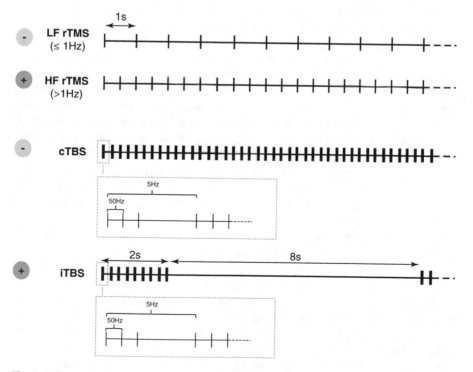

Fig. 2.4 Protocols of repetitive Transcranial Magnetic Stimulation (rTMS). Cf. text for details

able to induce long-term depression (LTD)-like plasticity, whereas HF rTMS and iTBS were considered excitatory protocols, able to induce long-term potentiation (LTP)-like plasticity [9]. However, it is now known that their effect is mixed and it depends on many variables, including the number of stimuli [46, 47], the intensity of stimulation, and the baseline cortical activation state [9, 48]. The after-effects of the different rTMS protocols are commonly described in terms of the changes that are produced in threshold or size of evoked MEPs, and the different protocols are simply classified as inhibitory or facilitatory, assuming that the physiological basis of all the inhibitory and of all the excitatory protocols are similar. However, epidural recordings in humans, performed before and after different rTMS protocols, have shown that, even though most protocols selectively modulate the late components of the corticospinal volleys, some of them could selectively modulate the earliest component or the inhibitory cortical circuits [25]. Thus, epidural recordings revealed that the effects of different protocols on cortical circuits are not homogeneous and that distinct protocols can modulate specific neural elements in distinct layers of the cortex. Different patterns of modulation have been demonstrated: (1) the most commonly observed change after rTMS is a selective modulation of late I-waves with no change in the amplitude of the I1-wave (i.e., inhibition is obtained after low-frequency rTMS (1 Hz), while a selective enhancement of late I-waves with no change in the amplitude of the I1-wave is observed after iTBS). This pattern indicates a more pronounced effect on cortico-cortical interneurons projecting on corticospinal cells with no change in the excitability of corticospinal cells; (2) after high-frequency rTMS (5 Hz), all the volleys are enhanced including the D-wave. This pattern highlights how that the excitability of corticospinal neurons is enhanced; (3) the cTBS protocol suppresses the I1-wave selectively, while later I-waves are much less affected. This suggests that cTBS has its major effect on a single source of inputs to corticospinal cells, which is responsible for the I1-wave production; (4) a very low-intensity and high-frequency stimulation has no effect on corticospinal volleys but suppresses intracortical inhibitory activity, as evaluated with paired-pulse stimulation, suggesting that this form of stimulation selectively modulates the excitability of GABAergic inhibitory networks in the motor cortex [25]. Thus, epidural recordings have shown that it might be possible to modulate specific cortical circuits using rTMS, and this could be extremely relevant because neural circuits that are differentially affected in various neuropsychiatric disorders can be targeted quite selectively with rTMS.

Extensive evidence supports the potential therapeutic applications of rTMS in specific neurological and psychiatric disorders [9].

The main clinical application of rTMS is drug-resistant unipolar major depression, for which rTMS received FDA approval in 2008. The optimal stimulation parameters for a safe and effective administration of rTMS in the treatment of depression have been recently reviewed [49]. The standard rTMS protocol used for the treatment of depression is the 10 Hz stimulation (trains of 4-second duration, with an intertrain interval of 26 seconds) delivered through a figure-of-eight coil, over the left DLPFC at an intensity of 120% relative to RMT. The total number of pulses per session is 3000. Each session lasts about 37 minutes. The total number of sessions is 20 (5 working days/week for 4 consecutive weeks).

In 2018, a randomized noninferiority trial, which included more than 400 patients (the largest trial of brain stimulation ever done), demonstrated that iTBS effectiveness is noninferior to that of the 10 Hz treatment, with very similar tolerability and safety profiles [50].

Since one iTBS session has a duration of about 3 minutes, approximately 10 times shorter than the standard 10 Hz rTMS session, the new protocol is advantageous in practical terms. However, the total number of sessions tested in the trial is still 20, which requires high patients' compliance.

Systematic clinical studies are still needed to define all the clinical indications of therapeutic rTMS and to identify effect predictors. Further research is also needed to clarify the mechanisms of action and to optimize the stimulation parameters.

References

1. Barker AT, Jalinous R, Freeston IL. Non-invasive magnetic stimulation of human motor cortex. Lancet. 1985;1(8437):1106–7.
2. Merton PA, Morton HB. Stimulation of the cerebral cortex in the intact human subject. Nature. 1980;285(5762):227.
3. Geddes LA. History of magnetic stimulation of the nervous system. J Clin Neurophysiol. 1991;8(1):3–9.
4. Di Lazzaro V, Rothwell J, Capogna M. Noninvasive stimulation of the human brain: activation of multiple cortical circuits. Neuroscientist. 2018;24(3):246–60.
5. Di Lazzaro V, Ziemann U. The contribution of transcranial magnetic stimulation in the functional evaluation of microcircuits in human motor cortex. Front Neural Circuits. 2013;7:18.
6. Siebner HR, Rothwell J. Transcranial magnetic stimulation: new insights into representational cortical plasticity. Exp Brain Res. 2003;148(1):1–16.
7. Hallett M. Transcranial magnetic stimulation: a primer. Neuron. 2007;55(2):187–99.
8. Hallett M, Di Iorio R, Rossini PM, Park JE, Chen R, Celnik P, et al. Contribution of transcranial magnetic stimulation to assessment of brain connectivity and networks. Clin Neurophysiol. 2017;128(11):2125–39.
9. Lefaucheur JP, Andre-Obadia N, Antal A, Ayache SS, Baeken C, Benninger DH, et al. Evidence-based guidelines on the therapeutic use of repetitive transcranial magnetic stimulation (rTMS). Clin Neurophysiol. 2014;125(11):2150–206.
10. Huang YZ, Edwards MJ, Rounis E, Bhatia KP, Rothwell JC. Theta burst stimulation of the human motor cortex. Neuron. 2005;45(2):201–6.
11. Rossi S, Hallett M, Rossini PM, Pascual-Leone A. Safety of TMSCG. Safety, ethical considerations, and application guidelines for the use of transcranial magnetic stimulation in clinical practice and research. Clin Neurophysiol. 2009;120(12):2008–39.
12. Rossini PM, Burke D, Chen R, Cohen LG, Daskalakis Z, Di Iorio R, et al. Non-invasive electrical and magnetic stimulation of the brain, spinal cord, roots and peripheral nerves: basic principles and procedures for routine clinical and research application. An updated report from an I.F.C.N. Committee. Clin Neurophysiol. 2015;126(6):1071–107.
13. Faraday M. Experimental researches in electricity. Second Series. Phil Trans Roy Soc London. 1832;122, 163.
14. Eldaief MC, Press DZ, Pascual-Leone A. Transcranial magnetic stimulation in neurology: a review of established and prospective applications. Neurol Clin Pract. 2013;3(6):519–26.

15. Holtzheimer PE, McDonald W. A clinical guide to transcranial magnetic stimulation. Oxford: Oxford University Press; 2014.
16. Peterchev AV, Wagner TA, Miranda PC, Nitsche MA, Paulus W, Lisanby SH, et al. Fundamentals of transcranial electric and magnetic stimulation dose: definition, selection, and reporting practices. Brain Stimul. 2012;5(4):435–53.
17. Deng ZD, Lisanby SH, Peterchev AV. Coil design considerations for deep transcranial magnetic stimulation. Clin Neurophysiol. 2014;125(6):1202–12.
18. Deng ZD, Lisanby SH, Peterchev AV. Electric field depth-focality tradeoff in transcranial magnetic stimulation: simulation comparison of 50 coil designs. Brain Stimul. 2013;6(1):1–13.
19. Di Lazzaro V, Oliviero A, Mazzone P, Insola A, Pilato F, Saturno E, et al. Comparison of descending volleys evoked by monophasic and biphasic magnetic stimulation of the motor cortex in conscious humans. Exp Brain Res. 2001;141(1):121–7.
20. Di Lazzaro V, Oliviero A, Pilato F, Saturno E, Insola A, Mazzone P, et al. Descending volleys evoked by transcranial magnetic stimulation of the brain in conscious humans: effects of coil shape. Clin Neurophysiol. 2002;113(1):114–9.
21. Di Lazzaro V, Oliviero A, Profice P, Insola A, Mazzone P, Tonali P, et al. Effects of voluntary contraction on descending volleys evoked by transcranial electrical stimulation over the motor cortex hand area in conscious humans. Exp Brain Res. 1999;124(4):525–8.
22. Di Lazzaro V, Restuccia D, Oliviero A, Profice P, Ferrara L, Insola A, et al. Magnetic transcranial stimulation at intensities below active motor threshold activates intracortical inhibitory circuits. Exp Brain Res. 1998;119(2):265–8.
23. Hess CW, Mills KR, Murray NM. Responses in small hand muscles from magnetic stimulation of the human brain. J Physiol. 1987;388:397–419.
24. Berardelli A, Inghilleri M, Cruccu G, Manfredi M. Descending volley after electrical and magnetic transcranial stimulation in man. Neurosci Lett. 1990;112(1):54–8.
25. Di Lazzaro V, Rothwell JC. Corticospinal activity evoked and modulated by non-invasive stimulation of the intact human motor cortex. J Physiol. 2014;592(19):4115–28.
26. Kiers L, Cros D, Chiappa KH, Fang J. Variability of motor potentials evoked by transcranial magnetic stimulation. Electroencephalogr Clin Neurophysiol. 1993;89(6):415–23.
27. Torrecillos F, Falato E, Pogosyan A, West T, Di Lazzaro V, Brown P. Motor cortex inputs at the optimum phase of beta cortical oscillations undergo more rapid and less variable corticospinal propagation. J Neurosci. 2019;40(2):369–81.
28. Adrian ED, Moruzzi G. Impulses in the pyramidal tract. J Physiol. 1939;97(2):153–99.
29. Patton HD, Amassian VE. Single and multiple-unit analysis of cortical stage of pyramidal tract activation. J Neurophysiol. 1954;17(4):345–63.
30. Kernell D, Chien-Ping WU. Responses of the pyramidal tract to stimulation of the baboon's motor cortex. J Physiol. 1967;191(3):653–72.
31. Di Lazzaro V, Profice P, Ranieri F, Capone F, Dileone M, Oliviero A, et al. I-wave origin and modulation. Brain Stimul. 2012;5(4):512–25.
32. Di Lazzaro V, Restuccia D, Oliviero A, Profice P, Ferrara L, Insola A, et al. Effects of voluntary contraction on descending volleys evoked by transcranial stimulation in conscious humans. J Physiol. 1998;508(Pt 2):625–33.
33. Tremblay S, Rogasch NC, Premoli I, Blumberger DM, Casarotto S, Chen R, et al. Clinical utility and prospective of TMS-EEG. Clin Neurophysiol. 2019;130(5):802–44.
34. Kujirai T, Caramia MD, Rothwell JC, Day BL, Thompson PD, Ferbert A, et al. Corticocortical inhibition in human motor cortex. J Physiol. 1993;471:501–19.
35. Ziemann U, Rothwell JC, Ridding MC. Interaction between intracortical inhibition and facilitation in human motor cortex. J Physiol. 1996;496(Pt 3):873–81.
36. Di Lazzaro V, Oliviero A, Meglio M, Cioni B, Tamburrini G, Tonali P, et al. Direct demonstration of the effect of lorazepam on the excitability of the human motor cortex. Clin Neurophysiol. 2000;111(5):794–9.

37. Di Lazzaro V, Pilato F, Dileone M, Profice P, Ranieri F, Ricci V, et al. Segregating two inhibitory circuits in human motor cortex at the level of GABAA receptor subtypes: a TMS study. Clin Neurophysiol. 2007;118(10):2207–14.
38. Hanajima R, Ugawa Y, Terao Y, Sakai K, Furubayashi T, Machii K, et al. Paired-pulse magnetic stimulation of the human motor cortex: differences among I waves. J Physiol. 1998;509(Pt 2):607–18.
39. Ziemann U, Reis J, Schwenkreis P, Rosanova M, Strafella A, Badawy R, et al. TMS and drugs revisited 2014. Clin Neurophysiol. 2015;126(10):1847–68.
40. Di Lazzaro V, Pilato F, Dileone M, Saturno E, Oliviero A, Marra C, et al. In vivo cholinergic circuit evaluation in frontotemporal and Alzheimer dementias. Neurology. 2006;66(7):1111–3.
41. Esser SK, Huber R, Massimini M, Peterson MJ, Ferrarelli F, Tononi G. A direct demonstration of cortical LTP in humans: a combined TMS/EEG study. Brain Res Bull. 2006;69(1):86–94.
42. Fitzgerald PB, Daskalakis ZJ. The mechanism of action of rTMS. Repetitive transcranial magnetic stimulation treatment for depressive disorders: a practical guide. Berlin: Springer; 2013. p. 13–27.
43. Soundara Rajan T, Ghilardi MFM, Wang HY, Mazzon E, Bramanti P, Restivo D, et al. Mechanism of action for rTMS: a working hypothesis based on animal studies. Front Physiol. 2017;8:457.
44. Diana M, Raij T, Melis M, Nummenmaa A, Leggio L, Bonci A. Rehabilitating the addicted brain with transcranial magnetic stimulation. Nat Rev Neurosci. 2017;18(11):685–93.
45. Anderson RJ, Hoy KE, Daskalakis ZJ, Fitzgerald PB. Repetitive transcranial magnetic stimulation for treatment resistant depression: re-establishing connections. Clin Neurophysiol. 2016;127(11):3394–405.
46. Gamboa OL, Antal A, Moliadze V, Paulus W. Simply longer is not better: reversal of theta burst after-effect with prolonged stimulation. Exp Brain Res. 2010;204(2):181–7.
47. Nettekoven C, Volz LJ, Kutscha M, Pool EM, Rehme AK, Eickhoff SB, et al. Dose-dependent effects of theta burst rTMS on cortical excitability and resting-state connectivity of the human motor system. J Neurosci. 2014;34(20):6849–59.
48. Silvanto J, Pascual-Leone A. State-dependency of transcranial magnetic stimulation. Brain Topogr. 2008;21(1):1–10.
49. McClintock SM, Reti IM, Carpenter LL, McDonald WM, Dubin M, Taylor SF, et al. Consensus recommendations for the clinical application of repetitive transcranial magnetic stimulation (rTMS) in the treatment of depression. J Clin Psychiatry. 2018;79(1).
50. Blumberger DM, Vila-Rodriguez F, Thorpe KE, Feffer K, Noda Y, Giacobbe P, et al. Effectiveness of theta burst versus high-frequency repetitive transcranial magnetic stimulation in patients with depression (THREE-D): a randomised non-inferiority trial. Lancet. 2018;391(10131):1683–92.

Neurophysiological Bases and Mechanisms of Action of Transcranial Direct Current Stimulation (tDCS)

3

Tommaso Bocci, Roberta Ferrucci, and Alberto Priori

3.1 Overview

Transcranial Direct Current Stimulation (tDCS) of the brain has emerged in the past two decades as a novel, noninvasive, cheap, and safe technique to modulate cortical excitability in humans, both in health and disease. Clinical applications ranged from post-stroke recovery [1] and movement disorders [2] to pain syndromes [3] and neuropsychiatric diseases [4, 5]. Recently, tDCS has also been proposed for pediatric use, showing promising results for the treatment of cerebral palsy [6, 7], refractory epilepsies [8], and Attention Deficit Hyperactivity Disorder [9].

tDCS commonly uses subthreshold currents (1.0–2.5 mA), too weak to induce neuronal activity independent from afferent input, but sufficient *per se* to alter both the excitability and spontaneous neuronal firing rate.

Despite a growing body of literature, putative mechanisms of action remain to be completely elucidated, both at molecular and cellular levels (see Fig. 3.1). Moreover, some questions are still unanswered: (1) whether tDCS can interfere with gene expression and protein folding; (2) how neuronal activity is modulated during and following tDCS (online effects versus offline aftereffects); and (3) how long neuronal and subsequent behavioral changes persist. In this chapter, we encompass the current knowledge about tDCS action in humans, suggesting novel mechanisms underlying its use in neuropsychiatric disorders and strengthening the importance of neurophysiological monitoring in human diseases.

T. Bocci (✉) · R. Ferrucci · A. Priori
"Aldo Ravelli" Research Center for Neurotechnology and Experimental Brain Therapeutics, Department of Health Sciences, Neurology Unit, University of Milan, San Paolo University Hospital, Milan, Italy
e-mail: tommaso.bocci@unimi.it; roberta.ferrucci@unimi.it; alberto.priori@unimi.it

© Springer Nature Switzerland AG 2020
B. Dell'Osso, G. Di Lorenzo (eds.), *Non Invasive Brain Stimulation in Psychiatry and Clinical Neurosciences*,
https://doi.org/10.1007/978-3-030-43356-7_3

Fig. 3.1 An overview of tDCS mechanisms of action. tDCS exerts both nonsynaptic and synaptic changes, modulating at the same time the inflammatory response and regional blood flow

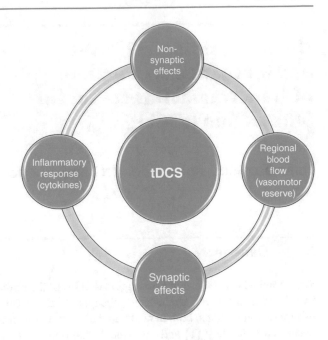

3.2   Basic tDCS Effects

Overall, tDCS effects are cumulative, nonlinear, and polarity-dependent [10–14]. From a molecular point of view, tDCS shows both short- and long-term effects; the first ones usually outlast the end of stimulation for only a few minutes and involve nonsynaptic mechanisms, comprising changes in membrane polarity, migration, and steric conformation of transmembrane proteins; conversely, the long-term after-effects are mainly mediated by synaptic modifications (Fig. 3.2). In particular, among synaptic changes, anodal and cathodal tDCS seem to have similar effects on different brain neurotransmitters: while anodal tDCS reduces GABA and increases myoinositol, cathodal tDCS decreases glutamate levels [15, 16], respectively, driving long-term potentiation and depression-like phenomena (LTP, LTD).

Nonetheless, the relationship between inhibition and stimulation is not so linear as previously described; the intra- and interindividual variability of tDCS action also depends on genetic polymorphisms [13], as well as on the preexisting excitability state of the cortex, a phenomenon referred to as "metaplasticity" and primed by N-methyl-D-aspartate receptors [17, 18]. In healthy humans, the existence of "metaplasticity" has been demonstrated by using neurophysiological methods, both in the primary motor [17] and visual cortex [18]. This kind of plasticity could explain, at least in part, some paradoxical effects, in that anodal tDCS can actually lead to dampened excitability when the stimulation time is increased [19], and cathodal tDCS can sometimes increase excitability when intensity is improved [20].

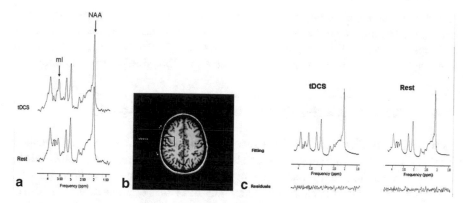

Fig. 3.2 tDCS and nonsynaptic effects. Active tDCS (anodal) over the right frontal lobe induces an increase in myoinositol (mI) content in healthy humans, as proved by the analysis of MRS spectra; given that tDCS alters biophysical properties of the membrane, it influences phospholipid's metabolism and, in turn, mI concentration (modified from Rango *et al.*, 2008, with permission)

From a cellular perspective, both synaptic and nonsynaptic effects of direct polarization ultimately lead to changes in phenotypic and functional aspects, such as morphology, orientation, migration, and cellular growth, as recognized for nearly a century [21]. The possibility to interfere with cells' migration is of particular interest for the development of nonneural cells (e.g., microglia) and for the modulation of immune responses in the human brain, even in adulthood, as discussed below in more detail.

Finally, although tDCS has been primarily studied for its cortical effects, recent animal data have suggested that direct polarization (1–4.16 A/m^2) may also affect subcortical white matter structures, such as the red nucleus, medial longitudinal fascicle [22, 23], and thalamus, likely through changes in regional blood flow and cerebral vasomotor reserve [24, 25].

3.3 Nonsynaptic Mechanisms

tDCS exerts nonsynaptic mechanisms of action. These effects involve changes at different levels, as proved in humans by historical neurophysiological evidence [11]. One of these is the ability to modify neuronal membrane polarity and its threshold for action potential generation, likely affecting the spike timing of individual neurons receiving suprathreshold inputs [26–28]. This effect critically depends on the orientation of the axons relative to the electric field [14, 29], thus driving the direction of tDCS modulation (excitation versus inhibition). For instance, when the electrical field is perpendicular to the axons, the physiological effects of stimulation are negligible, whereas if the current flows longitudinally, these effects are more pronounced, as larger membrane compartments are homogeneously polarized [30]. Together with the abovementioned "metaplasticity", this is another critical source of variability to predict behavioral effects of tDCS in humans, as in complex brain structures, synapses are not always oriented in the same direction.

3.4 Synaptic Mechanisms (Neuroplastic Changes)

Long-lasting tDCS aftereffects are recognized to be driven mainly by synaptic changes. GABA and glutamate, especially through NMDA receptors (NMDARs), are the most studied neurotransmitters regarding tDCS aftereffects in humans. This is of particular interest because a huge amount of evidence indicates abnormalities of glutamatergic neurotransmission or glutamatergic dysfunction as playing a key role in the development of schizophrenia, bipolar disorder, and major depressive disorder [31–33]. Moreover, changes in glutamatergic and GABAergic activity can be easily evaluated and monitored over time by using paired-pulse Transcranial Magnetic Stimulation (TMS) protocols [34–38].

Pharmacological studies have demonstrated that blockade of NMDA receptors prevents tDCS-induced excitability changes, for anodal as well as cathodal polarization, whereas NMDAR agonists improve anodal aftereffects [39, 40]. In particular, NMDARs regulate the influx of calcium ions (Ca^{2+}) into the neuron, a critical step to modulate the induction of both LTD and LTP plasticity [41, 42].

Regarding GABA modulation, a hierarchical model has been recently proposed: anodal tDCS also decreases GABA, thus leading to an increase in neuronal firing rates, which in turn enhances both local gamma-band oscillatory activity and functional connectivity among highly connected areas [43–45]. The possibility to modulate gamma-band, through a reduction in GABA release, is intriguing because this oscillatory activity seems to be selectively impaired in schizophrenia, although the exact relationship with disease mechanisms is not completely understood [46, 47].

3.5 New Frontiers in the tDCS Effects in Neuropsychiatric Diseases

In recent years, novel potential mechanisms have been explored, including a putative action on the inflammatory response. In particular, animal studies have proved that tDCS has a polarity-specific migratory effect on neural stem cells (NSC) in vivo, thus influencing the development and the distribution of microglia in the adult brain [48]. In addition, tDCS seems to directly modulate inflammatory response by downregulating pro-inflammatory cytokines [49].

Although not yet confirmed in humans, these results are intriguing for the use of tDCS in the treatment of neuropsychiatric disorders. In fact, recent evidence strengthens the role of inflammation in the pathophysiology of schizophrenia and other neurodegenerative diseases; in particular, the role of microglia in psychosis has been suggested, as the immune system plays not only an essential role in inflammatory processes but also in neurodevelopment and synapse refinement [50–53].

Further studies are needed to better understand the putative role of tDCS in modulating inflammatory responses, both in health and disease.

3.6   Contribution of Neurophysiology in the Study of tDCS Aftereffects

3.6.1   Transcranial Magnetic Stimulation (TMS)

Plastic changes induced by tDCS could be objectively assessed and monitored over time by using neurophysiological techniques, such as Transcranial Magnetic Stimulation (TMS). Single-pulse TMS has been used in the past to evaluate the effects of anodal and cathodal polarization of Motor Evoked Potentials (MEPs) in humans [10, 54], whereas paired-pulse TMS specifically investigates intracortical synaptic changes induced by tDCS [35–37]. Moreover, other TMS parameters can predict the response to tDCS modulation: in particular, the latency and duration of transcallosal inhibition (TI), as measured by single-pulse TMS, are significantly correlated to the extent of tDCS modulation [55]. That is of critical importance in the selection of patients who may benefit from early noninvasive neuromodulation strategies.

3.6.2   Electroencephalography (EEG) and Event-Related Potentials (ERPs)

EEG has been used to provide valuable information on the tDCS mechanisms of action. In particular, anodal tDCS has proved to increase alpha and beta power during and after stimulation, thus leading to a widespread activation of functionally connected brain areas [56]. This finding supports the use of tDCS for modulating the "resting state" of the brain, especially in cognitive and neurodegenerative disorders. Similarly, combined TMS-EEG studies have suggested that anodal tDCS specifically affects task-related functional networks, and the boost of specific circuits correlates with the observed clinical cognitive enhancement [57, 58]. Also, the endogenous event-related potentials (P3-ERPs) seem to be valuable markers for monitoring tDCS aftereffects on specific pathways involved in cognition; for instance, tDCS applied over the dorsolateral prefrontal cortex (DLPC) increases P3 amplitudes, supporting the role of DLPC both in preattentive and attentive functions [59–61]. In another study, Radman and co-workers have proved that tDCS applied over the DLPC also modulates language processing, without facilitating overt second language word production [62]. Similarly, Baptista and colleagues have shown that the stimulation of the medial prefrontal cortex modulates ironic information at the initial stage of irony comprehension [63], a phenomenon impaired in several neuropsychiatric disorders, such as autism [64, 65] and schizophrenia [66].

3.7 Novel Targets for Noninvasive DC Polarization in Humans

3.7.1 The Cerebellum

In the past decade, the cerebellum and the spinal cord have emerged as novel promising targets for tDCS action, also for the treatment of neuropsychiatric diseases [67]. For instance, recent modeling studies strengthen the spatial selectivity of either cerebellar or spinal stimulation [68–70].

Nonetheless, their mechanisms of action have been only partly elucidated.

Cerebellar tDCS has both online and offline effects on cerebellar excitability. Animal data suggest that the electrical stimulation of Purkinje cells mediates online effects [71], whereas depolarization of Golgi inhibitory neurons is responsible for long-lasting changes [72]. Purkinje cells represent the output from the cerebellar cortex, and their activation leads to the inhibition of the dentate nucleus, ultimately dampening motor cortex excitability, a phenomenon referred to as "cerebellar-brain inhibition", or CBI [73]. Cerebellar tDCS may ultimately interfere with this connectivity, with anodal stimulation likely increasing and cathodal polarization reducing CBI. From a molecular perspective, the cerebellum contains the same neurotransmitters of the cerebral cortex (e.g., GABA and glutamate); consequently, both synaptic and nonsynaptic changes induced by cerebellar tDCS should be similar to those previously discussed about brain tDCS.

Cerebellar tDCS has shown encouraging results for the treatment of movement disorders [74, 75] and pain syndromes [76], as well as for schizophrenia [77] and bipolar disorder [78].

3.7.2 Spinal Cord

As concerns spinal tDCS, anodal stimulation has probably an overall inhibitory effect on spinal cord activity [79–82]. Particularly, while anodal polarization could act directly on cortico-spinal descending pathways, cathodal stimulation interferes with interneuronal networks [3, 83, 84]. By analogy with the effects of direct currents on peripheral nerves, it has been hypothesized that anodal transcutaneous spinal DCS (tsDCS) leads to a hyperpolarizing "anodal block" [85]. Overall, as suggested for tDCS [15], rather than be simply specular, anodal and cathodal tsDCS may have similar effects on different targets.

Many studies have also shown possible supra-spinal mechanisms of action of spinal direct current stimulation, both in animals [86] and humans [3, 87], possibly synchronizing activity among different cortical areas and inducing neuroplasticity [88]. That is also not surprising, considering the literature about invasive current stimulation (Spinal Cord Stimulation, SCS), suggesting a possible modulation of glutamatergic cortical interneurons in patients with neuropathic pain [89]. Moreover, it is known that alternating currents epidurally delivered to the posterior columns of the spinal cord are able to modify sensory processing at thalamic relays and cortical levels [90]. Recently, studies from our laboratories have explored two main non-spinal targets, (1) GABA-A cortical interneurons, mediating so-called "short intracortical inhibition" (SICI) [3], and (2) interhemispheric processing [87].

Spinal tDCS has not been used for the treatment of neuropsychiatric disorders yet, but the possibility to modulate supra-spinal and cortical networks is intriguing for a combined cortico-spinal (or cerebello-spinal) stimulation, thus potentially increasing behavioral changes through different, but not mutually exclusive, mechanisms of action.

References

1. Sohn MK, Jee SJ, Kim YW. Effect of transcranial direct current stimulation on postural stability and lower extremity strength in hemiplegic stroke patients. Ann Rehabil Med. 2013;37(6):759–65.
2. Benninger DH, Lomarev M, Lopez G, Wassermann EM, Li X, Considine E, et al. Transcranial direct current stimulation for the treatment of Parkinson's disease. J Neurol Neurosurg Psychiatry. 2010;81(10):1105–11.
3. Bocci T, Marceglia S, Vergari M, Cognetto V, Cogiamanian F, Sartucci F, et al. Transcutaneous spinal direct current stimulation modulates human corticospinal system excitability. J Neurophysiol. 2015;114(1):440–6.
4. Andrade C. Once- to twice-daily, 3-year domiciliary maintenance transcranial direct current stimulation for severe, disabling, clozapine-refractory continuous auditory hallucinations in schizophrenia. J ECT. 2013;29(3):239–42.
5. Dell'Osso B, Zanoni S, Ferrucci R, Vergari M, Castellano F, D'Urso N, et al. Transcranial direct current stimulation for the outpatient treatment of poor-responder depressed patients. Eur Psychiatry. 2012;27(7):513–7.
6. Saleem GT, Crasta JE, Slomine BS, Cantarero GL, Suskauer SJ. Transcranial direct current stimulation in pediatric motor disorders: a systematic review and meta-analysis. Arch Phys Med Rehabil. 2019;100(4):724–38.
7. Kirton A, Ciechanski P, Zewdie E, Andersen J, Nettel-Aguirre A, Carlson H, et al. Transcranial direct current stimulation for children with perinatal stroke and hemiparesis. Neurology. 2017;88(3):259–67.
8. Lin LC, Ouyang CS, Chiang CT, Yang RC, Wu RC, Wu HC. Cumulative effect of transcranial direct current stimulation in patients with partial refractory epilepsy and its association with phase lag index—a preliminary study. Epilepsy Behav. 2018;84:142–7.
9. Sierawska A, Prehn-Kristensen A, Moliadze V, Krauel K, Nowak R, Freitag CM, et al. Unmet needs in children with attention deficit hyperactivity disorder-can transcranial direct current stimulation fill the gap? Promises and ethical challenges. Front Psychiatry. 2019;10:334.
10. Priori A, Berardelli A, Rona S, Accornero N, Manfredi M. Polarization of the human motor cortex through the scalp. Neuroreport. 1998;9(10):2257–60.
11. Ardolino G, Bossi B, Barbieri S, Priori A. Non-synaptic mechanisms underlie the after-effects of cathodal transcutaneous direct current stimulation of the human brain. J Physiol. 2005;568(Pt 2):653–63.
12. Cambiaghi M, Velikova S, Gonzalez-Rosa JJ, Cursi M, Comi G, Leocani L. Brain transcranial direct current stimulation modulates motor excitability in mice. Eur J Neurosci. 2010;31(4):704–9.
13. Fritsch B, Reis J, Martinowich K, Schambra HM, Ji Y, Cohen LG, et al. Direct current stimulation promotes BDNF-dependent synaptic plasticity: potential implications for motor learning. Neuron. 2010;66(2):198–204.
14. Kabakov AY, Muller PA, Pascual-Leone A, Jensen FE, Rotenberg A. Contribution of axonal orientation to pathway-dependent modulation of excitatory transmission by direct current stimulation in isolated rat hippocampus. J Neurophysiol. 2012;107(7):1881–9.

15. Stagg CJ, Best JG, Stephenson MC, O'Shea J, Wylezinska M, Kincses ZT, et al. Polarity-sensitive modulation of cortical neurotransmitters by transcranial stimulation. J Neurosci. 2009;29(16):5202–6.
16. Rango M, Cogiamanian F, Marceglia S, Barberis B, Arighi A, Biondetti P, et al. Myoinositol content in the human brain is modified by transcranial direct current stimulation in a matter of minutes: a 1H-MRS study. Magn Reson Med. 2008;60(4):782–9.
17. Siebner HR, Lang N, Rizzo V, Nitsche MA, Paulus W, Lemon RN, et al. Preconditioning of low-frequency repetitive transcranial magnetic stimulation with transcranial direct current stimulation: evidence for homeostatic plasticity in the human motor cortex. J Neurosci. 2004;24(13):3379–85.
18. Bocci T, Caleo M, Tognazzi S, Francini N, Briscese L, Maffei L, et al. Evidence for metaplasticity in the human visual cortex. J Neural Transm (Vienna). 2014;121(3):221–31.
19. Monte-Silva K, Kuo MF, Hessenthaler S, Fresnoza S, Liebetanz D, Paulus W, et al. Induction of late LTP-like plasticity in the human motor cortex by repeated non-invasive brain stimulation. Brain Stimul. 2013;6(3):424–32.
20. Batsikadze G, Moliadze V, Paulus W, Kuo MF, Nitsche MA. Partially non-linear stimulation intensity-dependent effects of direct current stimulation on motor cortex excitability in humans. J Physiol. 2013;591(7):1987–2000.
21. McCaig CD, Rajnicek AM, Song B, Zhao M. Controlling cell behavior electrically: current views and future potential. Physiol Rev. 2005;85(3):943–78.
22. Bolzoni F, Baczyk M, Jankowska E. Subcortical effects of transcranial direct current stimulation in the rat. J Physiol. 2013;591(16):4027–42.
23. Bolzoni F, Pettersson LG, Jankowska E. Evidence for long-lasting subcortical facilitation by transcranial direct current stimulation in the cat. J Physiol. 2013;591(13):3381–99.
24. Lang N, Siebner HR, Ward NS, Lee L, Nitsche MA, Paulus W, et al. How does transcranial DC stimulation of the primary motor cortex alter regional neuronal activity in the human brain? Eur J Neurosci. 2005;22(2):495–504.
25. Giorli E, Tognazzi S, Briscese L, Bocci T, Mazzatenta A, Priori A, et al. Transcranial direct current stimulation and cerebral vasomotor reserve: a study in healthy subjects. J Neuroimaging. 2015;25(4):571–4.
26. Liebetanz D, Nitsche MA, Tergau F, Paulus W. Pharmacological approach to the mechanisms of transcranial DC-stimulation-induced after-effects of human motor cortex excitability. Brain. 2002;125(Pt 10):2238–47.
27. Stagg CJ, Nitsche MA. Physiological basis of transcranial direct current stimulation. Neuroscientist. 2011;17(1):37–53.
28. Anastassiou CA, Perin R, Markram H, Koch C. Ephaptic coupling of cortical neurons. Nat Neurosci. 2011;14(2):217–23.
29. Purpura DP, McMurtry JG. Intracellular activities and evoked potential changes during polarization of motor cortex. J Neurophysiol. 1965;28:166–85.
30. Jefferys JG. Influence of electric fields on the excitability of granule cells in guinea-pig hippocampal slices. J Physiol. 1981;319:143–52.
31. Li CT, Lu CF, Lin HC, Huang YZ, Juan CH, Su TP, et al. Cortical inhibitory and excitatory function in drug-naive generalized anxiety disorder. Brain Stimul. 2017;10(3):604–8.
32. Li CT, Yang KC, Lin WC. Glutamatergic dysfunction and glutamatergic compounds for major psychiatric disorders: evidence from clinical neuroimaging studies. Front Psych. 2018;9:767.
33. Ohgi Y, Futamura T, Hashimoto K. Glutamate signaling in synaptogenesis and NMDA receptors as potential therapeutic targets for psychiatric disorders. Curr Mol Med. 2015; 15(3):206–21.
34. Kujirai T, Caramia MD, Rothwell JC, Day BL, Thompson PD, Ferbert A, et al. Corticocortical inhibition in human motor cortex. J Physiol. 1993;471:501–19.
35. Di Lazzaro V, Manganelli F, Dileone M, Notturno F, Esposito M, Capasso M, et al. The effects of prolonged cathodal direct current stimulation on the excitatory and inhibitory circuits of the ipsilateral and contralateral motor cortex. J Neural Transm (Vienna). 2012;119(12):1499–506.

36. Cengiz B, Murase N, Rothwell JC. Opposite effects of weak transcranial direct current stimulation on different phases of short interval intracortical inhibition (SICI). Exp Brain Res. 2013;225(3):321–31.
37. Vaseghi B, Zoghi M, Jaberzadeh S. The effects of anodal-tDCS on corticospinal excitability enhancement and its after-effects: conventional vs unihemispheric concurrent dual-site stimulation. Front Hum Neurosci. 2015;9:533.
38. Bocci T, Barloscio D, Vergari M, Di Rollo A, Rossi S, Priori A, et al. Spinal direct current stimulation modulates short intracortical inhibition. Neuromodulation. 2015;18(8):686–93.
39. Nitsche MA, Jaussi W, Liebetanz D, Lang N, Tergau F, Paulus W. Consolidation of human motor cortical neuroplasticity by D-cycloserine. Neuropsychopharmacology. 2004;29(8):1573–8.
40. Nitsche MA, Fricke K, Henschke U, Schlitterlau A, Liebetanz D, Lang N, et al. Pharmacological modulation of cortical excitability shifts induced by transcranial direct current stimulation in humans. J Physiol. 2003;553(Pt 1):293–301.
41. Malenka RC, Bear MF. LTP and LTD: an embarrassment of riches. Neuron. 2004;44(1):5–21.
42. Lisman JE. Three Ca2+ levels affect plasticity differently: the LTP zone, the LTD zone and no man's land. J Physiol. 2001;532(Pt 2):285.
43. Polania R, Nitsche MA, Paulus W. Modulating functional connectivity patterns and topological functional organization of the human brain with transcranial direct current stimulation. Hum Brain Mapp. 2011;32(8):1236–49.
44. Venkatakrishnan A, Contreras-Vidal JL, Sandrini M, Cohen LG. Independent component analysis of resting brain activity reveals transient modulation of local cortical processing by transcranial direct current stimulation. Conf Proc IEEE Eng Med Biol Soc. 2011;2011:8102–5.
45. Polania R, Paulus W, Nitsche MA. Modulating cortico-striatal and thalamo-cortical functional connectivity with transcranial direct current stimulation. Hum Brain Mapp. 2012;33(10):2499–508.
46. Grent-'t-Jong T, Rivolta D, Sauer A, Grube M, Singer W, Wibral M, et al. MEG-measured visually induced gamma-band oscillations in chronic schizophrenia: evidence for impaired generation of rhythmic activity in ventral stream regions. Schizophr Res. 2016;176(2–3):177–85.
47. Leicht G, Vauth S, Polomac N, Andreou C, Rauh J, Mussmann M, et al. EEG-informed fMRI reveals a disturbed gamma-band-specific network in subjects at high risk for psychosis. Schizophr Bull. 2016;42(1):239–49.
48. Rueger MA, Keuters MH, Walberer M, Braun R, Klein R, Sparing R, et al. Multi-session transcranial direct current stimulation (tDCS) elicits inflammatory and regenerative processes in the rat brain. PLoS One. 2012;7(8):e43776.
49. Leffa DT, Bellaver B, Salvi AA, de Oliveira C, Caumo W, Grevet EH, et al. Transcranial direct current stimulation improves long-term memory deficits in an animal model of attention-deficit/hyperactivity disorder and modulates oxidative and inflammatory parameters. Brain Stimul. 2018;11(4):743–51.
50. Fillman SG, Cloonan N, Miller LC, Weickert CS. Markers of inflammation in the prefrontal cortex of individuals with schizophrenia. Mol Psychiatry. 2013;18(2):133.
51. Fillman SG, Cloonan N, Catts VS, Miller LC, Wong J, McCrossin T, et al. Increased inflammatory markers identified in the dorsolateral prefrontal cortex of individuals with schizophrenia. Mol Psychiatry. 2013;18(2):206–14.
52. Sekar A, Bialas AR, de Rivera H, Davis A, Hammond TR, Kamitaki N, et al. Schizophrenia risk from complex variation of complement component 4. Nature. 2016;530(7589):177–83.
53. Ormel PR, van Mierlo HC, Litjens M, Strien MEV, Hol EM, Kahn RS, et al. Characterization of macrophages from schizophrenia patients. NPJ Schizophr. 2017;3(1):41.
54. Jamil A, Batsikadze G, Kuo HI, Labruna L, Hasan A, Paulus W, et al. Systematic evaluation of the impact of stimulation intensity on neuroplastic after-effects induced by transcranial direct current stimulation. J Physiol. 2017;595(4):1273–88.
55. Davidson TW, Bolic M, Tremblay F. Predicting modulation in corticomotor excitability and in transcallosal inhibition in response to anodal transcranial direct current stimulation. Front Hum Neurosci. 2016;10:49.

56. Mangia AL, Pirini M, Cappello A. Transcranial direct current stimulation and power spectral parameters: a tDCS/EEG co-registration study. Front Hum Neurosci. 2014;8:601.
57. Pisoni A, Mattavelli G, Papagno C, Rosanova M, Casali AG, Romero Lauro LJ. Cognitive enhancement induced by anodal tDCS drives circuit-specific cortical plasticity. Cereb Cortex. 2018;28(4):1132–40.
58. Wirth M, Rahman RA, Kuenecke J, Koenig T, Horn H, Sommer W, et al. Effects of transcranial direct current stimulation (tDCS) on behaviour and electrophysiology of language production. Neuropsychologia. 2011;49(14):3989–98.
59. Cespon J, Rodella C, Rossini PM, Miniussi C, Pellicciari MC. Anodal transcranial direct current stimulation promotes frontal compensatory mechanisms in healthy elderly subjects. Front Aging Neurosci. 2017;9:420.
60. Weigl M, Mecklinger A, Rosburg T. Transcranial direct current stimulation over the left dorsolateral prefrontal cortex modulates auditory mismatch negativity. Clin Neurophysiol. 2016;127(5):2263–72.
61. Bersani FS, Minichino A, Fattapposta F, Bernabei L, Spagnoli F, Mannarelli D, et al. Prefrontocerebellar transcranial direct current stimulation increases amplitude and decreases latency of P3b component in patients with euthymic bipolar disorder. Neuropsychiatr Dis Treat. 2015;11:2913–7.
62. Radman N, Britz J, Buetler K, Weekes BS, Spierer L, Annoni JM. Dorsolateral prefrontal transcranial direct current stimulation modulates language processing but does not facilitate overt second language word production. Front Neurosci. 2018;12:490.
63. Baptista NI, Manfredi M, Boggio PS. Medial prefrontal cortex stimulation modulates irony processing as indexed by the N400. Soc Neurosci. 2018;13(4):495–510.
64. Nuber S, Jacob H, Kreifelts B, Martinelli A, Wildgruber D. Attenuated impression of irony created by the mismatch of verbal and nonverbal cues in patients with autism spectrum disorder. PLoS One. 2018;13(10):e0205750.
65. Zalla T, Amsellem F, Chaste P, Ervas F, Leboyer M, Champagne-Lavau M. Individuals with autism spectrum disorders do not use social stereotypes in irony comprehension. PLoS One. 2014;9(4):e95568.
66. Rossetti I, Brambilla P, Papagno C. Metaphor comprehension in schizophrenic patients. Front Psychol. 2018;9:670.
67. Priori A, Ciocca M, Parazzini M, Vergari M, Ferrucci R. Transcranial cerebellar direct current stimulation and transcutaneous spinal cord direct current stimulation as innovative tools for neuroscientists. J Physiol. 2014;592(16):3345–69.
68. Parazzini M, Rossi E, Ferrucci R, Liorni I, Priori A, Ravazzani P. Modelling the electric field and the current density generated by cerebellar transcranial DC stimulation in humans. Clin Neurophysiol. 2014;125(3):577–84.
69. Parazzini M, Fiocchi S, Liorni I, Rossi E, Cogiamanian F, Vergari M, et al. Modeling the current density generated by transcutaneous spinal direct current stimulation (tsDCS). Clin Neurophysiol. 2014;125(11):2260–70.
70. Fiocchi S, Ravazzani P, Priori A, Parazzini M. Cerebellar and spinal direct current stimulation in children: computational modeling of the induced electric field. Front Hum Neurosci. 2016;10:522.
71. Chan CY, Nicholson C. Modulation by applied electric fields of Purkinje and stellate cell activity in the isolated turtle cerebellum. J Physiol. 1986;371:89–114.
72. Hull CA, Chu Y, Thanawala M, Regehr WG. Hyperpolarization induces a long-term increase in the spontaneous firing rate of cerebellar Golgi cells. J Neurosci. 2013;33(14):5895–902.
73. Ugawa Y, Day BL, Rothwell JC, Thompson PD, Merton PA, Marsden CD. Modulation of motor cortical excitability by electrical stimulation over the cerebellum in man. J Physiol. 1991;441:57–72.
74. Ferrucci R, Cortese F, Bianchi M, Pittera D, Turrone R, Bocci T, et al. Cerebellar and motor cortical transcranial stimulation decrease levodopa-induced dyskinesias in Parkinson's disease. Cerebellum. 2016;15(1):43–7.

75. Alizad V, Meinzer M, Frossard L, Polman R, Smith S, Kerr G. Effects of transcranial direct current stimulation on gait in people with Parkinson's disease: study protocol for a randomized, controlled clinical trial. Trials. 2018;19(1):661.
76. Bocci T, De Carolis G, Ferrucci R, Paroli M, Mansani F, Priori A, et al. Cerebellar transcranial direct current stimulation (ctDCS) ameliorates phantom limb pain and non-painful phantom limb sensations. Cerebellum. 2019;18(3):527–35.
77. Gupta T, Dean DJ, Kelley NJ, Bernard JA, Ristanovic I, Mittal VA. Cerebellar transcranial direct current stimulation improves procedural learning in nonclinical psychosis: a double-blind crossover study. Schizophr Bull. 2018;44(6):1373–80.
78. Martin DM, Chan HN, Alonzo A, Green MJ, Mitchell PB, Loo CK. Transcranial direct current stimulation to enhance cognition in euthymic bipolar disorder. Bipolar Disord. 2015;17(8):849–58.
79. Cogiamanian F, Vergari M, Pulecchi F, Marceglia S, Priori A. Effect of spinal transcutaneous direct current stimulation on somatosensory evoked potentials in humans. Clin Neurophysiol. 2008;119(11):2636–40.
80. Cogiamanian F, Vergari M, Schiaffi E, Marceglia S, Ardolino G, Barbieri S, et al. Transcutaneous spinal cord direct current stimulation inhibits the lower limb nociceptive flexion reflex in human beings. Pain. 2011;152(2):370–5.
81. Lim CY, Shin HI. Noninvasive DC stimulation on neck changes MEP. Neuroreport. 2011;22(16):819–23.
82. Truini A, Vergari M, Biasiotta A, La Cesa S, Gabriele M, Di Stefano G, et al. Transcutaneous spinal direct current stimulation inhibits nociceptive spinal pathway conduction and increases pain tolerance in humans. Eur J Pain. 2011;15(10):1023–7.
83. Ahmed Z. Effects of cathodal trans-spinal direct current stimulation on mouse spinal network and complex multijoint movements. J Neurosci. 2013;33(37):14949–57.
84. Bocci T, Vannini B, Torzini A, Mazzatenta A, Vergari M, Cogiamanian F, et al. Cathodal transcutaneous spinal direct current stimulation (tsDCS) improves motor unit recruitment in healthy subjects. Neurosci Lett. 2014;578:75–9.
85. Bhadra N, Kilgore KL. Direct current electrical conduction block of peripheral nerve. IEEE Trans Neural Syst Rehabil Eng. 2004;12(3):313–24.
86. Aguilar J, Pulecchi F, Dilena R, Oliviero A, Priori A, Foffani G. Spinal direct current stimulation modulates the activity of gracile nucleus and primary somatosensory cortex in anaesthetized rats. J Physiol. 2011;589(Pt 20):4981–96.
87. Bocci T, Caleo M, Vannini B, Vergari M, Cogiamanian F, Rossi S, et al. An unexpected target of spinal direct current stimulation: interhemispheric connectivity in humans. J Neurosci Methods. 2015;254:18–26.
88. Song W, Truong DQ, Bikson M, Martin JH. Transspinal direct current stimulation immediately modifies motor cortex sensorimotor maps. J Neurophysiol. 2015;113(7):2801–11.
89. Schlaier JR, Eichhammer P, Langguth B, Doenitz C, Binder H, Hajak G, et al. Effects of spinal cord stimulation on cortical excitability in patients with chronic neuropathic pain: a pilot study. Eur J Pain. 2007;11(8):863–8.
90. Paradiso C, De Vito L, Rossi S, Setacci C, Battistini N, Cioni R, et al. Cervical and scalp recorded short latency somatosensory evoked potentials in response to epidural spinal cord stimulation in patients with peripheral vascular disease. Electroencephalogr Clin Neurophysiol. 1995;96(2):105–13.

Repetitive Magnetic and Low-Intensity Electric Transcranial Stimulation in the Interventional Psychiatry: Summary of Safety Issues

4

Simone Rossi and Andrea Antal

4.1   Introduction

The aim of this review is to give a short but informative summary of the safety of repetitive transcranial magnetic stimulation (rTMS) and low-intensity transcranial electric stimulation (TES) based on available published research and clinical data in the interventional psychiatry, including animal models and human studies.

The current approach in the clinical field is to estimate the potential of a stimulation protocol becoming a hazard that could result in safety problems. Hazard and risks should be considered separately: hazard is a potential for an Adverse Event (AE) (e.g., using too high stimulations intensities). Risk is a measure of the combination of the hazard, the likelihood of occurrence of the AE and the severity [1, 2] (See also: http://www.who.int/medical_devices/publications/en/MD_Regulations.pdf).

Risk is not the same as burden: a stimulation procedure may be burdensome, e.g., resulting in much discomfort (e.g., face muscle twitching during rTMS), but nevertheless safe, without relevant risk for permanent damage.

In brain stimulation research and related clinical applications, safety can only be considered in relative terms [3]. According to the definition of the European Medical Device Directive (MDD), "safe" is a condition where all risks are accepted risks

S. Rossi (✉)
Siena Brain Investigation and Neuromodulation Lab (Si-BIN Lab), Unit of Neurology and Clinical Neurophysiology, Department of Medicine, Surgery and Neuroscience, University of Siena, Siena, Italy
e-mail: simone.rossi@unisi.it

A. Antal
Institute of Medical Psychology, Otto-von-Guericke University Magdeburg, Magdeburg, Germany

Department of Clinical Neurophysiology, University Medical Center Göttingen, Göttingen, Germany
e-mail: aantal@gwdg.de

© Springer Nature Switzerland AG 2020
B. Dell'Osso, G. Di Lorenzo (eds.), *Non Invasive Brain Stimulation in Psychiatry and Clinical Neurosciences*,
https://doi.org/10.1007/978-3-030-43356-7_4

(MDD; Annex I; § I. General Requirements). We have to keep in mind that all stimulation protocols could carry a certain degree of risk and could cause problems in specific circumstances, e.g., when medicated patients or children are treated with stimulation.

Generally, the assumption that a stimulation protocol is safe is based on a full and unprejudiced documentation of all AEs that may occur during application of a given protocol. However, it should be underlined here that the prevalence of published AEs in the brain stimulation studies is higher in studies specifically assessing AEs, compared to those not assessing them. Furthermore, in these studies AEs are frequently reported by subjects receiving placebo stimulation.

AEs are undesirable or harmful effects that are observed after a medical intervention that may or may not be causally related to it (https://evs.nci.nih.gov/ftp1/ CTCAE/Archive/CTCAE_4.02_2009-09-15_QuickReference_5x7_Locked.pdf). A mild AE (grade 1) is defined as involving mild symptoms, for which no medical treatment is necessary (i.e., transient local discomfort during rTMS or skin redness after tDCS), while a moderate AE (grade 2) indicates the need of noninvasive treatment (e.g., transient but persistent pain after rTMS needing an analgesic, or in the case of tDCS local application of a cream after a skin burn). Serious AEs (SAE) (grade 3) are medically significant but not immediately life-threatening events: they include the requirement for inpatient hospitalization (or prolongation of it). *Life-threatening SAEs* include events that are life threatening (grade 4) or death (grade 5).

Special stimulation conditions that have been increasingly used during the last few years, e.g., combination of rTMS and TES with other methods, such as stimulating patients with intracranial implants or combination of TES with functional magnetic resonance imaging (fMRI) or EEG, or other types of noninvasive stimulation (magnetic seizure therapy, trans-spinal and transorbital stimulation) should require different and many times deeper and individually tailored safety considerations, and therefore will not be mentioned and discussed in this paper (but see [3]).

4.2   Transcranial Magnetic Stimulation

An impressive growing of scientific publications has appeared in the last 20 years concerning the use of rTMS, including theta burst (TBS) stimulation, in the psychiatric field. New coils for stimulation have been presented, able to stimulate deeper than conventional ones, and new protocols—as "high-density rTMS"— have been introduced. Meanwhile, the use of rTMS has been cleared by regulatory agencies in many countries for treatment of depression and obsessive-compulsive disorder. So, constant updating of safety issues remains a crucial point, and this is why the International Federation of Clinical Neurophysiology (IFCN) supported a further consensus meeting 10 years later the last available safety guidelines [4, 5]. The meeting has been held again in Siena during October 2018, and a new release of the safety guideline was scheduled for the end of 2019, as a result of that meeting.

4.2.1   A General Short Summary Related to the Safety Aspects of rTMS, and Basic Procedures to Limit AEs

If safety recommendations in terms of intensity, frequency, and timing of stimulation are adhered to, rTMS and TBS stimulation can be considered overall safe. Currently available safety limits are reported in [5]. These limits are not mandatory, but just reflect proven safety limits in healthy subjects. In fact, they are meant not to prevent the development of new protocols of stimulation, as indeed it has been done since their publication.

Therefore, in case of new protocols, it is advisable to use all precautions that might alert the treating physician on the occurrence of an incoming seizure, the most SAE that might take place during an rTMS intervention. These include: (1) adjustment of the parameters of the stimulation according to the resting motor threshold (RMT); (2) the neurophysiological monitoring during the rTMS application.

Regarding the RMT, it is traditionally considered as the minimum intensity required to elicit an electromyographic (EMG) response (motor evoked potential, MEP) of at least 50 μV with a probability of 50% in a hand muscle at rest [6]. RMT can also be determined by observing the clinical motor responses (finger or arm movement) rather than recording the MEP by surface EMG. Such a visual method, which is often used in private clinics to save time, overestimates the minimum intensity required to activate the motor cortex; therefore, it potentially increases the danger of TMS. During a treatment course, the RMT has to be searched every day of stimulation, as it may change from day to day and due to the intervention itself [7].

Neurophysiological monitoring is strongly recommended either for all those studies that are based on new TMS protocols that are not fully tested yet by a safety point of view, or for all those protocols based on a combination of parameters of stimulation (including new coils or multiple-site intervention) that are close to upper safety limits of the published tables. This applies to both healthy subjects for research use and, even more, for patients' populations.

In studies where rTMS is not expected to generate MEPs (as during motor cortex stimulation below motor threshold or stimulation outside the motor cortex), the session can be monitored by recording MEPs in a hand muscle contralateral to the stimulated hemisphere: hand muscles are generally used to these purposes as they have the lowest threshold of excitation. The occurrence of TMS-evoked EMG activity during the rTMS application reflects an increase in cortical excitability, taking place at the motor cortex. The appearance of MEPs under these circumstances may indicate a lowering of the threshold in the subthreshold stimulated motor cortex, or the spread of excitation from neighboring areas to the motor cortex itself.

In studies where the stimulus is supposed to produce hand MEPs, EMG monitoring can be performed on a more proximal arm muscle, like the deltoid or the biceps muscle. If EMG recording is not available, a visual monitoring of the patients by a qualified person is mandatory, although it is less sensitive and objective [8].

Theoretically, the most appropriate method to detect an emerging seizure during rTMS could be represented by electroencephalographic (EEG) recordings. Indeed, EEG post-discharge after the cessation of cortical stimulation is classically considered to be the first indicator of an occurring seizure [9], as demonstrated for a variety of cortical targets [10–12] and for variable periods after the intervention [13, 14]. However, EEG monitoring is not feasible in the routine practice of rTMS, mostly because of the need for expensive specialized equipment to enable EEG recording during rTMS without artifacts due to magnetic pulses.

4.2.2 Illness-Therapy-Stimulation Interactions in Psychiatry

In a recent survey of the 5-year period 2012–2016, over 300,000 TMS sessions were applied with various frequencies and 21 seizures were reported (standardized risk 7/100,000): 14 of these occurred in subjects considered to have an elevated risk, such as taking medications, having brain lesions, or epilepsy (standardized risk: 24/100,000 sessions) [15]. However, the same survey reported that the concurrent use of psychotropic medications did not modify so much the risk of seizure occurrence (less than 0.02% of all treatment sessions; 8/45,000 sessions) [15]. Of these, only three—all psychiatric patients—were free from anatomical lesions and on medications suspected of lowering the seizure threshold. Two seizures were reported in depressed individuals without concurrent pharmacological treatment.

Regarding deep-coils, a recent review reported 31 seizures on 35,443 treated patients (seizure frequency of 0.00087) [16]. Of these, 29 occurred in depressed patients, one seizure in a schizophrenic patient and one in a post-traumatic stress disorder patient. In most cases, patients took one or more psychopharmacological agent(s) (amitriptyline, aripiprazole, bupropion, citalopram, clomipramine, desvenlafaxine, duloxetine, escitalopram, fluoxetine, lithium, lurasidone, mianserin, mirtazapine, olanzapine, sertraline, trazodone, venlafaxine, vortioxetine). It remains difficult to answer whether these drugs have had a causal role or not, as seizures occurred either with high-risk drugs (e.g., clomipramine) or during treatment with drugs whose favoring seizure role is negligible [17].

Another AE potentially relevant in psychiatric patients undergoing TMS interventions is treatment-emergent mania, which has been reported after stimulation of the left prefrontal cortex, either with low- or high-frequency rTMS in patients with unipolar and bipolar depression [18]. However, the overall rate of 0.84% for active rTMS versus 0.73% for sham rTMS is even lower than the natural switch rate in bipolar patients under mood stabilizers treatment (2.3–3.45%) [18].

Suicidal ideation has never been described in healthy subjects during or after rTMS, and there is even evidence for an anti-suicidal effect of rTMS in depression [19, 20]. Psychotic symptoms, or anxiety, agitation, and insomnia have been occasionally reported: they were transient and resolved spontaneously or with light pharmacological treatment [21, 22], but it is unknown whether their frequency is higher during rTMS interventions than during the natural course of the disease.

Even if these AEs are minor and transient, it is advisable that psychiatric patients undergoing rTMS are clearly informed about the risk of psychiatric side effects, as they are not uncommon.

4.2.3   Conclusions and Recommendations

Patients undergoing rTMS intervention should be screened for suitability, as with magnetic resonance procedures [23]. When reviewing rTMS and TBS applications in human applications and clinical trials, no reports of an SAE or irreversible injury attributable to these interventions were found, despite the thousands of patients treated. Epileptic seizures induced by rTMS are a rare, but possible phenomenon: the most recent estimate shows a standardized risk of 7/100,000, which seems however not increased in psychiatric patient populations [15].

Mild AEs are instead quite frequent, but they are very mild, transitory, and do not require pharmacological treatment in most cases [5]: the most common are transient headache, local or neck pain, toothache, paresthesia, and transient hearing changes if earplugs are not properly positioned. Anxiety is possible, especially at the beginning of treatment, but it is likely an unspecific effect.

Although there is no evidence suggesting that AEs in psychiatric patients are significantly higher and different in magnitude in comparison to healthy subjects, care has to be taken to evaluate the concomitant treatment, as many of the drugs acting on the central nervous system may lower the excitability threshold. However, even in such a population of patients, the risk remains low [5].

For every new trial, stimulation parameters must always be chosen with safety considerations in mind, and be accepted by the Ethical Committee/IRB before initiation of a study.

4.3   Low-Intensity TES Methods

Low-intensity TES methods, which are used in psychiatry, are encompassing transcranial direct current (tDCS—most frequently), transcranial alternating current (tACS), and transcranial random noise (tRNS) stimulation or their combinations. "Low intensity" is defined as intensities <4 mA (at the case of tACS and tRNS peak-to-peak,) a total stimulation duration of up to 60 minutes per day, applied through at least 2 electrodes, using electrode sizes between 1 and 100 cm^2 (delivering $\leq$7.2 coulombs of charge) [3, 24]. With regard to tACS and tRNS, the applied frequency range is between 0.1 and 10,000 Hz.

4.3.1   A General Short Summary Related to the Safety Aspects of TES

The TES dose is defined by the parameters delivered by the stimulation device, generating an electric field (EF) in the body (in units of V/m or mV/mm) [25]. These parameters can be well defined (intensity, duration of the stimulation, size of the electrodes); however, other parameters, including physiological factors such as individual anatomy, age, gender, baseline neurotransmitter concentrations, genetics, and dynamic state of the brain before and during stimulation are barely controllable (this, of course, applies to every brain stimulation protocol). Therefore, the current state of knowledge concerning the physiological mechanisms (and related safety aspects) of low-intensity TES still remains limited.

In most recent studies, the stimulation parameters are chosen based on previously published research and clinical data, computational modeling, and safety considerations based on human and animal experimental data. Finding the "optimal" dose for a given application still represents a challenge. With regard to the safe use of low-intensity TES for research and clinical purposes, it is recommended to consider the following issues.

1. EF modeling for targeting predefined areas for stimulation, including subject-specific current optimization can be helpful and results in increased safety. The current density is much higher in the skin than in the brain; therefore, the lack of skin injury indirectly supports the claim that the brain current flow is safe (assuming equal sensitivity to injury of skin and brain) [24–26]. It is suggested that the predicted EF strength is about 0.4–0.6 V/m in the cortex when the traditional stimulation protocols are used (up to 2 mA). The maximal value that was so far reported in a normal brain is 1.6 V/m [27]. Nevertheless, anatomical variations can lead to differences by a factor of ~2 for a fixed stimulation intensity [28–31]. The abovementioned data are very similar to those recorded in epilepsy patients with EF strengths of 0.6–1.6 V/m [32] and $\leq$ 0.5 V/m using 1 mA [33]. Of course, these small EFs are below the intensity required to elicit action potentials [34]; nevertheless, they can modify ongoing brain processes, inducing molecular or structural changes [35–38]. No irreversible electrochemical products are known to accumulate at the electrode with such low current densities. Conductive rubber electrodes are convenient for TES; they are not placed directly on the skin; an electrolyte that is saline or gel always separates the two [39]. Tap water is not recommended, and care should be taken, even when using a saline solution in longer-lasting experiments as increased contact resistance may also arise from the drying of the sponges [40]. Abrading the skin before electrode placement is not recommended [41].

2. Modeling studies can be just an estimation of the EF. However, the relation of this to time-integrated EF on the cortex is not simple [42, 43]. The other possibility is testing a given protocol in animal models; nevertheless, there are still many uncertainties in the translation of animal studies to human experiments. In humans, tDCS with 1 mA intensity using standard contact electrodes (16–35 cm^2) results in charge densities ranging from 170 to 480 C/m^2. In animal studies, at current densities between 14.3 and 28.7 mA/cm^2, corresponding to a charge density threshold below 52,400 C/m^2, no histologically detectable brain lesions were induced [44]. Threshold approximation obtained from rat experiments was estimated to be over one order of magnitude higher compared to current clinical protocols [24].

3. In clinical practice, safety of low-intensity TES (mainly tDCS) is mostly derived from an analysis assessing efficacy as the primary outcome; the number of trials targeting only "safety" is limited. In general, these human studies evaluated parameters of neuronal damage, such as neuron-specific enolase (NSE), magnetic resonance imaging (MRI) [45], electroencephalography (EEG), and neuropsychological tests [46, 47] and they all support the safety of TES.

Concerning human studies, the most typical events during stimulation are slight transient tingling sensations, very rarely local pain under the electrodes or light flashes when the stimulation was switched on or off abruptly, or when tACS is used in the EEG frequency range, with an intensity of 1–2 mA. Following the stimulation, light headache and erythema or contact dermatitis under the stimulation electrodes were reported [3]. It was repeatedly documented that the profile of AEs in terms of frequency, magnitude, and type is comparable in healthy and clinical populations, and this is also the case for more vulnerable populations, such as children, elderly persons, or pregnant women [3]. With regard to skin irritations, the contributing factors are pre-existing conditions, such as allergies to skin creams, high impedance (e.g., electrode dry or defect, inappropriate contact solution, nonuniform contact pressure of electrodes to skin), prolonged duration or repeated sessions, and too high current density (high current, small electrode) [3]. Therefore, irritation of the skin can be prevented by the best possible preparation of skin and stimulation electrode (without abrading the skin). The application of the stimulation over non-homogenous (e.g., scars) or inflamed skin areas should be avoided. During and after treatment, participants should be instructed to report discomfort immediately.

4.3.2 Illness-Therapy-Stimulation Interactions

TES, similarly to rTMS, can be combined with basically any other therapeutic intervention, including motor or cognitive training, behavioral interventions or the application of medications [48–50]. Combinations of TES with motor or cognitive training or behavioral interventions appear to be safe (e.g., in the neurorehabilitation). However, some pharmacological interventions might increase the risk of AEs, e.g., when they amplify cortical excitability changes. On the other side, anticonvulsant medications can decrease or abolish anodal tDCS effects [51]. In the following section, we concentrate on reported AEs in one of the most frequently TES-treated patient groups in interventional psychiatry: major depressive disorder (MDD).

Generally, the burden associated with TES in MDD trials was basically the same as in all other trials with tDCS, i.e., cutaneous symptoms and sensations occurring with the same frequency [52]. Several RCTs [50, 53–55] described treatment-emergent mania/hypomania cases (generally, less than 15 patients until 2019). Only two occurred in patients with bipolar disorder. Five patients out of these cases started receiving tDCS and sertraline simultaneously. In a meta-analysis on the topic [56], it was found that the treatment-emergent hypomania/mania rates were not statistically different between active and sham stimulation, although they were higher in active (3.5%) vs. sham (0.5%) stimulation.

Treatment-emergent suicidal ideation or behavior is a risk in the treatment of any depressed patient. According to available data, one patient committed suicide during a clinical tDCS trial, but this was most likely unrelated to tDCS intervention [54].

In summary, patients should be carefully assessed for a history of bipolar disorder or of switching into mania with past antidepressant treatments, as these factors may indicate a higher risk of manic switch with tDCS; yet, a causal relationship is difficult to prove because of the low incidence rate and limited numbers of subjects in controlled trials. In these patients, concurrent treatment with mood stabilizer medications during the tDCS treatment course should be considered.

4.3.3 Conclusions and Recommendations

When reviewing only conventional bipolar tDCS in human applications and clinical trials, no reports of an SAE or irreversible injury attributable to low-intensity TES were found in over 33,200 sessions and 1000 subjects with repeated sessions [24]. About 400 publications using low-intensity TES between 2000 and 2019 reported mild AEs, mainly in the category of skin sensations; however, several studies were not placebo controlled and double blinded. At present, there is no direct evidence suggesting that the AEs in patients or in vulnerable populations are significantly higher and different in magnitude in comparison to healthy subjects. Generally, in a systematic review of 64 tDCS trials [52], it was found that the quality of AEs reporting in neuropsychiatry was quite low. Lack of adequate AEs reporting is a problem because this usually leads to an underestimation of the true rate of AEs.

Stimulation parameters should always be chosen with safety considerations in mind, and be accepted by the Ethical Committee/IRB before initiation of a study. Alterations during applications should always be documented. We suggest using standard questionnaires for screening and reporting [3] (http://www.neurologie.uni-goettingen.de/downloads.html). Additional questions and information can be inserted according to particular experimental or clinical demands. Furthermore, reporting each patient's guess for type of stimulation and reporting the researcher's assessment of the patient's propensity to complain [57, 58] should be required in future studies. As mentioned above, AEs have been rare and minor in the course of thousands of hours of TES in controlled settings, using CE certified stimulation devices around the world. There is little reliable data on the safety of direct-to-consumer brain stimulation devices. Therefore, we warn against the use of devices and methods unless they have shown both efficacy and safety in appropriately designed clinical trials.

References

1. Altenstetter C. EU and member state medical devices regulation. Int J Technol Assess Health Care. 2003;19:228–48.
2. McAllister P, Jeswiet J. Medical device regulation for manufacturers. P I Mech Eng H. 2003;217:459–67.
3. Antal A, Alekseichuk I, Bikson M, et al. Low intensity transcranial electric stimulation: safety, ethical, legal regulatory and application guidelines. Clin Neurophysiol. 2017;128:1774–809.

4. Wassermann EM. Risk and safety of repetitive transcranial magnetic stimulation: report and suggested guidelines from the International Workshop on the Safety of Repetitive Transcranial Magnetic Stimulation, June 5-7, 1996. Electroencephalogr Clin Neurophysiol. 1988;108:1–16.
5. Rossi S, Hallett M, Rossini PM, Pascual-Leone A, Safety of TMS Consensus Group. Safety, ethical considerations, and application guidelines for the use of transcranial magnetic stimulation in clinical practice and research. Clin Neurophysiol. 2009;120:2008–39.
6. Rossini PM, Burke D, Chen R, et al. Non-invasive electrical and magnetic stimulation of the brain, spinal cord, roots and peripheral nerves: basic principles and procedures for routine clinical and research application. An updated report from an I.F.C.N. Committee. Clin Neurophysiol. 2015;126:1071–107.
7. Mantovani A, Rossi S, Bassi BD, et al. Modulation of motor cortex excitability in obsessive-compulsive disorder: an exploratory study on the relations of neurophysiology measures with clinical outcome. Psychiatry Res. 2013;210:1026–32.
8. Lorenzano C, Gilio F, Inghilleri M, et al. Spread of electrical activity at cortical level after repetitive magnetic stimulation in normal subjects. Exp Brain Res. 2002;147:186–92.
9. Aimone-Marsan C. Focal electrical stimulation. In: Purpura DP, Penry JK, Tower DB, Woodbury DM, Walter RD, editors. Experimental models of epilepsy. New York: Raven Press; 1972. p. 147–72.
10. Rossi S, Pasqualetti P, Rossini PM, et al. Effects of repetitive transcranial magnetic stimulation on movement-related cortical activity in humans. Cereb Cortex. 2000;10:802–8.
11. Hansenne M, Laloyaux O, Mardaga S, Ansseau M. Impact of low frequency transcranial magnetic stimulation on event-related brain potentials. Biol Psychol. 2004;67:331–41.
12. Holler I, Siebner HR, Cunnington R, Gerschlager W. 5 Hz repetitive TMS increases anticipatory motor activity in the human cortex. Neurosci Lett. 2006;392:221–5.
13. Enomoto H, Ugawa Y, Hanajima R, et al. Decreased sensory cortical excitability after 1 Hz rTMS over the ipsilateral primary motor cortex. Clin Neurophysiol. 2001;112:2154–8.
14. Tsuji T, Rothwell JC. Long lasting effects of rTMS and associated peripheral sensory input on MEPs, SEPs and transcortical reflex excitability in humans. J Physiol (London). 2002;540:367–76.
15. Lerner AJ, Wassermann EM, Tamir D. Non-invasive electrical and magnetic stimulation of the brain, spinal cord, roots and peripheral nerves: Basic principles and procedures for routine clinical and research application. An updated report from an I.F.C.N. Committee. Clin Neurophysiol. 2019;130:1409–16.
16. Tendler A, Roth Y, Zangen A. Rate of inadvertently induced seizures with deep repetitive transcranial magnetic stimulation. Brain Stimul. 2018;11:1410–4.
17. Steinert T, Fröscher W. Epileptic seizures under antidepressive drug treatment: systematic review. Pharmacopsychiatry. 2018;51:121–35.
18. Xia G, Gajwani P, Muzina DJ, Kemp DE, Gao K, Ganocy SJ, Calabrese JR. Treatment-emergent mania/hypomania during antidepressant monotherapy in patients with rapid cycling bipolar disorder. Int J Neuropsychopharmacol. 2008;11:119–30.
19. George MS, Raman R, Benedek DM, et al. A two-site pilot randomized 3 day trial of high dose left prefrontal repetitive transcranial magnetic stimulation (rTMS) for suicidal inpatients. Brain Stimul. 2014;7:421–31.
20. Weissman CR, Blumberger DM, Brown PE, et al. Bilateral repetitive transcranial magnetic stimulation decreases suicidal ideation in depression. J Clin Psychiatry. 2018;79. pii:17m11692.
21. Zwanzger P, Ella R, Keck ME, Rupprecht R, Padberg F. Occurrence of delusions during repetitive transcranial magnetic stimulation (rTMS) in major depression. Biol Psychiatry. 2002;51:602–3.
22. Janicak PG, O'Reardon JP, Sampson SM, et al. Transcranial magnetic stimulation in the treatment of major depressive disorder: a comprehensive summary of safety experience from acute exposure, extended exposure, and during reintroduction treatment. J Clin Psychiatry. 2008;69:222–32.
23. Rossi S, Hallett M, Rossini PM, Pascual-Leone A. Screening questionnaire before TMS: an update. Clin Neurophysiol. 2011;122:1866.

24. Bikson M, Grossman P, Thomas C, Zannou AL, Jiang J, Adnan T, et al. Safety of transcranial direct current stimulation: evidence based update 2016. Brain Stimul. 2016;9:641–61.
25. Peterchev AV, Wagner TA, Miranda PC, et al. Fundamentals of transcranial electric and magnetic stimulation dose: definition, selection, and reporting practices. Brain Stimul. 2012;5:435–53.
26. Saturnino GB, Antunes A, Thielscher A. On the importance of electrode parameters for shaping electric field patterns generated by tDCS. Neuroimage. 2015;120:25–35.
27. Parazzini M, Fiocchi S, Rossi E, Paglialonga A, Ravazzani P. Transcranial direct current stimulation: estimation of the electric field and of the current density in an anatomical human head model. IEEE Trans Biomed Eng. 2011;58:1773–80.
28. Datta A, Truong D, Minhas P, Parra LC, Bikson M. Inter-individual variation during transcranial direct current stimulation and normalization of dose using MRI-derived computational models. Front Psych. 2012;3:e91.
29. Kessler SK, Minhas P, Woods AJ, Rosen A, Gorman C, Bikson M. Dosage considerations for transcranial direct current stimulation in children: a computational modeling study. PLoS One. 2013;8:e76112.
30. Laakso I, Tanaka S, Koyama S, De Santis V, Hirata A. Inter-subject variability in electric fields of motor cortical tDCS. Brain Stimul. 2015;8:906–13.
31. Truong DQ, Magerowski G, Blackburn GL, Bikson M, Alonso-Alonso M. Computational modeling of transcranial direct current stimulation (tDCS) in obesity: impact of head fat and dose guidelines. NeuroImage Clinical. 2013;2:759–66.
32. Dymond AM, Coger RW, Serafetinides EA. Intracerebral current levels in man during electrosleep therapy. Biol Psychiatry. 1975;10:101–4.
33. Opitz A, Falchier A, Yan CG, et al. Spatiotemporal structure of intracranial electric fields induced by transcranial electric stimulation in humans and nonhuman primates. Sci Rep. 2016;6:31236.
34. Radman T, Ramos RL, Brumberg JC, Bikson M. Role of cortical cell type and morphology in subthreshold and suprathreshold uniform electric field stimulation in vitro. Brain Stimul. 2009;2:215–28.
35. Fritsch B, Reis J, Martinowich K, Schambra HM, Ji Y, Cohen LG, et al. Direct current stimulation promotes BDNF-dependent synaptic plasticity: potential implications for motor learning. Neuron. 2010;66:198–204.
36. Jackson MP, Rahman A, Lafon B, et al. Animal models of transcranial direct current stimulation: methods and mechanisms. Clin Neurophysiol. 2016;127:3425–54.
37. Ranieri F, Podda MV, Riccardi E, et al. Modulation of LTP at rat hippocampal CA3-CA1 synapses by direct current stimulation. J Neurophysiol. 2012;107:1868–80.
38. Frohlich F, McCormick DA. Endogenous electric fields may guide neocortical network activity. Neuron. 2010;67:129–43.
39. Minhas P, Bansal V, Patel J, et al. Electrodes for high-definition transcutaneous DC stimulation for applications in drug delivery and electrotherapy, including tDCS. J Neurosci Methods. 2010;190:188–97.
40. Woods AJ, Antal A, Bikson M, et al. A technical guide to tDCS, and related non-invasive brain stimulation tools. Clin Neurophysiol. 2016;127:1031–48.
41. Loo CK, Martin DM, Alonzo A, et al. Avoiding skin burns with transcranial direct current stimulation: preliminary considerations. Int J Neuropsychopharmacol. 2011;14:425–6.
42. Miranda PC, Faria P, Hallett M. What does the ratio of injected current to electrode area tell us about current density in the brain during tDCS? Clin Neurophysiol. 2009;120:1183–7.
43. Ruffini G, Wendling F, Merlet I, et al. Transcranial current brain stimulation (tCS): models and technologies. IEEE Transa Neural Syst Rehabil Eng. 2013;21:333–45.
44. Liebetanz D, Koch R, Mayenfels S, Konig F, Paulus W, Nitsche MA. Safety limits of cathodal transcranial direct current stimulation in rats. Clin Neurophysiol. 2009;120:1161–7.
45. Nitsche MA, Niehaus L, Hoffmann KT, et al. MRI study of human brain exposed to weak direct current stimulation of the frontal cortex. Clin Neurophysiol. 2004;115:2419–23.

46. Iyer MB, Mattu U, Grafman J, Lomarev M, Sato S, Wassermann EM. Safety and cognitive effect of frontal DC brain polarization in healthy individuals. Neurology. 2005;64:872–5.

47. Tadini L, El-Nazer R, Brunoni AR, et al. Cognitive, mood, and electroencephalographic effects of noninvasive cortical stimulation with weak electrical currents. J ECT. 2011;27:134–40.

48. Bajbouj M, Padberg F. A perfect match: noninvasive brain stimulation and psychotherapy. Eur Arch Psy Neurosci. 2014;264(Suppl 1):S27–33.

49. Wessel MJ, Zimerman M, Hummel FC. Non-invasive brain stimulation: an interventional tool for enhancing behavioral training after stroke. Front Hum Neurosci. 2015;9:265.

50. Brunoni AR, Valiengo L, Baccaro A, et al. The sertraline vs electrical current therapy for treating depression clinical study results from a factorial, randomized, controlled trial. JAMA Psychiatry. 2013;70:383–91.

51. Brunoni AR, Ferrucci R, Bortolomasi M, Scelzo E, Boggio PS, Fregni F, et al. Interactions between transcranial direct current stimulation (tDCS) and pharmacological interventions in the Major Depressive Episode: findings from a naturalistic study. Eur Psychiatry. 2013;28:356–61.

52. Aparicio LV, Guarienti F, Razza LB, Carvalho AF, Fregni F, Brunoni AR. A systematic review on the acceptability and tolerability of transcranial direct current stimulation treatment in neuropsychiatry trials. Brain Stimul. 2016;9:671–81.

53. Bennabi D, Nicolier M, Monnin J, et al. Pilot study of feasibility of the effect of treatment with tDCS in patients suffering from treatment-resistant depression treated with escitalopram. Clin Neurophysiol. 2014;126:1185–9.

54. Loo CK, Sachdev P, Martin D, Pigot M, Alonzo A, Malhi GS, et al. A double-blind, sham-controlled trial of transcranial direct current stimulation for the treatment of depression. Int J Neuropsychopharmacol. 2010;13:61–9.

55. Loo CK, Alonzo A, Martin D, Mitchell PB, Galvez V, Sachdev P. Transcranial direct current stimulation for depression: 3-week, randomised, sham-controlled trial. Br J Psychiatry. 2012;200:52–9.

56. Brunoni AR, Moffa AH, Sampaio-Junior B, Galvez V, Loo CK. Treatment-emergent mania/hypomania during antidepressant treatment with transcranial direct current stimulation (tDCS): a systematic review and meta-analysis. Brain Stimul. 2016;10:260–2.

57. Fertonani A, Ferrari C, Miniussi C. What do you feel if I apply transcranial electric stimulation? Safety, sensations and secondary induced effects. Clin Neurophysiol. 2015;126:2181–8.

58. Wallace D, Cooper NR, Paulmann S, Fitzgerald PB, Russo R. Perceived comfort and blinding efficacy in randomised sham-controlled transcranial direct current stimulation (tDCS) trials at 2 mA in young and older healthy adults. PLoS One. 2016;11:e0149703.

NIBS as a Research Tool in Clinical and Translational Neuroscience

Asif Jamil, Fatemeh Yavari, Min-Fang Kuo, and Michael A. Nitsche

5.1 Introduction

To understand the foundation of central nervous system diseases in humans, the exploration of human brain physiology is of utmost importance. In the last 40 years, numerous tools that allow the exploration of respective mechanisms in health and disease have been developed. Two main groups of tools are neuroimaging and non-invasive brain stimulation (NIBS) approaches. Neuroimaging allows to identify areas activated during psychological and behavioral processes, including not only regional but also network activations, as well as process-related alterations of transmitter and neuromodulator systems. Noninvasive brain stimulation has been developed based on the findings that sufficiently strong electrical stimulation over the scalp is able to activate cortical neurons [1]. Based on these initial findings, numerous tools have been developed, which enable not only global activation of specific target areas but also monitoring the central nervous system conduction time, activation of cortical subsystems defined by neurotransmitters and modulators, and network activation. Because of these specific functions and the high spatial and temporal specificity of some protocols, NIBS allows revealing aspects of human brain physiology, which we cannot obtain by functional imaging alone. Furthermore, brain stimulation approaches are able to modulate task-related cerebral activity.

A. Jamil · F. Yavari · M.-F. Kuo
Department of Psychology and Neurosciences, Leibniz Research Centre for Working Environment and Human Factors, Dortmund, Germany
e-mail: yavari@ifado.de; Kuo@ifado.de

M. A. Nitsche (✉)
Department of Psychology and Neurosciences, Leibniz Research Centre for Working Environment and Human Factors, Dortmund, Germany

Department of Neurology, University Hospital Bergmannsheil, Bochum, Germany
e-mail: nitsche@ifado.de

© Springer Nature Switzerland AG 2020
B. Dell'Osso, G. Di Lorenzo (eds.), *Non Invasive Brain Stimulation in Psychiatry and Clinical Neurosciences*,
https://doi.org/10.1007/978-3-030-43356-7_5

This allows for deriving causal relations about the involvement of specific physiological activity during psychological and behavioral processes, based on intervention-dependent performance alterations. In addition, based on respective alterations, therapeutic interventions have been developed, which aim to counteract pathologically altered cortical activity, neuroplasticity, and oscillatory activity. Some of these interventions, e.g., repetitive transcranial magnetic stimulation (rTMS), have already been approved for routine clinical treatment of psychiatric disorders, while others may also soon reach approval. In this chapter, we provide an overview of the main NIBS tools available at present, which are transcranial magnetic stimulation (TMS) and transcranial electrical stimulation (tES), and discuss their application as a research tool for understanding cognition and behavior, and their potential for treating diseases of the brain. This includes exploration of disease-relevant pathological alterations of brain physiology. Improving the knowledge in this field not only enhances our mechanistic understanding but may also lead to the identification of biomarkers for a specific disease, or therapeutic progress, and thereby guide individualization of therapeutic approaches in the future. Moreover, with both TMS and tES approaches, it is possible to generate plasticity in the human brain. As such, these tools allow us not only to identify plasticity-related pathological alterations in central nervous system diseases, but also to counteract pathological alterations in respective diseases. In the last part of this chapter, we will give examples of how these tools can be used to improve comprehension of disease-specific pathophysiology, and based on this, to develop therapeutic approaches. Finally, we will give a short overview of future developments in the field, which might help to further improve the utility of NIBS.

5.2   Using NIBS to Monitor Brain Physiology

For the exploration of human brain physiology, NIBS is used to study cortical excitability, cerebral connectivity, and neuroplasticity. These methods help to clarify the physiological foundation of cognitive processes and behavior and are also relevant to identify pathological alterations in clinical syndromes, and mechanistic effects of interventions dedicated to reducing clinical symptoms. In the following, we refer primarily to protocols relevant to psychological and behavioral processes. For determination of central conduction time, mapping procedures, and related protocols, which are relevant for clinical diagnostics of neurological diseases, refer to the respective literature [2].

5.2.1   Monitoring Cortical Excitability by NIBS

For the exploration of cerebral excitability, TMS is the main stimulation paradigm used for application in humans. Numerous TMS protocols have been developed, including single- and double-pulse stimulation of cerebral target regions, as well as peripheral–central stimulus combinations, to explore the functional state of cortical, corticocortical, and corticospinal pathways. These protocols also allow for a more detailed understanding of the specific functionality of pharmacologically defined subsystems. TMS alone can probe the reactivity of the motor and visual cortex, and when coupled with other neuroimaging techniques such as electroencephalography (EEG), can be used to assess the response of other cortical targets as well. Respective measures are valuable for the identification of neurophysiological and pathophysiological aspects of CNS diseases, and for the exploration of disease dynamics, including the impact of interventions. Thus, TMS-based monitoring approaches, which we describe below, may be powerful co-adjuvants for the early diagnosis and grading of diseases.

Motor Threshold (MT), Motor Evoked Potential (MEP) amplitude and latency, and the recruitment curve are the main protocols to investigate corticospinal excitability by TMS. MT is a summated index of neuronal membrane excitability of corticospinal neurons, the interneurons projecting onto these neurons along the corticospinal tract, as well as the excitability of motor neurons in the spinal cord, neuromuscular junctions, and muscles [3]. MT is increased by drugs that block voltage-gated sodium channels in the motor cortex but is not altered by the block of glutamatergic or enhancement of GABAergic activity [4]. Thus, MT reflects mainly neuronal membrane, but not synaptic, excitability. The electromyographic amplitude of MEP responses elicited by suprathreshold single-pulse TMS reflects the excitability of motor cortex neurons, the integrity of the corticospinal tract, and conduction along the peripheral motor pathway to the muscles. Here, the recruitment curve describes the sigmoidal input–output properties of the corticospinal system. MEPs elicited by low TMS intensities—similar to MT—reflect primarily neuronal membrane excitability, whereas larger MEPs generated by higher TMS intensities are also partially controlled by glutamatergic synaptic effects [5].

Additional protocols have also been developed for detecting more specific alterations of cortical excitability. The Cortical Silent Period (CSP), Short-Latency Afferent Inhibition (SAI), Short-Latency Intracortical Inhibition (SICI), Long-Interval Intracortical Inhibition (LICI), and I-wave facilitation are neurophysiological measures, which assess intracortical inhibitory processes. CSP refers to a temporary suppression of ongoing electromyographic activity in an active muscle caused by a TMS pulse. It mainly originates from inhibitory mechanisms at the level of the motor cortex and is mediated by $GABA_A$ and $GABA_B$ receptors in low- and high-stimulus intensities, respectively [4]. SAI is obtained by combination of a peripheral electrical stimulus of a mixed nerve with a subsequent TMS pulse over the motor cortex. Within specific interstimulus intervals, the peripheral nerve stimulus has an inhibitory effect on the TMS-elicited MEP, which is controlled by $GABA_A$ receptors and central cholinergic transmission [6]. SICI reflects the inhibitory effect of a subthreshold TMS pulse on the MEP amplitude generated by a subsequent suprathreshold TMS pulse, which is observed at interstimulus intervals (ISIs) between 1 and 6 ms. It is primarily controlled by $GABA_A$ receptors but also affected by glutamatergic and dopaminergic systems [4, 7]. LICI is tested by application of two suprathreshold TMS pulses with ISIs of 20–300 ms and controlled by $GABA_B$ receptors [8]. Another suprathreshold/subthreshold paired-pulse TMS paradigm to assess intracortical excitability is I-wave facilitation. I-waves or indirect waves are repetitive discharges of corticospinal fibers elicited by a suprathreshold TMS pulse over the motor cortex. I-wave facilitation is attributed to intracortical interactions between circuits responsible for the production of these waves, and depends on $GABA_A$-related neuronal circuits, with later I-waves being more affected by intracortical inhibition than early ones [9, 10].

At the intracortical level, beyond inhibitory mechanisms, facilitation can also be probed by combination of a subthreshold TMS conditioning pulse with a suprathreshold test pulse. For interstimulus intervals of 7–20 ms, the conditioning pulse enhances MEP amplitudes evoked by the test pulse (intracortical facilitation (ICF)), which is primarily controlled by the glutamatergic system [4].

Beyond monitoring motor cortex excitability through TMS, specific protocols have also been developed for probing excitability of other brain areas. Visual cortex excitability can be probed by the TMS threshold for the generation of phosphenes, which are light flashes perceived, in this case, by application of TMS over the respective target area. Furthermore, integration of TMS with neuroimaging techniques such as EEG extends TMS excitability measures to additional cortical regions. Single- and paired-pulse TMS protocols have been integrated into TMS-EEG paradigms to study excitation/inhibition mechanisms at the cortical level in both motor and nonmotor areas. The combination of TMS with EEG has identified novel and useful measures of evoked activity that index inhibitory (e.g., GABAergic) and excitatory neurotransmission (see [11] for a review). LICI-related inhibition of cortical evoked activity, for instance, has been identified for DLPFC and parietal TMS-EEG protocols and is associated with GABA-B receptor activity in these areas [12, 13]. In contrast, the amplitudes of the P30 and P60 components of TEPs were reduced by SICI and increased by ICF protocols in both M1 and DLPFC stimulation, which suggests a dependency of these TEP components from GABAergic and glutamatergic synaptic mechanisms [14]. Considering the ability of paired-pulse TMS-EEG protocols to obtain neurophysiological readouts for nonmotor regions, they might also be suited to characterize healthy versus pathological brain states of these regions and introduce novel electrophysiological diagnostic and prognostic markers in clinical populations.

One relevant limitation of the abovementioned TMS-derived measures is the appreciable level of the observed variability of most of them, which is caused by various biological and methodological factors. This variability compromises the reliability of TMS-derived neurophysiological markers, especially at the level of the individual, which, in addition to difficulties in defining normative values, challenges their use as standard diagnostic protocols. Further studies are required to enhance the sensitivity and specificity of these metrics to translate them into clinical applications.

5.2.2 Monitoring Network Connectivity by NIBS

Beyond alterations of cortical activity and excitability of regional areas, the pathophysiology underlying psychiatric and neurological disorders is increasingly attributed to dysfunctional networks, involving abnormal interactions between multiple brain regions. NIBS techniques alone, and in combination with neuroimaging methods, promote our understanding of the network activity underlying both healthy human brain functions as well as connectivity changes associated with dysfunctional states.

Two TMS pulses applied to different regions of the brain can be used to probe both intra- and interhemispheric corticocortical interactions. Double-pulse techniques have been especially explored for motor control and movement disorders. One example is the exploration of transcallosal inhibition, where a conditioning TMS stimulus is applied over one motor cortex, and the inhibitory effect is explored on the contralateral homolog [15]. Similarly, a conditioning TMS stimulus over the cerebellum inhibits subsequent motor cortex excitability through cerebellar-cortical pathways [16].

Application of NIBS over a specific region affects not only neural activity of the respective target area but also the evoked activity that propagates to anatomically and functionally interconnected regions. Integration of brain stimulation and neuroimaging tools enables evaluation of these dynamic network interactions. Depending on the neuroimaging modality, different aspects of NIBS-induced changes in brain activity can be captured. EEG is suited to monitor TMS/tES-evoked/altered cortical activity not just at the stimulation site, but also across remote, but interconnected areas. Tracing the spatiotemporal propagation pattern of NIBS evoked potentials with EEG allows determining corticocortical excitability and functional connectivity. The high temporal resolution of the EEG enables tracking of the temporal sequence of communication between regions and, combined with NIBS, can identify effective (causal) connectivity patterns in the brain. Moreover, NIBS techniques can trigger oscillatory rhythms or perturb/enhance ongoing oscillations. NIBS-EEG approaches thus make it possible to study the functional/causal specificity of brain rhythms for distinct cognitive and motor functions/malfunctions. Altered amplitudes, synchronization, and propagation of TMS-induced natural frequencies in different cortical areas have the potential to act as diagnostic and prognostic electrophysiological markers—for a review, see [17].

Besides EEG, use of fMRI in combination with NIBS may also deliver relevant additional information about brain connectivity. Although its temporal resolution is inferior in comparison with EEG measures, important advantages include its superior spatial resolution as well as the opportunity to monitor activity alterations across larger and deeper brain areas, including subcortical regions [18].

5.3   Using NIBS to Modulate Neurophysiological Processes

In addition to the value provided as a monitoring technique, NIBS is increasingly being used in diverse research and clinical settings as a means to directly *modulate* neural processes. Researchers wishing to study the causal nature of cognitive functions or neurological disorders may consider NIBS to complement traditional neurophysiological techniques such as electrophysiological recordings in animals, which are often invasive, or functional neuroimaging techniques such as fMRI, or

EEG/MEG, which are typically limited in disentangling associative/epiphenomenal observations of neural activity from direct causal relations. NIBS as a neuromodulatory technique is not limited to causing acute or short-lasting effects but may also be used to induce aftereffects that extend beyond the duration of application for up to several minutes or hours. These effects share features that are consistent with synaptic plasticity mechanisms, such as long-term depression/potentiation (LTD/LTP). Respective protocols can thus be used to explore the relevance of plasticity for psychological processes, including the involvement of pathological plasticity in psychiatric and neurological diseases, or to counteract respective pathological plasticity for therapeutic reasons.

5.3.1 Transcranial Magnetic Stimulation (TMS)

Direct-effects: Single stimuli or short bursts of TMS can be used to induce a "virtual brain lesion" whereby local neural activity is disrupted within a specific brain region during a task, allowing inference on the functional *role* of a particular region, and also *when* it may become involved during a task (chronometry studies) [19]. Extending the duration of the disruption can be achieved by repeating pulses of TMS (rTMS) at 5–10 Hz, lasting for a few seconds [20]. Short-lasting rTMS protocols have also been shown to transiently induce and synchronize neural firing, leading to changes in neuronal oscillations [21]. As practical examples of these approaches, Amassian et al. [22] demonstrated the dependence of timing TMS to successful vs. unsuccessful processing of visual stimuli relative to delivery intervals.

    After-effects: Short- and long-term aftereffects of TMS have been observed with longer duration repetitive TMS protocols (more than 50 pulses), which induce changes in cortical excitability beyond the stimulation period [23]. Understanding the mechanistic and physiological bases for these effects remains a topic of ongoing research; however, synaptic plasticity is assumed to be the likely model, since (1) the direction of plasticity (LTP or LTD) appears to be dependent on the induction protocol, (2) the effects appear related to the activity of gene-encoded proteins that are active during early stages of synaptic plasticity [24, 25], and (3) among other molecular activity, aftereffects are dependent on neurotransmitter release and NMDA receptor-dependent activity [26, 27]. Specifically, low-frequency stimulation such as rTMS in the range between 0.9 and 1 Hz leads to a reduction in cortical excitability, while higher frequency rTMS above 5 Hz increases cortical excitability [28]. Patterned rTMS, such as continuous or intermittent theta-burst stimulation (c/iTBS), whereby 3 pulses are delivered at 50 Hz and repeated at 5 Hz [29], or quadripulse stimulation, which delivers 4 pulses repeated at a rate of 0.2 Hz [30], also induce lasting effects on cortical excitability. Finally, paired associative stimulation (PAS), which combines stimulation of a mixed peripheral nerve with motor cortex TMS, induces—dependent on the interval between respective stimuli—LTP—or LTD-like plasticity, which is similar to spike-timing-dependent plasticity developed in animal models [31]. However, the strength and duration of these effects are not, in all cases, homogeneous. They depend on the physiological state of the brain prior to and during the stimulation [32], as well as on stimulation parameters such as intensity, number of pulses, and repetition of stimulation [33, 34]. In healthy adults, rTMS, TBS, and QPS have been used to induce functional alterations offline, such as in working memory, motor reaction time, visual attention, and tactile discrimination, among other cognitive paradigms (see review by [35]).

5.3.2   Transcranial Direct Current Stimulation (tDCS)

Direct-effects: tDCS does not induce firing of action potentials but results in polarity-dependent shifts in the resting membrane potential of neurons. Similarly to TMS, the characterization of the specific cell compartments polarized by tDCS critically depends on the neuronal morphology relative to the induced electric field, as well as stimulation intensity and duration [36]. The polarity of the stimulation (anodal or cathodal) is conventionally termed by the respective type of electrode (surface positive or surface negative) placed over the target cortical area on the scalp. Current flows from the anode to the cathode and must flow into and out of the cell in order to exert effects [37]. Animal studies demonstrated that application of weak DC fields delivered epidurally induced polarity-dependent changes in excitability and spontaneous activity during and after the course of stimulation [38]. In animal and human studies, anodal tDCS applied over the motor cortex results in simultaneous enhancement of motor cortical excitability while cathodal tDCS diminishes it [39]. The neuronal effects depend on membrane polarization changes since pharmacological blockage of voltage-dependent sodium and calcium ion channels abolished the respective effects [40].

After-effects: Neuroplastic aftereffects of tDCS are also mediated by changes in synaptic efficacy, and thereby share properties of LTP/LTD. In the seminal animal study by Bindman et al. [38], anodal stimulation led to enhanced cortical activity and excitability lasting for hours while cathodal stimulation led to reduced activity. In humans, respective identically directed polarity-dependent effects were also observed [39, 41]. These effects depend on NMDA receptor activity, which involves regulation of neuronal calcium [40, 42, 43]. Similarly to TMS mechanisms of synaptic plasticity, aftereffects induced by tDCS are not linear and depend on intrinsic cortical activity [44, 45], as well as stimulation parameters, such as current intensity, stimulation duration, and repetition [46–48]. Moreover, physiological effects of tDCS are not limited to the cortical region directly stimulated by the electrode montage, but may also extend to regional and remote loci, either due to the diffuse spatial focality of the induced electric field (depending on the montage—[49]) or by functional connectivity-driven changes [50–52]. Similarly to rTMS effects, tDCS induces long-lasting functional changes in target regions and networks, such as in motor learning (see review by [53]), as well as in neuropsychological processes such as emotion, attention, and working memory [54].

5.3.3   Transcranial Alternating Current Stimulation (tACS)

Direct-effects: tACS is a variant of tDCS, which differs mainly in that tACS is applied with an alternating waveform at a specific frequency (or multiple superimposed frequencies). Therefore, the main rationale of applying tACS is to rhythmically alter cortical activity, which is accomplished by frequency-pulsed subthreshold changes in membrane polarization leading to entrainment of intrinsic oscillatory activity with the applied waveform. In classic montages consisting of two electrodes, oscillatory synchronization between the two sites will become anti-phasic since the electric field should alternate unidirectionally. However, by including more than two electrodes with multichannel stimulators, researchers can synchronize oscillatory activity between two or more regions in-phase by specifying the precise phase of the oscillatory cycle individually for each electrode, while ensuring that the net electric field is conserved [55]. The online physiological effects of tACS on neuronal oscillations have been demonstrated by animal studies [56], as well as human studies using EEG, where alpha frequency stimulation increased the power of the respective frequency band [57]. Stimulation at a specific frequency may also entrain harmonic multiples of that frequency or interact with other frequencies due to cross-frequency coupling. Recent studies supporting the functional relevance of these effects have demonstrated that working memory processes can be facilitated with either theta [58] or theta-gamma coupled tACS [59]. Therefore, tACS provides a customizable approach to investigate the causal dependence of oscillatory activity with cognitive functions.

After-effects: Beyond the direct effects of oscillatory entrainment, a few studies have also reported neuroplastic aftereffects in cortical excitability [60–62]. Available evidence suggests that the induction of plasticity might partially depend on the stimulation parameters (e.g., frequency and intensity/amplitude), since high- but not low-intensity tACS induced aftereffects up to 60 minutes after stimulation [61, 62], and since tACS was more effective when applied at the beta frequency, which is the predominant frequency band in the resting motor cortex [63]. In the same way, aftereffects in occipital alpha have been observed when tACS was applied within the alpha range [57, 64]. Since a direct association between excitability alterations and oscillatory changes was not observed, whether the observed aftereffects in oscillatory rhythms reflect LTP/LTD-like plasticity mechanisms, such as spike-timing-dependent plasticity (STDP), remains unclear [62, 65, 66].

To summarize, NIBS offers various means to directly modulate and induce aftereffects in neurophysiological processes, such as cortical excitability, neuronal oscillations, and hemodynamic activity, among others. However, these effects are not linearly related to stimulation parameters, may be heterogeneous between individuals due to anatomical or physiological profiles, and may be nontrivially affected by cognitive state, due to metaplastic or homeostatic regulatory mechanisms. The goal of ongoing research and development of NIBS is to understand how these factors interact with each other, in order to develop better-suited stimulation protocols that deliver state-of-the-art efficacy in research and clinical settings.

5.4 Translation of NIBS Techniques from Basic to Clinical Applications

NIBS may also be applied in clinical settings to treat psychiatric and neurological diseases. In one perspective, they may be used to explore the pathophysiology of these diseases, which include the development of diagnostic measures and relevant biomarkers to track the efficacy of therapeutic interventions, as well as evaluation of therapeutic effects, and their foundations. In a second approach, NIBS protocols may be applied for therapeutic purposes in order to counteract pathological alterations in brain physiology. They may also serve as adjuvants to support therapeutic activities in other domains, e.g., re-learning or rehabilitative approaches, which profit from enhanced plasticity. In the following, we will give examples of how respective NIBS tools can be employed for these purposes.

5.4.1 Application of NIBS for Identification of Disease-Related Pathophysiology

NIBS techniques have contributed relevantly in enhancing our understanding of the pathophysiology of neurological and psychiatric diseases. In numerous psychiatric diseases, pathological alterations of cortical excitability have been identified. For example, decreased GABAergic inhibition, as obtained by SICI, has been shown for major depression (MDD), schizophrenia (SCZ), and obsessive-compulsive disorder (OCD). Additionally, enhanced intracortical facilitation has been shown in OCD by ICF protocols (for a review, see [67]). These results suggest an imbalance of corresponding neurotransmitters in the respective diseases, mainly of the glutamatergic and GABAergic systems. Moreover, these findings show that respective alterations differ between disease entities. In Alzheimer's disease (AD), reduced SAI has been shown in patients at the initial stage of disease, which is expected according to the cholinergic hypothesis of AD, and makes this parameter a potential adjunctive tool for early diagnosis of the disease. This deficit was abolished by cholinergic medication, which further suggests such an approach being promising to explore mechanisms of action of respective pharmacological treatment approaches [6].

Beyond the evaluation of regional excitability alterations in psychiatric diseases, network connectivity analysis based on TMS–EEG has emerged recently as a new option to explore respective pathophysiological alterations in psychiatric and neurological diseases. Here, abnormal functional and effective connectivity have been shown to be relevant in disease populations, e.g., patients with SCZ having reduced amplitude and synchrony of frontal and prefrontal gamma oscillations, which was associated with disrupted effective connectivity, as assessed by TMS-EEG [68]. Another important physiological measure of disease-related pathological alterations is neuroplasticity, which has been extensively studied in neuropsychiatric disorders. PAS-generated LTP-like plasticity is impaired in Parkinson's disease in the off state but restored by dopaminergic treatment, which underscores the relevance of dopamine for plasticity, and might help to explain the cognitive deficits in these patients [69]. For SCZ, a decrease in LTP-like plasticity was demonstrated via tDCS [70], possibly due to pathological alterations of dopaminergic and glutamatergic activity [71]. In accordance with the importance of plasticity for cognitive functions, the respective plasticity reduction is correlated with cognitive decline in these patients [72], supporting the concept of employing alterations in NIBS-induced plasticity as a biomarker of disease or symptom manifestation [70].

These exemplary studies show that NIBS is not only an important tool to explore different aspects of disease-related pathophysiological alterations in the human brain but also potentially relevant to enhance diagnostic efficiency or predict clinical prognosis, e.g., of pharmacological treatment responses. So far, only TMS measures, including central motor conduction time and the triple stimulation technique, have been clinically adopted for the diagnosis of diseases of the motor system. In principle, the abovementioned protocols might also be valuable for these purposes, including monitoring of not only regional excitability, but also plasticity and connectivity. One current drawback of these techniques, which limits their use at individual level, is the relatively large intra- and interindividual variability. However, new paradigms are under development, which might help to overcome these limitations.

5.4.2 Application of NIBS as Therapeutic Intervention

Given their capability to induce neuroplasticity, and taking into account pathological alterations of plasticity, and cortical excitability in psychiatric diseases, as well as the importance of neuroplasticity for psychotherapeutic and rehabilitative treatments, NIBS techniques have been implemented in numerous treatment studies. As one of the first clinically approved NIBS interventions, rTMS was shown to be efficient for the treatment of MDD. Based on findings of pathological hypo-activation of the left and a relative hyper-activation of the right dorsolateral prefrontal cortex in depression, and a systemic reduction of LTP, which goes along with cognitive deficits, excitability-enhancing left prefrontal or excitability-reducing right prefrontal rTMS and tDCS have successfully demonstrated to reduce symptoms (see [73] for an overview). This application can be taken as a paradigmatic example for the therapeutic application of NIBS, which has since then extended to a larger disease spectrum with similar underlying concepts. In stroke rehabilitation, upregulation of the lesioned area and downregulation of the nonlesioned contralateral homolog have been proposed as an important therapeutic aim to rebalance the motor system, thereby improving functions. Similarly, tDCS has been shown to improve poststroke recovery through this concept [74]. In addition, NIBS based on similar principles has been applied in numerous neuropsychiatric disorders such as neuropathic pain and SCZ (for an overview, see [75, 76]).

Beyond the sole application of NIBS as a therapeutic option, its combination with conventional treatment has also been probed. The conceptual background is to enhance plasticity and/or functions via synergistic effects of dual interventions. For instance, tDCS has been adopted as an adjunctive therapeutic option for stroke reha-bilitation or MDD, as it allows combination with simultaneous occupational/physi-cal therapy or psychotherapy, respectively, and thereby further facilitates the recovery process [77, 78]. Likewise, conventional pharmaceutical treatment, with NIBS as an add-on treatment, has revealed synergistic effects. It has been demon-strated that co-application of a serotonergic antidepressant with bilateral prefrontal tDCS significantly improved depression symptoms as compared to treatment with medication or stimulation alone [73].

Apart from the pathological plasticity, neuropsychiatric symptoms can also be associated with abnormal oscillatory activities of specific brain areas. Here tACS is a potentially valuable approach. tACS was shown to suppress Parkinsonian tremor via phase cancellation when an antagonizing stimulation phase was applied over the motor cortex [79]. A similar principle might be considered for other clini-cal symptoms. For example, consciousness states are associated with specific brain oscillations of prefrontal areas. Gamma oscillations are specifically relevant for the so-called secondary consciousness states, which allow the separation of inner and outer reality, including, but probably not restricted to, the perceived sense of reality during dreams. Here, enhancing gamma activity not only improved secondary consciousness during dreams [80] but also improved symptoms in a pilot study in OCD. In this condition, symptoms are at least partially caused by an unsurmountable drive to perform activities, which are known to be intellectu-ally senseless by the patients, but cannot be completely suppressed, which may be partially due to a missing cognitive dissociation to respective impulses [81]. However, apart from these approaches, therapeutic tACS studies remain scarce at present.

In general, the therapeutic application of neuromodulatory NIBS techniques shows potential as a clinical intervention, and implementation of some protocols into routine therapy is already showing promising efficacy. Nevertheless, beyond numerous pilot studies in various diseases, there is still a long way to go for many applications to be transferred to routine clinical treatment, due to a relative lack of systematic studies to identify optimal protocols. Moreover, pivotal studies are still required in many fields, and interindividual differences in efficacy require a nuanced approach in study designs and analyses, which has largely not been tackled system-atically so far.

5.5 Conclusions

Noninvasive brain stimulation relevantly enriches the arsenal of methods available to explore the physiological foundation of neurological and psychiatric diseases, including not only pathological alterations but also dynamic changes relevant for treatment effects. Moreover, specific variants of these methods are suited to induce or modulate prolonged alterations of respective physiological processes, which have therapeutic potential. This especially includes NIBS-generated plasticity and alterations of oscillatory brain activity.

For exploration of physiological processes, it is evident that NIBS helps in obtaining a more enriched understanding of the physiological bases of respective diseases at the group level, and thereby insightful knowledge about the general pathophysiology of respective syndromes, as well as physiological alterations which are associated with therapeutic success (although the latter has been explored less extensively). These kinds of studies, especially when combined with imaging methods, might help to develop innovative physiology-based therapeutic regimens and also to evaluate the potential of new treatment options based on their physiological effects. However, a relatively scarce amount of protocols has been used so far as diagnostic procedure for individual patients. Exceptions are central conductance measures, measures of MEP amplitudes under specific conditions (i.e., the triple stimulation technique), and mapping procedures. One reason for this shortcoming is the relevant trial-to-trial variability of TMS-evoked outcome measures. While it might be possible to reduce certain methodologically caused foundations of this variability by sophisticated stimulation protocols, e.g., neuronavigation or robot-assisted procedures, some aspects of this variability are intrinsic, i.e., the partially asynchronous activation of target neurons, and differences in conduction velocity between respective neurons. Thus, usage of respective tools to extract biomarkers at the individual level, and/or tools for personalized medicine, might be somewhat limited with presently available procedures.

For therapeutic applications, plasticity-inducing and plasticity-modulating tools are available at present. These include mainly rTMS and tDCS, but new techniques are emerging, including oscillatory electrical stimulation (tACS, tRNS), stimulation with static magnets, or ultrasound stimulation. These tools have been investigated as viable treatment options for numerous psychiatric and neurological diseases, and conclusive evidence for therapeutic effects in a couple of syndromes is available, such as for rTMS in major depression, which has FDA approval. However, here also, systematic studies are required at the group level to identify protocols with optimized efficacy, as well as protocols that allow a sophisticated and individualized adaptation. Achieving these objectives is not trivial because the effects of these techniques are neuromodulatory, and therefore nonlinear, and state-dependent. Newly developing approaches might combine specific intervention concepts, e.g., by combinations of stimulation with pharmacotherapy, and psychotherapy, to achieve more targeted effects of therapeutic plasticity alterations.

A common limitation of both diagnostic and therapeutic approaches is the restriction of the direct effects of respective interventions to only superficial cortical targets. This might be partially overcome by network stimulation approaches; however, some emerging techniques offer the promise to also allow subcortical stimulation selectively, which would open completely new avenues for NIBS. These include techniques such as ultrasound stimulation and more specialized forms of oscillatory electric brain stimulation protocols.

Taken together, NIBS has been developed into a valuable tool for exploring the physiological underpinning of brain diseases, monitoring therapeutic effects, and also as an interventional method for modulating neurophysiological activity. The combination of NIBS with other approaches and the development of these tools might help to further enhance the utility of respective techniques.

Acknowledgments This work was supported by the BMBF GCBS project (grant 01EE1403C).

References

1. Merton PA, Morton HB. Stimulation of the cerebral cortex in the intact human subject. Nature [Internet]. 1980 May 22 [cited 2016 Nov 26];285(5762):227. Available from: http://www.ncbi.nlm.nih.gov/pubmed/7374773.
2. Committee IFCN, Rossini PM, Burke D, Chen R, Cohen LG, Daskalakis Z, et al. Non-invasive electrical and magnetic stimulation of the brain, spinal cord, roots and peripheral nerves: basic principles and procedures for routine clinical and research application: an updated report from an I.F.C.N. Committee. Clin Neurophysiol [Internet]. 2015;126(6):1071–107. https://doi.org/10.1016/j.clinph.2015.02.001.
3. Ziemann U, Lönnecker S, Steinhoff BJ, Paulus W. Effects of antiepileptic drugs on motor cortex excitability in humans: a transcranial magnetic stimulation study. Ann Neurol. 1996;40(3):367–78.
4. Paulus W, Classen J, Cohen LG, Large CH, Di Lazzaro V, Nitsche M, et al. State of the art: pharmacologic effects on cortical excitability measures tested by transcranial magnetic stimulation. Brain Stimul [Internet]. 2008;1(3):151–63. Available from: http://linkinghub.elsevier.com/retrieve/pii/S1935861X08000387.
5. Prout AJ, Eisen AA. The cortical silent period and amyotrophic lateral sclerosis. Muscle Nerve. 1994;17(2):217–23.
6. Nardone R, Bergmann J, Kronbichler M, Kunz A, Klein S, Caleri F, et al. Abnormal short latency afferent inhibition in early Alzheimer's disease: a transcranial magnetic demonstration. J Neural Transm. 2008;115(11):1557–62.
7. Ziemann U, Tergau F, Bruns D, Baudewig J, Paulus W. Changes in human motor cortex excitability induced by dopaminergic and anti-dopaminergic drugs. Electroencephalogr Clin Neurophysiol. 1997;105(6):430–7.
8. Siebner HR, Dressnandt J, Auer C, Conrad B. Continuous intrathecal baclofen infusions induced a marked increase of the transcranially evoked silent period in a patient with generalized dystonia. Muscle Nerve. 1998;21(9):1209–12.
9. Hanajima R, Ugawa Y, Terao Y, Enomoto H, Shiio Y, Mochizuki H, et al. Mechanisms of intracortical I-wave facilitation elicited with paired-pulse magnetic stimulation in humans. J Physiol. 2002;538(1):253–61.
10. Ziemann U, Tergau F, Wischer S, Hildebrandt J, Paulus W. Pharmacological control of facilitatory I-wave interaction in the human motor cortex. A paired transcranial magnetic stimulation study. Electroencephalogr Clin Neurophysiol. 1998;109(4):321–30.
11. Farzan F, Vernet M, Shafi M, Rotenberg A, Daskalakis ZJ, Pascual-Leone A. Characterizing and modulating brain circuitry through transcranial magnetic stimulation combined with electroencephalography. Front Neural Circuits. 2016;10:73.
12. Fitzgerald PB, Daskalakis ZJ, Hoy K, Farzan F, Upton DJ, Cooper NR, et al. Cortical inhibition in motor and non-motor regions: a combined TMS-EEG study. Clin EEG Neurosci. 2008;39(3):112–7.
13. Fitzgerald PB, Maller JJ, Hoy K, Farzan F, Daskalakis ZJ. GABA and cortical inhibition in motor and non-motor regions using combined TMS–EEG: a time analysis. Clin Neurophysiol. 2009;120(9):1706–10.
14. Cash RFH, Noda Y, Zomorrodi R, Radhu N, Farzan F, Rajji TK, et al. Characterization of glutamatergic and GABA A-mediated neurotransmission in motor and dorsolateral prefrontal cortex using paired-pulse TMS–EEG. Neuropsychopharmacology. 2017;42(2):502.

15. Meyer B-U, Röricht S, Von Einsiedel HG, Kruggel F, Weindl A. Inhibitory and excitatory interhemispheric transfers between motor cortical areas in normal humans and patients with abnormalities of the corpus callosum. Brain. 1995;118(2):429–40.

16. Werhahn KJ, Taylor J, Ridding M, Meyer B-U, Rothwell JC. Effect of transcranial magnetic stimulation over the cerebellum on the excitability of human motor cortex. Electroencephalogr Clin Neurophysiol. 1996;101(1):58–66.

17. Thut G, Miniussi C. New insights into rhythmic brain activity from TMS–EEG studies. Trends Cogn Sci. 2009;13(4):182–9.

18. Siebner HR, Bergmann TO, Bestmann S, Massimini M, Johansen-Berg H, Mochizuki H, et al. Consensus paper: combining transcranial stimulation with neuroimaging. Brain Stimul [Internet]. 2009;2(2):58–80. Available from: http://www.sciencedirect.com/science/article/pii/S1935861X08003616.

19. Pascual-Leone A, Walsh V, Rothwell J. Transcranial magnetic stimulation in cognitive neuroscience what does it do and when does it do it? A causal chronometry of brain function. Curr Opin Neurobiol. 2000;10:232–7.

20. Hallett M. Transcranial magnetic stimulation: a primer. Neuron. 2007;55(2):187–99.

21. Veniero D, Vossen A, Gross J, Thut G. Lasting EEG/MEG aftereffects of rhythmic transcranial brain stimulation: level of control over oscillatory network activity. Front Cell Neurosci [Internet]. 2015;9:477. Available from: http://www.pubmedcentral.nih.gov/articlerender.fcgi?artid=4678227&tool=pmcentrez&rendertype=abstract.

22. Amassian VE, Cracco RQ, Maccabee PJ, Cracco JB, Rudell A, Eberle L. Suppression of visual perception by magnetic coil stimulation of human occipital cortex. Electroencephalogr Clin Neurophysiol Potentials Sect [Internet]. 1989;74(6):458–62. Available from: https://linkinghub.elsevier.com/retrieve/pii/0168559789900361.

23. Ziemann U, Paulus W, Nitsche MA, Pascual-Leone A, Byblow WD, Berardelli A, et al. Consensus: motor cortex plasticity protocols. Brain Stimul [Internet]. 2008;1(3):164–82. Available from: http://linkinghub.elsevier.com/retrieve/pii/S1935861X08000429.

24. Hoppenrath K, Funke K. Time-course of changes in neuronal activity markers following iTBS-TMS of the rat neocortex. Neurosci Lett [Internet]. 2013 Mar 1 [cited 2019 Jul 1];536:19–23. Available from: http://www.ncbi.nlm.nih.gov/pubmed/23328445.

25. Volz LJ, Benali A, Mix A, Neubacher U, Funke K. Dose-dependence of changes in cortical protein expression induced with repeated transcranial magnetic theta-burst stimulation in the rat. Brain Stimul [Internet]. 2013 Jul [cited 2019 Jul 1];6(4):598–606. Available from: http://www.ncbi.nlm.nih.gov/pubmed/23433874.

26. Cirillo G, Di Pino G, Capone F, Ranieri F, Florio L, Todisco V, et al. Neurobiological aftereffects of non-invasive brain stimulation. Brain Stimul [Internet]. 2017;10(1):1–18. https://doi.org/10.1016/j.brs.2016.11.009.

27. Rajan TS, Ghilardi MFM, Wang HY, Mazzon E, Bramanti P, Restivo D, et al. Mechanism of action for rTMS: a working hypothesis based on animal studies [Internet]. Front Physiol. 2017;8 [cited 2019 Jul 2]. Available from: http://journal.frontiersin.org/article/10.3389/fphys.2017.00457/full.

28. Lenz M, Müller-Dahlhaus F, Vlachos A. Cellular and molecular mechanisms of rTMS-induced neural plasticity. In: Therapeutic rTMS in neurology [Internet]. Cham: Springer International Publishing; 2016. p. 11–22. Available from: http://link.springer.com/10.1007/978-3-319-25721-1_2.

29. Huang YZ, Edwards MJ, Rounis E, Bhatia KP, Rothwell JC. Theta burst stimulation of the human motor cortex. Neuron. 2005;45(2):201–6.

30. Hamada M, Terao Y, Hanajima R, Shirota Y, Nakatani-Enomoto S, Furubayashi T, et al. Bidirectional long-term motor cortical plasticity and metaplasticity induced by quadripulse transcranial magnetic stimulation. J Physiol. 2008;586(16):3927–47.

31. Stefan K, Kunesch E, Cohen LG, Benecke R, Classen J. Induction of plasticity in the human motor cortex by paired associative stimulation. Brain. 2000;123(Pt 3):572–84.

32. Karabanov A, Ziemann U, Hamada M, George MS, Quartarone A, Classen J, et al. Consensus paper: probing homeostatic plasticity of human cortex with non-invasive transcranial

brain stimulation. Brain Stimul [Internet]. 2015;8(5):993–1006. https://doi.org/10.1016/j.brs.2015.01.404.

33. Tse NY, Goldsworthy MR, Ridding MC, Coxon JP, Fitzgerald PB, Fornito A, et al. The effect of stimulation interval on plasticity following repeated blocks of intermittent theta burst stimulation. Sci Rep [Internet]. 2018 Jun 4 [cited 2019 Jul 2];8(1):8526. Available from: http://www.nature.com/articles/s41598-018-26791-w.

34. Bäumer T, Lange R, Liepert J, Weiller C, Siebner HR, Rothwell JC, et al. Repeated premotor rTMS leads to cumulative plastic changes of motor cortex excitability in humans. NeuroImage. 2003;20(1):550–60.

35. Luber B, Lisanby SH. Enhancement of human cognitive performance using transcranial magnetic stimulation (TMS). Neuroimage [Internet]. 2014;85(2):961–70. Available from: https://linkinghub.elsevier.com/retrieve/pii/S1053811913006447.

36. Nitsche MA, Cohen LG, Wassermann EM, Priori A, Lang N, Antal A, et al. Transcranial direct current stimulation: state of the art 2008. Brain Stimul [Internet]. 2008;1(3):206–23. Available from: http://www.sciencedirect.com/science?_ob=ArticleURL&_udi=B8JBG-4SWGB96-1&_user=10&_coverDate=07%2F31%2F2008&_rdoc=11&_fmt=high&_orig=browse&_srch=doc-info(%23toc%2343558%232008%23999989996%2369643 8%23FLA%23display%23Volume)&_cdi=43558&_sort=d&_docanchor=&.

37. Rahman A, Reato D, Arlotti M, Gasca F, Datta A, Parra LC, et al. Cellular effects of acute direct current stimulation: somatic and synaptic terminal effects. J Physiol [Internet]. 2013;591(Pt 10):2563–78. Available from: http://www.pubmedcentral.nih.gov/articlerender.fcgi?artid=3678043&tool=pmcentrez&rendertype=abstract.

38. Bindman LJ, Lippold OCJ, Redfearn JWT. The action of brief polarizing currents on the cerebral cortex of the rat (1) during current flow and (2) in the production of long-lasting after-effects. J Physiol [Internet]. 1964;172(1):369–82. Available from: http://www.ncbi.nlm.nih.gov/pubmed/14199369%5Cn, http://www.pubmedcentral.nih.gov/articlerender.fcgi?artid=PMC136885.

39. Nitsche MA, Paulus W. Excitability changes induced in the human motor cortex by weak transcranial direct current stimulation. J Physiol [Internet]. 2000;527(Pt 3):633–9. Available from: http://www.ncbi.nlm.nih.gov/pubmed/10990547%5Cn, http://www.pubmedcentral.nih.gov/articlerender.fcgi?artid=2270099&tool=pmcentrez&rendertype=abstract.

40. Nitsche MA, Fricke K, Henschke U, Schlitterlau A, Liebetanz D, Lang N, et al. Pharmacological modulation of cortical excitability shifts induced by transcranial direct current stimulation in humans. J Physiol [Internet]. 2003;553(1):293–301. Available from: http://www.jphysiol.org/cgi/doi/10.1113/jphysiol.2003.049916.

41. Nitsche MA, Nitsche MS, Klein CC, Tergau F, Rothwell JC, Paulus W. Level of action of cathodal DC polarisation induced inhibition of the human motor cortex. Clin Neurophysiol [Internet]. 2003;114(4):600–4. Available from: http://ac.els-cdn.com/S1388245702004121/1-s2.0-S1388245702004121-main.pdf?_tid=d330e68c-b706-11e2-b24b-00000aab0f02&acdnat=1367925251_049960c317c14dbb692895176e623ccd.

42. Malenka RC, Bear MF. LTP and LTD: an embarrassment of riches. Neuron [Internet]. 2004 Sep 30 [cited 2016 Nov 25];44(1):5–21. Available from: http://www.ncbi.nlm.nih.gov/pubmed/15450156.

43. Liebetanz D, Nitsche MA, Tergau F, Paulus W. Pharmacological approach to the mechanisms of transcranial DC-stimulation-induced after-effects of human motor cortex excitability. Brain. 2002;125(10):2238–47.

44. Antal A, Terney D, Poreisz C, Paulus W. Towards unravelling task-related modulations of neuroplastic changes induced in the human motor cortex. Eur J Neurosci. 2007;26(9):2687–91.

45. Thirugnanasambandam N, Sparing R, Dafotakis M, Meister IG, Paulus W, Nitsche MA, et al. Isometric contraction interferes with transcranial direct current stimulation (tDCS) induced plasticity: evidence of state-dependent neuromodulation in human motor cortex. Restor Neurol Neurosci [Internet]. 2011 [cited 2019 Jul 2];29(5):311–20. Available from: http://www.ncbi.nlm.nih.gov/pubmed/21697590.

46. Batsikadze G, Moliadze V, Paulus W, Kuo M-F, Nitsche MA. Partially non-linear stimulation intensity-dependent effects of direct current stimulation on motor cortex excitability in humans. J Physiol [Internet]. 2013;591(7):1987–2000. Available from: http://doi.wiley.com/10.1113/jphysiol.2012.249730.

47. Monte-Silva K, Kuo M-FF, Hessenthaler S, Fresnoza S, Liebetanz D, Paulus W, et al. Induction of late LTP-like plasticity in the human motor cortex by repeated non-invasive brain stimulation. Brain Stimul [Internet]. 2013 May [cited 2014 Feb 27];6(3):424–32. Available from: http://www.ncbi.nlm.nih.gov/pubmed/22695026.

48. Monte-Silva K, Kuo M-F, Liebetanz D, Paulus W, Nitsche MA. Shaping the optimal repetition interval for cathodal transcranial direct current stimulation (tDCS). J Neurophysiol. 2010;103(4):1735–40.

49. Nitsche MA, Doemkes S, Karakose T, Antal A, Liebetanz D, Lang N, et al. Shaping the effects of transcranial direct current stimulation of the human motor cortex shaping the effects of transcranial direct current stimulation of the human motor cortex. J Neurophysiol [Internet]. 2007;97:3109–17. Available from: http://jn.physiology.org/cgi/doi/10.1152/jn.01312.2006.

50. Polanía R, Paulus W, Antal A, Nitsche MA. Introducing graph theory to track for neuroplastic alterations in the resting human brain: a transcranial direct current stimulation study. Neuroimage [Internet]. 2011;54(3):2287–96. https://doi.org/10.1016/j.neuroimage.2010.09.085.

51. Polanía R, Nitsche MA, Paulus W. Modulating functional connectivity patterns and topological functional organization of the human brain with transcranial direct current stimulation. Hum Brain Mapp [Internet]. 2011 Aug [cited 2014 Feb 25];32(8):1236–49. Available from: http://www.ncbi.nlm.nih.gov/pubmed/20607750.

52. Kunze T, Hunold A, Haueisen J, Jirsa V, Spiegler A. Transcranial direct current stimulation changes resting state functional connectivity: a large-scale brain network modeling study. Neuroimage [Internet]. 2016;140:174–87. Available from: http://www.sciencedirect.com/science/article/pii/S1053811916001221.

53. Buch ER, Santarnecchi E, Antal A, Born J, Celnik PA, Classen J, et al. Effects of tDCS on motor learning and memory formation: a consensus and critical position paper. Clin Neurophysiol [Internet]. 2017;128(4):589–603. Available from: https://linkinghub.elsevier.com/retrieve/pii/S1388245717300263.

54. Shin Y-I, Foerster Á, Nitsche MA. Transcranial direct current stimulation (tDCS)—application in neuropsychology. Neuropsychologia [Internet]. 2015;69:154–75. Available from: http://www.sciencedirect.com/science/article/pii/S0028393215000639.

55. Saturnino GB, Madsen KH, Siebner HR, Thielscher A. How to target inter-regional phase synchronization with dual-site transcranial alternating current stimulation. Neuroimage [Internet]. 2017;163:68–80. https://doi.org/10.1016/j.neuroimage.2017.09.024.

56. Fröhlich F, McCormick DA. Endogenous electric fields may guide neocortical network activity. Neuron. 2010;67(1):129–43.

57. Zaehle T, Rach S, Herrmann CS. Transcranial alternating current stimulation enhances individual alpha activity in human EEG. PLoS One. 2010;5(11):1–7.

58. Polanía R, Nitsche MA, Korman C, Batsikadze G, Paulus W. The importance of timing in segregated theta phase-coupling for cognitive performance. Curr Biol [Internet]. 2012 Jul 5 [cited 2014 Jan 21];22(14):1–5. Available from: http://wwdw.ncbi.nlm.nih.gov/pubmed/22683259.

59. Alekseichuk I, Turi Z, De Lara GA, Antal A, Alekseichuk I, Turi Z, et al. Spatial working memory in humans depends on theta and high gamma synchronization in the prefrontal cortex article spatial working memory in humans depends on theta and high gamma synchronization in the prefrontal cortex. Curr Biol [Internet]. 2016;26(12):1513–1521. https://doi.org/10.1016/j.cub.2016.04.035.

60. Moliadze V, Antal A, Paulus W. Boosting brain excitability by transcranial high frequency stimulation in the ripple range. J Physiol. 2010;588(24):4891–904.

61. Antal A, Boros K, Poreisz C, Chaieb L, Terney D, Paulus W. Comparatively weak after-effects of transcranial alternating current stimulation (tACS) on cortical excitability in humans. Brain Stimul [Internet]. 2008 Apr [cited 2015 Jan 6];1(2):97–105. Available from: http://www.ncbi.nlm.nih.gov/pubmed/20633376.

62. Wischnewski M, Engelhardt M, Salehinejad MA, Schutter DJLG, Kuo M-F, Nitsche MA. NMDA receptor-mediated motor cortex plasticity after 20 hz transcranial alternating current stimulation. Cereb Cortex [Internet]. 2019;29(7):2924–2931. Available from: https://academic.oup.com/cercor/advance-article/doi/10.1093/cercor/bhy160/5051079.

63. St. Louis EK, Frey LC, Britton JW, Frey LC, Hopp JL, Korb P, et al. The Normal EEG. 2016 [cited 2019 Jul 2]. Available from: https://www.ncbi.nlm.nih.gov/books/NBK390343/.

64. Kasten FH, Dowsett J, Herrmann CS. Sustained aftereffect of α -tACS lasts up to 70 min after stimulation. Front Hum Neurosci. 2016;10:245.

65. Thut G, Miniussi C, Gross J. The functional importance of rhythmic activity in the brain. Curr Biol [Internet]. 2012;22(16):R658–63. https://doi.org/10.1016/j.cub.2012.06.061.

66. Vossen A, Gross J, Thut G. Alpha power increase after transcranial alternating current stimulation at alpha frequency (α-tACS) reflects plastic changes rather than entrainment. Brain Stimul [Internet]. 2015 May [cited 2019 Jul 2];8(3):499–508. Available from: http://www.ncbi.nlm.nih.gov/pubmed/25648377.

67. Radhu N, de Jesus DR, Ravindran LN, Zanjani A, Fitzgerald PB, Daskalakis ZJ. A meta-analysis of cortical inhibition and excitability using transcranial magnetic stimulation in psychiatric disorders. Clin Neurophysiol. 2013;124(7):1309–20.

68. Hui J, Tremblay S, Daskalakis ZJ. The current and future potential of transcranial magnetic stimulation with electroencephalography in psychiatry. Clin Pharmacol Ther. 2019;106(4):734–46. https://doi.org/10.1002/cpt.1541. Epub 2019 Aug 30. PMID: 31179533.

69. Morgante F, Espay AJ, Gunraj C, Lang AE, Chen R. Motor cortex plasticity in Parkinson's disease and levodopa-induced dyskinesias. Brain. 2006;129(Pt 4):1059–69.

70. Hasan A, Falkai P, Wobrock T. Transcranial brain stimulation in schizophrenia: targeting cortical excitability, connectivity and plasticity. Curr Med Chem. 2013;20(3):405–13.

71. Balu DT, Coyle JT. Neuroplasticity signaling pathways linked to the pathophysiology of schizophrenia. Neurosci Biobehav Rev. 2011;35(3):848–70.

72. Frantseva MV, Fitzgerald PB, Chen R, Möller B, Daigle M, Daskalakis ZJ. Evidence for impaired long-term potentiation in schizophrenia and its relationship to motor skill learning. Cereb Cortex. 2008;18(5):990–6.

73. Brunoni AR, Sampaio-Junior B, Moffa AH, Aparício LV, Gordon P, Klein I, et al. Noninvasive brain stimulation in psychiatric disorders: a primer. Braz J Psychiatry. 2019;41(1):70–81.

74. Fregni F, Boggio PS, Mansur CG, Wagner T, Ferreira MJ, Lima MC, et al. Transcranial direct current stimulation of the unaffected hemisphere in stroke patients. Neuroreport. 2005;16(14):1551–5.

75. Lefaucheur JP, André-Obadia N, Antal A, Ayache SS, Baeken C, Benninger DH, et al. Evidence-based guidelines on the therapeutic use of repetitive transcranial magnetic stimulation (rTMS). Clin Neurophysiol. 2014;125(11):2150–206.

76. Lefaucheur JP. Cortical neurostimulation for neuropathic pain: state of the art and perspectives. Pain. 2016;157(Suppl):S81–9.

77. Jung IY, Lim JY, Kang EK, Sohn HM, Paik NJ. The factors associated with good responses to speech therapy combined with transcranial direct current stimulation in post-stroke aphasic patients. Ann Rehabil Med. 2011;35(4):460–9.

78. Welch ES, Weigand A, Hooker JE, Philip NS, Tyrka AR, Press DZ, et al. Feasibility of computerized cognitive-behavioral therapy combined with bifrontal transcranial direct current stimulation for treatment of major depression. Neuromodulation. 2019;22(8):898–903.

79. Brittain JS, Probert-Smith P, Aziz TZ, Brown P. Tremor suppression by rhythmic transcranial current stimulation. Curr Biol. 2013;23(5):436–40.

80. Voss U, Holzmann R, Hobson A, Paulus W, Koppehele-Gossel J, Klimke A, et al. Induction of self awareness in dreams through frontal low current stimulation of gamma activity. Nat Neurosci. 2014;17(6):810–2.

81. Klimke A, Nitsche MA, Maurer K, Voss U. Case report: successful treatment of therapy-resistant OCD with application of transcranial alternating current stimulation (tACS). Brain Stimul. 2016;9(3):463–5.

Part II

TMS and Its Applications in Neuropsychiatry and Clinical Neuroscience

Depressive Disorders

6

Anna-Katharine Brem, Chris Baeken, Martijn Arns,
Andre R. Brunoni, Igor Filipčcić, Ana Ganho-Ávila,
Berthold Langguth, Soili M. Lehto, Frank Padberg,
Emmanuel Poulet, Fady Rachid, Alexander T. Sack,
Marie-Anne Vanderhasselt, and Djamila Bennabi

On behalf of the Scientific Committee of the European Conference on Brain Stimulation in Psychiatry.

A.-K. Brem
Max-Planck Institute of Psychiatry, Munich, Germany

Division of Cognitive Neurology, Department of Neurology, Berenson-Allen Center for Noninvasive Brain Stimulation, Beth Israel Deaconess Medical Center, Harvard Medical School, Boston, MA, USA

C. Baeken (✉)
Department of Head and Skin, Ghent University, Brussels, Belgium

Ghent Experimental Psychiatry (GHEP) Lab, Brussels, Belgium

Department of Psychiatry, Vrije Universiteit Brussel (VUB), Universitair Ziekenhuis Brussel (UZBrussel), Brussels, Belgium
e-mail: Chris.Baeken@UGent.be

M. Arns
Research Institute Brainclinics, Nijmegen, The Netherlands

Department of Experimental Psychology, Utrecht University, Utrecht, The Netherlands

A. R. Brunoni
Departments of Internal Medicine and Psychiatry, Faculdade de Medicina da Universidade de São Paulo, São Paulo, Brazil

I. Filipčcić
Psychiatric Hospital 'Sveti Ivan', Zagreb, Croatia

School of Medicine, University of Zagreb, Zagreb, Croatia

Faculty of Dental Medicine and Health, Josip Juraj Strossmayer University of Osijek, Osijek, Croatia

A. Ganho-Ávila
Faculty of Psychology and Educational Sciences, Center for Research in Neuropsychology and Cognitive Behavioral Intervention, University of Coimbra, Coimbra, Portugal

© Springer Nature Switzerland AG 2020
B. Dell'Osso, G. Di Lorenzo (eds.), *Non Invasive Brain Stimulation in Psychiatry and Clinical Neurosciences*,
https://doi.org/10.1007/978-3-030-43356-7_6

B. Langguth
Department of Psychiatry and Psychotherapy, University of Regensburg,
Regensburg, Germany

S. M. Lehto
Psychiatry, University of Helsinki and Helsinki University Hospital, Helsinki, Finland

Faculty of Medicine, Department of Psychology and Logopedics, University of Helsinki,
Helsinki, Finland

Institute of Clinical Medicine, University of Eastern Finland, Kuopio, Finland

Department of Psychiatry, Kuopio University Hospital, Kuopio, Finland

F. Padberg
Department of Psychiatry and Psychotherapy, University Hospital, LMU Munich,
Munich, Germany

E. Poulet
INSERM, U1028, CNRS, UMR5292, Lyon Neuroscience Research Center, PSY-R2 Team,
University Claude Bernard Lyon1, Lyon, France

F. Rachid
Private Practice, Geneva, Switzerland

A. T. Sack
Faculty of Psychology and Neuroscience, Department of Cognitive Neuroscience, Maastricht
University, Maastricht, The Netherlands

M.-A. Vanderhasselt
Department of Experimental Clinical and Health Psychology, Ghent University,
Ghent, Belgium

Department of Head and Skin, Unit of Psychiatry and Medical Psychology, Ghent University,
Ghent, Belgium

D. Bennabi
Department of Clinical Psychiatry, CHU de Besancon, CIC-1431 INSERM, CHU de
Besançon, EA481 Neurosciences, University Bourgogne Franche-Comte, FondaMental
Foundation, Creteil, France

6.1   Introduction

Major depressive disorder (MDD) is the leading cause of mental health related disability worldwide, with an increase in prevalence of more than 18% in the past
decade. Clinical treatment based on pharmacotherapy, psychotherapy, or both is
limited in its effectiveness, particularly if therapy-resistance, chronicity, or adverse
effects come into play. Repetitive transcranial magnetic stimulation (rTMS) has
undergone intensive research, becoming one of the most important nonpharmaco-
logical treatment options in MDD. In 2008, rTMS was approved by the FDA as a
therapy for treatment-resistant depression (TRD) in the USA and since then it has
been approved in other countries, including Canada, Australia, Brazil, and several
European countries [1]. Moreover, rTMS is considered a first-line treatment according to current North American and European guidelines. Besides the initial rTMS

treatment protocols, recently, theta burst stimulation (TBS) and H1-coil TMS have been FDA-cleared for the treatment of MDD.

In this chapter, we discuss current state-of-the-art treatment of depression with rTMS and summarize findings from trials focusing on efficacy, maintenance treatment and long-term outcomes in MDD, combinatory treatments, and personalized and stratified treatment, including treatment of MDD subpopulations and vulnerable populations, as an avenue to precision medicine.

6.2   The Rationale of Using rTMS in Depression

The causes of depression are manifold, including neurophysiological dysregulation, genetic vulnerability, and impaired mood regulation. One of the key findings that are relevant for the application of TMS is the observation of distinct changes in the prefrontal cortex (PFC) of patients with depression. The rationale of using noninvasive brain stimulation applied to the PFC for depression is based on the premise that certain stimulation parameters can enhance, or at least modify, brain activity in the targeted brain area. The dorsolateral PFC (DLPFC) has become the most prominent rTMS target area in MDD, not only since early rTMS studies, but also in more recent, pivotal trials [2]. The DLPFC is part of the frontoparietal network (FPN), which is implicated in the regulation of a multitude of processes such as decision-making, working memory, and attention. The DLPFC is thought to be hypoactive in clinically depressed patients [3]. Moreover, hypoconnectivity of the FPN is associated with hyperconnectivity of the default mode network (DMN), which may promote negative emotional bias, dysfunctional self-referential processing, and rumination [4]. Stimulation of the left DLPFC with high-frequency rTMS (HF-rTMS) has been suggested to normalize the functional balance between neural networks, e.g., downregulate connectivity within the DMN, the left DLPFC and insula, and between the salience network and the hippocampus, which has been shown to be associated with an improvement of depressive symptoms. This rationale has been supported, to some extent, by neuroimaging studies in depressed patients receiving rTMS although replication is warranted [5, 6]. Furthermore, reaching a "normal" homeostasis again between cortico-subcortical networks may normalize the known endocrinological disturbances documented in MDD [7].

6.3   The Role of Cognition in rTMS Applications

So far, cognitive outcomes in the context of rTMS depression treatment have primarily been explored to confirm that rTMS is safe. Indeed, with few exceptions, most single session studies showed no adverse cognitive effects of rTMS [8]. Interestingly, MDD itself is often characterized by specific cognitive deficits, including attention, memory, and executive function deficits, and recent meta-analyses not only showed that rTMS techniques are cognitively safe but also that rTMS may even be associated with specific cognitive improvements in MDD patients. Hence, the rTMS depression treatment targeting the PFC may exert pro-cognitive effects, enhancing cognitive performance specifically in specifically in those functions that are considered vulnerability factors to MDD. Nevertheless, although some studies reported such cognitive improvements in depression after rTMS [9], others failed to find such beneficial cognitive changes [10]. In any case, systematically evaluating and tracking cognitive changes may provide valuable insights into the mechanisms of action by which DLPFC rTMS exerts its antide-pressant effects. It may, e.g., be the case that the cognitive changes induced by rTMS drive or, at least, mediate the improvement in depression symptoms, rather than being an independent side effect or a consequence of the antidepressant treat-ment. In line with this, Harty and colleagues [11] recently described how variability in neural circuits, for example, associated with cognitive functioning, may play a critical role in mediating or moderating the influence of brain stimulation on behav-ioral changes, such as depression.

6.4 State-of-the-Art rTMS Treatment for MDD

6.4.1 Treatment Recommendations for TMS Therapy

Over the past three decades, two different rTMS approaches for the treatment of major depressive episodes have emerged based on some older theories on the hemi-spheric lateralization of emotional processes: either high-frequency rTMS (HF-rTMS) delivered to the left DLPFC (aimed at correcting an alleged hypoactiv-ity) or low-frequency rTMS (LF-rTMS) applied to the right DLPFC (aimed at reducing an alleged hyperactivity) [12]. However, current insights into the working mechanisms of rTMS do not follow these lateralization assumptions anymore. Although LF-rTMS or bilateral rTMS (delivering sequentially HF-rTMS over the left DLPFC and LF-rTMS over the right DLPFC) may not have the FDA approval yet or have not reached the Level A in the European guideline recommendations, both rTMS approaches have shown significantly better results than sham in the majority of studies and future large, randomized, controlled studies may indicate similar efficacy as with HF-rTMS over the left DLPFC. Indeed, a recent network meta-analysis showed a higher response to real vs. sham stimulation condition for bilateral prefrontal rTMS (and intermittent TBS or iTBS), LF-rTMS of the right DLPFC, and HF-rTMS of the left DLPFC [13].

Notably, response and remission to rTMS alone have similar efficacy compared to antidepressant medication, and the magnitude of clinical effects remains modest. In a recent network meta-analysis, the efficacy and tolerability of 8 rTMS modali-ties and sham, including 81 studies and 4233 patients, were evaluated. Some rTMS strategies were more effective than sham [14]. However, none of the active rTMS strategies was significantly superior to another. This highlights the need for identi-fying subgroups of patients more prone to respond to specific rTMS strategies and better understanding TMS' mechanisms of action.

6.4.2 Intensifying rTMS Protocols

One major drawback of current treatment options is the extended time of up to 2 weeks that is needed for effects to unfold. This has led to the development of accelerated high-frequency rTMS (aHF-rTMS) and accelerated intermittent Theta Burst Stimulation (aiTBS), novel stimulation protocols that apply multiple daily sessions (with at least 600 pulses per session), thereby reducing the total treatment time [15]. From a clinical perspective, the aim was also to challenge response and remission rates as observed with electroconvulsive therapy (ECT). Using excitatory stimulation paradigms over the left DLPFC, aHF-rTMS and aiTBS seem to yield similar remission and response rates as daily rTMS, but still do not reach the remission and response rates of ECT. Increasing the number of rTMS sessions over the left DLPFC may further improve clinical outcomes and reduce treatment time. Furthermore, increasing the number of stimulation sessions over the dorsomedial PFC (dmPFC) is associated with a similar clinical response, adding to a significantly faster onset [16]. This agrees not only with clinical observations using aHF-rTMS [15] and aiTBS [17] but also with a recent pilot study [18] showing that high dose aHF-rTMS (i.e., 10 sessions per day) over the left DLPFC for 5 days results in acute response and remission in high TRD.

These recent findings underline the value of novel protocols in terms of a much faster alleviation of depressive symptoms with respect to time (note that the number of sessions remains the same). The most important clinical challenge will therefore be to validate and further optimize the stimulation parameters while still reaching comparable response and remission rates at or beyond the level that is observed with ECT.

6.4.3 TMS Coil Geometry, Orientation, and Position

The geometry of a coil determines stimulation focality as well as depth of the electric field. Since the beginning of TMS, many different coil geometries have been investigated. For the treatment of depression, the most prevalent coil to date is the figure-of-eight coil; however, recent developments suggest the use of novel coil geometries, including the double cone coil and the H-coil. These latter two coils allow modulation of deeper brain areas such as the dorsomedial prefrontal cortex (dmPFC) or anterior cingulate, albeit also being less focal.

The double cone coil features two windings that are set apart at a defined angle (e.g., 120°): its specific geometry is thought to lead to higher current in the central fissure resulting in a more efficient stimulation targeting the dmPFC and/or the more dorsal parts of the ACC. The rationale behind this approach lies in the involvement of the dmPFC in affective, sensory autonomic, cognitive, and salience regulation. The double cone coil has also been used to target the right orbitofrontal cortex in depression [19], where it was shown that 30% of nonresponders to DMPFC rTMS did respond to stimulation at this target, offering hope for stepped-care approaches in TMS, which could enhance efficacy.

The "H-coil" is thought to stimulate up to a depth of 4–6 cm and was therefore introduced as deep TMS (dTMS). Phantom measurements have shown that while H-coils (e.g., the H1 coil for depression) reach deeper targets, they also provide less focal stimulation, following the well-known trade-off between depth (or intensity) and focality of TMS [20]. In 2013, based on the findings by Levkovitz and colleagues [21], the FDA approved the first dTMS device (featuring an H1-coil) for the use in patients with TRD. In this RCT with 212 MDD outpatients, remission rates were higher in the dTMS (32.6%) compared to the sham group (14.6%), and were stable during the 12-week maintenance phase. Moreover, dTMS appears to be well tolerated and efficacious in late-life depression [22] and showed to be potentially effective as add-on treatment in resistant bipolar depressed patients [23]. To date, there is only one randomized head-to-head comparison of effectiveness between dTMS and standard rTMS using the figure-of-eight coil [24]. Here, the authors demonstrated that, when depressed patients did not respond, or only partly responded, to classical antidepressant medications, neurostimulation add-on or augmentation could be beneficial for the majority of them, with a slightly better outcome for the H1 dTMS coil compared to the more commonly used figure-of-eight coil. Of course, this finding warrants replication.

An often underexplored aspect in the application of rTMS is the orientation of the coil. It is known from primary motor cortex stimulation that a deviation of the 45° orientation of the coil can make a significant difference ("angular sensitivity"), for instance, in observing or not a motor evoked potential (MEP) [25]. Similar research investigating the relevance of coil orientation over the DLPFC using Near Infra-Red Spectroscopy (NIRS) showed that a blood-oxygenation response could only be measured at an angle of 45° to the midline [26], confirming the approach that has been adopted in most clinical trials to date.

The correct positioning of the coil is critical in terms of which underlying brain area is stimulated. Even slight changes in coil positioning can lead to large variations in clinical response. In order to ensure reliable stimulation of the identified targets throughout the treatment period, different coil positioning methods are used, with varying levels of cost versus clinical effectiveness: (1) the 5-cm-rule; (2) stimulation over F3 in accordance with the 10–20 EEG system; (3) the Beam F3 method and (4) MRI-based TMS guided by individual fiducials or neuronavigation. The 5-cm-rule has been the standard approach used for almost two decades. Here, the administrator applies a single TMS pulse to the primary motor cortex to cause an observable muscle twitch or a motor evoked potential (MEP) for indexing the exact coil position within the motor system (the so-called motor hotspot). The TMS depression treatment target is then defined relative to this "functional marker" by simply shifting the TMS coil in the anterior direction, parallel to the midline, by 5 cm (sometimes also 6 cm). However, this approach is critically viewed, as it does not account for interindividual anatomical differences. Stimulation over F3 follows the 10–20 EEG system and therefore considers individual differences in head size. Here, the TMS coil is positioned at EEG electrode position F3, which is thought to correspond to the DLPFC. Recently, the Beam-F3 method has been proposed as a new method [27], which does take individual differences in skull size into account and is based on the 10–20 EEG location F3 or F4. Free software to easily apply this method can be found at: http://www.clinicalresearcher.org/software.htm. This method has been shown to lead to an adequate determination, with a minimal discrepancy, compared to MRI-neuronavigated location determination [28].

However, MRI-based TMS is thought to be the most precise coil positioning approach, as it is based on the neuroimaging data of individual patients or a template. Frameless stereotactic systems allow precise (online) neuronavigation of a predefined brain area. However, the question of whether higher precision is associated with increased clinical efficacy continues to be discussed.

6.5   Real-Life Outcomes, Durability and Maintenance rTMS (mTMS)

Concerning the effectiveness of clinical outcomes, several large open-label studies have addressed the real-life clinical effects of rTMS. It seems that rTMS can be considered an effective treatment within research and naturalistic settings, with clinical benefits translating well into clinical practice. Additionally, in combination with psychotherapy or other treatment modalities, response and remission rates may have the potential to further increase and lead to sustained and durable effects.

Several large open-label studies have addressed the long-term effects of rTMS. In a large multicenter study with 307 treatment-resistant MDD patients applying HF L-DLPFC TMS, Carpenter and colleagues [29] reported response rates of 58% and 37% remission. Another large open-label study in 1132 patients demonstrated similar effects to Carpenter et al. with 46% response and 31% remission rates using several TMS protocols, mainly HF L-DLPFC and LF R-DLPFC rTMS [30]. In an extension of the Carpenter et al. study, good long-term effects were observed [31], the majority of patients (62.5%) continued to meet response criteria at a 12-month follow-up.

Although guidelines on the topic are lacking to date, maintenance rTMS (mTMS) has been suggested to prolong positive clinical effects. mTMS consists of an ongoing treatment at a lower rate—a similar approach that is used in ECT—and is used after a successful response to an acute course of rTMS. The frequency of mTMS varies from distributed single sessions (weekly, biweekly, bimonthly, or monthly) during the first 2–3 months after the end of the main treatment course, to short treatment periods of daily mTMS (e.g., 1 week per month) or so-called clustered mTMS (e.g., 5 sessions over a two-and-a-half-day period per month or every fifth week) applied over 1, 2, 3, 9, 12 months and up to several years. Studies are highly heterogeneous in terms of design, with rather small sample sizes and lacking placebo controls. Nonetheless, most patients show moderate to clear benefits with mTMS compared to no treatment, achieving remission for up to 3 months to 5 years [32]. While applying clustered mTMS, Wang and colleagues [33] showed significantly reduced relapse rates compared to a previous study that applied clustered mTMS [34]. To date, there are no guidelines for mTMS. Although the protocol should be individualized clinically, a tentative maintenance protocol following a rTMS taper (4 times weekly for 1 week, 3 times weekly for 1 week, 2 times weekly for 1–2 weeks) could consist of 1 session every 2 or 3 weeks for several months up to several years, depending on the nature of the mood disorder, although this schedule may not be sufficient for certain patients [35].

6.6   Combinatory Treatments

The rationale behind combining rTMS with other treatment approaches lies in the assumption that concomitant stimulation on different levels (i.e., physiological, cognitive, affective, behavioral) may result in synergistic effects.

6.6.1   Combining rTMS with Psychopharmacotherapy

An important issue concerns the relationship between rTMS efficacy and antidepressant intake. In general, patients undergoing rTMS continue to receive antidepressants. However, little is known about the impact of pharmacotherapy on rTMS efficacy. Preclinical studies suggest that antidepressants, anticonvulsants, and benzodiazepines influence cortical excitability. In humans, antidepressants appear to facilitate neuroplastic effects of brain stimulation, whereas anticonvulsants and benzodiazepines seem to have an inhibitory effect [36]. So far, rTMS studies in MDD are very heterogeneous concerning concomitant pharmacotherapy, precluding a comparison. Two questions are imminent: firstly, is there a difference between rTMS and antidepressants in terms of therapeutic efficacy? And secondly, is there an augmenting effect when under stable antidepressant therapy or is there an additive effect when introduced concomitantly as add-on therapy? However, currently, it has not been clearly demonstrated that there is a differential antidepressant efficacy between rTMS therapy performed alone vs. combined with antidepressants or that there is a clear superiority of an "add-on" effect of the combined procedure (Lefaucheur et al., in revision). It has to be noted that while in some studies patients were unmedicated, other studies only allowed benzodiazepines or other specific antidepressant medications to be continued during rTMS treatment, or medication could be freely chosen, but had to be kept stable. As psychopharmacological treatment is known to exert effects on both cortical excitability and neuroplasticity, potential interactions of specific pharmacological regimes and rTMS should be further investigated and henceforward exploited to achieve better clinical outcomes.

6.6.2   Combining rTMS with Psychotherapy

Within a naturalistic setting, rTMS can be considered an effective treatment and clinical benefit appears to translate well into clinical practice. Additionally, in combination with psychotherapy, response and remission rates may have the potential to increase further and sustain durable effects. In a large naturalistic study, Donse and colleagues [37] reported that the simultaneous application of rTMS and psycho-therapy in TRD resulted in a 66% response and a 56% remission rate at the end of treatment with 60% sustained remission at a 6-month follow-up. Though promising, randomized controlled clinical trials, as well as systematic research on combined rTMS-psychotherapy approaches, are needed.

6.6.3 Combining rTMS with Cognitive Training

Cognitive impairments can be observed in over 50% of depressed patients. They are thought to be predictive for poor socio-occupational outcomes and to persist beyond depression symptoms [38]. The persistence of cognitive symptoms and largely lack-ing effects of pharmacological treatment on cognitive symptoms implies that the two phenomena are dissociated and therefore require a more holistic treatment approach. Cognitive training of working memory used on its own has shown prom-ising effects [39]. However, it might be more effective when used as an add-on to rTMS. This assumes that the application of rTMS during cognitively relevant brain activity induces synergistic effects and therefore enhances cognitive training out-comes. From a perspective of practicability, it appears feasible, as patients are usu-ally unengaged during rTMS treatment.

6.6.4 Combining rTMS with Other (Non)invasive Brain Stimulation Techniques

Although in the field of brain stimulation it is discussed to combine or to prime rTMS treatment with other (non)invasive brain stimulation techniques, for example, (1) in order to increase clinical outcome, or (2) to use it as a maintenance treatment, currently, no systematic studies have been conducted to investigate these assumptions.

6.7 Personalized and Stratified Treatment as an Avenue to Precision Medicine

A general issue in the field is the high interindividual variability of rTMS response not only in clinical applications but also in experimental paradigms. Though not allowing one-size-fits-all approaches, such variability may pave the way to person-alized treatment: (1) adjusting rTMS to individualized targets and predictors based on structural or functional connectivity [40, 41], see target engagement below; and (2) applying closed-loop rTMS protocols targeting individual neurophysiological markers. Furthermore, cognitive and clinical indices could be leveraged for several purposes: (1) use as predictors to response to rTMS [42]; (2) cognitive changes can provide insights on rTMS mechanisms of action, for instance, by exploring whether they mediate depression improvement. Unfortunately, to date, no reliable predictors exist for response to rTMS in a clinically meaningful manner. Many individual studies have reported older age, high MDD severity, high anxiety, etc. to be predictors of poor response; however, a recent large scale study using a strict discovery-replication approach could not replicate any of these associations, albeit only high anhedonia was associated with a lower response, but this did not meet prediction accuracies suitable for clinical practice [42].

A complementary approach for addressing precision in psychiatry is stratification with machine learning approaches and other advanced statistics. In the rTMS field, such approaches have been conducted for symptom clustering and to define subtypes of MDD. Based on clustering according to anxiety and anhedonia dimensions and associated resting-state fMRI connectivity patterns, Drysdale and colleagues [43] identified and validated four biotypes, two of which were more responsive to rTMS than the others. In contrast to standard protocols, however, rTMS was applied over the DMPFC using a double cone coil. Furthermore, a very recent study failed to replicate the biotype solution of the prior report [44]. Kaster et al. [45] published a secondary analysis of a noninferiority trial comparing 10 Hz rTMS and iTBS applying group-based trajectory modeling. Four response trajectories were identified: nonresponse; rapid response; higher baseline symptoms—linear response; and lower baseline symptoms—linear response. The nonresponse trajectory was associated with higher depression scores at baseline, and the rapid response trajectory with older age, lower depression scores (i.e., self-rating) and lack of benzodiazepine use. A recent meta-analysis, investigating EEG predictors for antidepressant treatments, including rTMS, concluded that EEG is not clinically reliable, mainly due to publication bias and lack of replication [46]. In conclusion, while treatment prediction is a promising avenue and in line with notions of personalized medicine and Research Domain Criteria (RDoC), replication and focus on clinical relevance (opposed to "statistical significance" only) need to be further addressed in future studies [42, 46]. Besides true "prediction of response", another possibility is to optimize the stimulation targets by means of a focus on "target engagement".

6.7.1 Target Engagement

Target engagement comprises the use of a direct functional outcome measure as a validation for targeting the optimal TMS location, whereby it can be demonstrated that said location is activated, either directly or transsynaptically. In the same way, as the motor cortex is identified by thumb movement as a demonstration of primary motor cortex activation, such functional outcome measures are thus far lacking for the prefrontal cortex or, more specifically, the DLPFC. One proposed method is by extracting connectivity patterns to frontal areas using the sgACC as a seed region [47]. Other studies hypothesize that the DLPFC could be more accurately targeted with the aid of heart rate, so-called Neuro-Cardiac-Guided TMS (NCG-TMS) [48]. The depression network and the brain–heart axis are interconnected, and a recent meta-analysis demonstrated that stimulation of the DLPFC systematically resulted in reduced heart rate [49]. Iseger et al. [48] recently demonstrated that rTMS applied to F4 and F3 locations resulted in the most significant heart rate decelerations, followed by FC3 and FC4, whereas heart rate accelerations were found for central sites overlying the primary motor cortex. Individual variation was also found, indicating that the NCG-TMS method could be used to individualize stimulation targets, under the assumption that transsynaptic activation of the sgACC indeed activates the whole DLPFC-sgACC-Vagal nerve pathway that is involved in MDD. However, it remains yet to be established how this correlates with treatment outcome and if such targeting methods result in increased clinical efficacy.

6.7.2 Treatment of MDD Subpopulations and Vulnerable Populations

Knowledge about the relevance of the type of depression for rTMS efficacy is rather limited. In many rTMS studies, patients with both unipolar and bipolar disorder were included, without resulting in any clear indication of differential response. Notably, out of four RCTs [50] that included only patients with bipolar disorder, only one was positive. Regarding bipolar depression, the published data appear to be generally insufficient to draw definitive conclusions about its efficacy for this condition. Albeit a major reason not to include bipolar patients in clinical trials, there is currently no evidence to suggest that rTMS is associated with an increased risk of hypomanic switch. Importantly, rTMS seems to be ineffective in cases of MDD with psychotic features, a condition which is, on the other hand, a major clinical indication of ECT. The application of rTMS in children and adolescents, as well as in the elderly has not been studied extensively. However, the available studies, mostly comprising relatively small samples, do not seem to differ in clinical efficacy nor in tolerability or safety. Another vulnerable population is elderly individuals for whom efficacy of pharmacological treatment is known to be reduced and for whom polypharmacy and interactions of medications pose additional health risks. Some moderating factors possibly influencing clinical response to rTMS in the elderly depressed include but are not limited to: (1) brain atrophy; (2) the intensity and number of pulses (dose–response relationship); and (3) the clinical profile of patients (including treatment resistance, somatic/melancholic and psychotic features, a higher degree of cognitive impairment/dementia and medical comorbidity) [51]. Furthermore, although the current data suggest that the clinical effects, safety, and tolerability of TMS in adolescents may be similar to what has been described in adults, one has to consider neurodevelopmental factors and the unknowns associated with TMS exposure in this particular group [52]. For patients with MDD and Parkinson's disease, a recent meta-analysis has shown clear antidepressant efficacy of rTMS [52], indicating that medical comorbidities have no negative influence on the antidepressant efficacy of rTMS.

rTMS seems especially suited for the treatment of patients with contraindications for pharmacologic treatment, e.g., pregnant and breastfeeding women, or patients with polypharmacotherapy or comorbid somatic disorders. The application of rTMS in pregnant and breastfeeding women, for whom ECT or pharmacological treatment poses larger risks and side effects than rTMS, is of specific importance. Importantly, no negative pregnancy or fetal outcomes were found except for the potential association with preterm birth and mild headache for mothers [53]. A follow-up study of 30 mothers who had received rTMS for treatment of depression during pregnancy in an open trial setting investigated possible long-term effects of rTMS on offspring neurocognitive development [54]. No impairments were observed in cognitive or motor development in children who were aged 18–62 months at the time of the follow-up. The use of rTMS in postnatal depression was also recently analyzed in a systematic review that extracted data between 1999 and 2018, summing up 49 women [55]. Whereas higher frequencies correspond to increased discomfort and potential increased dropout rates, decreased frequencies seem to lead to less robust results.

6.8   Current Challenges and Future Directions

The main challenge in the treatment of depression lies in the large interindividual variability in treatment response. Researchers worldwide are focused on identifying personalized predictive factors and underlying mechanisms associated with response and remission rates. Further challenges include the extended time it takes for clinical effects to emerge and the lack of successful preventative strategies.

Future clinical research should therefore include large, controlled, noninferiority rTMS treatment studies comparing different stimulation localizations and the further development of novel stimulation patterns, such as accelerated rTMS protocols, that are thought to achieve a faster response. Moreover, our increasing knowledge of underlying neuronal mechanisms of MDD and network interactions should not only fuel the investigation of novel stimulation targets and development of coil designs that allow reaching deeper brain structures but could also be key to the development of more fine-tuned individualized treatment approaches. Future studies should further investigate synergistic effects of combinatory approaches, such as the combination with psychotherapy, cognitive training, and pharmacological treatment, to further enhance clinical outcomes and medium- to long-term antidepressant effects of this technique.

6.9   Conclusions

Despite the worldwide application of rTMS in depressed patients, there is still a large heterogeneity in the published data concerning the populations included and the stimulation settings. They mostly apply to patients in an acute phase of a drug-resistant MDD episode in the context of unipolar depression. A definite antidepressant efficacy of HF-rTMS of the left DLPFC (using either a focal figure-of-eight coil or a deep H-coil) and a probable antidepressant efficacy of LF-rTMS of the right DLPFC is currently the most evidence-based documented treatment proposal. Efficacy does not seem to differ significantly whether patients are concomitantly treated by antidepressant medication. At this point, it has to be acknowledged that rTMS is an acute antidepressant intervention and that beyond the acute phase data are limited with the exception of maintenance sessions [33].

Acknowledgments The Center for Research in Neuropsychology and Cognitive Behavioral Intervention of the Faculty of Psychology and Educational Sciences of the University of Coimbra is supported by the Portuguese Foundation for Science and Technology and the Portuguese Ministry of Education and Science through national funds and co-financed by FEDER through COMPETE2020 under the PT2020 Partnership Agreement [UID/PSI/01662/2013]. This work was also supported by the German Center for Brain Stimulation (GCBS) research consortium (grant number 01EE1403), funded by the Federal Ministry of Education and Research (BMBF), and by a BOF16/GOA/017 grant for a Concerted Research Action of Ghent University (Belgium).

Financial support and sponsorship: None.

Conflicts of interest: CB, FP, and EP are members of the European Scientific Advisory Board of Brainsway Inc., Jerusalem, Israel. FP has received speaker's honoraria from Mag&More GmbH and the neuroCare Group. His lab has received support with equipment from neuroConn GmbH, Ilmenau, Germany, and Mag&More GmbH and Brainsway Inc., Jerusalem, Israel. MA reports unpaid director and owner of Research Institute Brainclinics, a minority shareholder in neuroCare Group (Munich, Germany), and a coinventor on 4 patent applications related to EEG, neuromodulation and psychophysiology, but receives no royalties related to these patents; Research Institute Brainclinics received research funding from Brain Resource (Sydney, Australia) and neuroCare Group (Munich, Germany), and equipment support from Deymed, neuroConn, Brainsway, and Magventure.

References

1. Brunoni AR, Sampaio-Junior B, Moffa AH, Aparício LV, Gordon P, Klein I, et al. Noninvasive brain stimulation in psychiatric disorders: a primer. Braz J Psychiatry. 2019;41(1):70–81.
2. Blumberger DM, Vila-Rodriguez F, Thorpe KE, Feffer K, Noda Y, Giacobbe P, et al. Effectiveness of theta burst versus high-frequency repetitive transcranial magnetic stimulation in patients with depression (THREE-D): a randomised non-inferiority trial. Lancet. 2018;391(10131):1683–92.
3. Kaiser RH, Andrews-Hanna JR, Wager TD, Pizzagalli DA. Large-scale network dysfunction in major depressive disorder: a meta-analysis of resting-state functional connectivity. JAMA Psychiatry. 2015;72(6):603–11.
4. Williams LM. Precision psychiatry: a neural circuit taxonomy for depression and anxiety. Lancet Psychiatry. 2016;3(5):472–80.
5. Philip NS, Barredo J, Aiken E, Carpenter LL. Neuroimaging mechanisms of therapeutic transcranial magnetic stimulation for major depressive disorder. Biol Psychiatry Cogn Neurosci Neuroimaging. 2018;3(3):211–22.
6. Philip NS, Barredo J, van't Wout-Frank M, Tyrka AR, Price LH, Carpenter LL. Network mechanisms of clinical response to transcranial magnetic stimulation in posttraumatic stress disorder and major depressive disorder. Biol Psychiatry. 2018;83(3):263–72.
7. Baeken C, De Raedt R. Neurobiological mechanisms of repetitive transcranial magnetic stimulation on the underlying neurocircuitry in unipolar depression. Dialogues Clin Neurosci. 2011;13(1):139–45.
8. Kim TD, Hong G, Kim J, Yoon S. Cognitive enhancement in neurological and psychiatric disorders using transcranial magnetic stimulation (TMS): a review of modalities, potential mechanisms and future implications. Exp Neurobiol. 2019;28(1):1–16.

9. Martin DM, McClintock SM, Forster JJ, Lo TY, Loo CK. Cognitive enhancing effects of rTMS administered to the prefrontal cortex in patients with depression: a systematic review and meta-analysis of individual task effects. Depress Anxiety. 2017;34(11):1029–39.
10. Tortella G, Selingardi PML, Moreno ML, Veronezi BP, Brunoni AR. Does non-invasive brain stimulation improve cognition in major depressive disorder? A systematic review. CNS Neurol Disord Drug Targets. 2014;13(10):1759–69.
11. Harty S, Sella F, Cohen KR. Transcranial electrical stimulation and behavioral change: the intermediary influence of the brain. Front Hum Neurosci. 2017;11:112.
12. De Raedt R, Vanderhasselt M-A, Baeken C. Neurostimulation as an intervention for treatment resistant depression: from research on mechanisms towards targeted neurocognitive strategies. Clin Psychol Rev. 2015;41:61–9.
13. Mutz J, Vipulananthan V, Carter B, Hurlemann R, Fu CHY, Young AH. Comparative efficacy and acceptability of non-surgical brain stimulation for the acute treatment of major depressive episodes in adults: systematic review and network meta-analysis. BMJ. 2019;364:l1079.
14. Brunoni AR, Chaimani A, Moffa AH, Razza LB, Gattaz WF, Daskalakis ZJ, et al. Repetitive transcranial magnetic stimulation for the acute treatment of major depressive episodes: a systematic review with network meta-analysis. JAMA Psychiatry. 2017;74(2):143–52.
15. Baeken C. Accelerated rTMS: a potential treatment to alleviate refractory depression. Front Psychol. 2018;9:2017.
16. Schulze L, Feffer K, Lozano C, Giacobbe P, Daskalakis ZJ, Blumberger DM, et al. Number of pulses or number of sessions? An open-label study of trajectories of improvement for once-vs twice-daily dorsomedial prefrontal rTMS in major depression. Brain Stimulat. 2018;11(2):327–36.
17. Duprat R, Desmyter S, Rudi DR, van Heeringen K, Van den Abbeele D, Tandt H, et al. Accelerated intermittent theta burst stimulation treatment in medication-resistant major depression: a fast road to remission? J Affect Disord. 2016;200:6–14.
18. Williams NR, Sudheimer KD, Bentzley BS, Pannu J, Stimpson KH, Duvio D, et al. High-dose spaced theta-burst TMS as a rapid-acting antidepressant in highly refractory depression. Brain J Neurol. 2018;141(3):e18.
19. Feffer K, Fettes P, Giacobbe P, Daskalakis ZJ, Blumberger DM, Downar J. 1Hz rTMS of the right orbitofrontal cortex for major depression: safety, tolerability and clinical outcomes. Eur Neuropsychopharmacol. 2018;28(1):109–17.
20. Fadini T, Matthäus L, Rothkegel H, Sommer M, Tergau F, Schweikard A, et al. H-coil: induced electric field properties and input/output curves on healthy volunteers, comparison with a standard figure-of-eight coil. Clin Neurophysiol. 2009;120(6):1174–82.
21. Levkovitz Y, Isserles M, Padberg F, Lisanby SH, Bystritsky A, Xia G, et al. Efficacy and safety of deep transcranial magnetic stimulation for major depression: a prospective multicenter randomized controlled trial. World Psychiatry. 2015;14(1):64–73.
22. Kaster TS, Daskalakis ZJ, Noda Y, Knyahnytska Y, Downar J, Rajji TK, et al. Efficacy, tolerability, and cognitive effects of deep transcranial magnetic stimulation for late-life depression: a prospective randomized controlled trial. Neuropsychopharmacology. 2018;43(11):2231–8.
23. Tavares DF, Myczkowski ML, Alberto RL, Valiengo L, Rios RM, Gordon P, et al. Treatment of bipolar depression with deep TMS: results from a double-blind, randomized, parallel group, sham-controlled clinical trial. Neuropsychopharmacology. 2017;42(13):2593–601.
24. Filipčić I, Šimunović Filipčić I, Milovac Ž, Sučić S, Gajšak T, Ivezić E, et al. Efficacy of repetitive transcranial magnetic stimulation using a figure-8-coil or an H1-Coil in treatment of major depressive disorder; a randomized clinical trial. J Psychiatr Res. 2019;114:113–9.
25. Rotem A, Neef A, Neef NE, Agudelo-Toro A, Rakhmilevitch D, Paulus W, et al. Solving the orientation specific constraints in transcranial magnetic stimulation by rotating fields. PLoS One. 2014;9(2):e86794.
26. Thomson RH, Cleve TJ, Bailey NW, Rogasch NC, Maller JJ, Daskalakis ZJ, et al. Blood oxygenation changes modulated by coil orientation during prefrontal transcranial magnetic stimulation. Brain Stimulat. 2013;6(4):576–81.

27. Beam W, Borckardt JJ, Reeves ST, George MS. An efficient and accurate new method for locating the F3 position for prefrontal TMS applications. Brain Stimulat. 2009;2(1):50–4.
28. Mir-Moghtadaei A, Caballero R, Fried P, Fox MD, Lee K, Giacobbe P, et al. Concordance between beamF3 and MRI-neuronavigated target sites for repetitive transcranial magnetic stimulation of the left dorsolateral prefrontal cortex. Brain Stimulat. 2015;8(5):965–73.
29. Carpenter LL, Janicak PG, Aaronson ST, Boyadjis T, Brock DG, Cook IA, et al. Transcranial magnetic stimulation (TMS) for major depression: a multisite, naturalistic, observational study of acute treatment outcomes in clinical practice. Depress Anxiety. 2012;29(7):587–96.
30. Fitzgerald PB, Hoy KE, Anderson RJ, Daskalakis ZJ. A study of the pattern of response to rtms treatment in depression. Depress Anxiety. 2016;33(8):746–53.
31. Dunner DL, Aaronson ST, Sackeim HA, Janicak PG, Carpenter LL, Boyadjis T, et al. A multisite, naturalistic, observational study of transcranial magnetic stimulation for patients with pharmacoresistant major depressive disorder: durability of benefit over a 1-year follow-up period. J Clin Psychiatry. 2014;75(12):1394–401.
32. Rachid F. Maintenance repetitive transcranial magnetic stimulation (rTMS) for relapse prevention in with depression: a review. Psychiatry Res. 2018;262:363–72.
33. Wang H-N, Wang X-X, Zhang R-G, Wang Y, Cai M, Zhang Y-H, et al. Clustered repetitive transcranial magnetic stimulation for the prevention of depressive relapse/recurrence: a randomized controlled trial. Transl Psychiatry. 2017;7(12):1292.
34. Fitzgerald PB, Grace N, Hoy KE, Bailey M, Daskalakis ZJ. An open label trial of clustered maintenance rTMS for patients with refractory depression. Brain Stimulat. 2013;6(3):292–7.
35. Benadhira R, Thomas F, Bouaziz N, Braha S, Andrianisaina PS-K, Isaac C, et al. A randomized, sham-controlled study of maintenance rTMS for treatment-resistant depression (TRD). Psychiatry Res. 2017;258:226–33.
36. Hunter AM, Minzenberg MJ, Cook IA, Krantz DE, Levitt JG, Rotstein NM, et al. Concomitant medication use and clinical outcome of repetitive Transcranial Magnetic Stimulation (rTMS) treatment of major depressive disorder. Brain Behav. 2019;9(5):e01275.
37. Donse L, Padberg F, Sack AT, Rush AJ, Arns M. Simultaneous rTMS and psychotherapy in major depressive disorder: clinical outcomes and predictors from a large naturalistic study. Brain Stimulat. 2018;11(2):337–45.
38. Evans VC, Iverson GL, Yatham LN, Lam RW. The relationship between neurocognitive and psychosocial functioning in major depressive disorder: a systematic review. J Clin Psychiatry. 2014;75(12):1359–70.
39. Motter JN, Pimontel MA, Rindskopf D, Devanand DP, Doraiswamy PM, Sneed JR. Computerized cognitive training and functional recovery in major depressive disorder: a meta-analysis. J Affect Disord. 2016;189:184–91.
40. Fox MD, Buckner RL, White MP, Greicius MD, Pascual-Leone A. Efficacy of transcranial magnetic stimulation targets for depression is related to intrinsic functional connectivity with the subgenual cingulate. Biol Psychiatry. 2012;72(7):595–603.
41. Weigand A, Horn A, Caballero R, Cooke D, Stern AP, Taylor SF, et al. Prospective validation that subgenual connectivity predicts antidepressant efficacy of transcranial magnetic stimulation sites. Biol Psychiatry. 2018;84(1):28–37.
42. Krepel N, Rush AJ, Iseger TA, Sack AT, Arns M. Can psychological features predict antidepressant response to rTMS? A discovery-replication approach. Psychol Med. 2019;50(2):264–72.
43. Drysdale AT, Grosenick L, Downar J, Dunlop K, Mansouri F, Meng Y, et al. Resting-state connectivity biomarkers define neurophysiological subtypes of depression. Nat Med. 2017;23(1):28–38.
44. Dinga R, Schmaal L, Penninx BWJH, van Tol MJ, Veltman DJ, van Velzen L, et al. Evaluating the evidence for biotypes of depression: methodological replication and extension of. NeuroImage Clin. 2019;22:101796.
45. Kaster TS, Downar J, Vila-Rodriguez F, Thorpe KE, Feffer K, Noda Y, et al. Trajectories of response to dorsolateral prefrontal rTMS in major depression: a THREE-D study. Am J Psychiatry. 2019;176(5):367–75.

46. Widge AS, Bilge MT, Montana R, Chang W, Rodriguez CI, Deckersbach T, et al. Electroencephalographic biomarkers for treatment response prediction in major depressive illness: a meta-analysis. Am J Psychiatry. 2019;176(1):44–56.
47. Fox MD, Liu H, Pascual-Leone A. Identification of reproducible individualized targets for treatment of depression with TMS based on intrinsic connectivity. NeuroImage. 2013;66:151–60.
48. Iseger TA, Padberg F, Kenemans JL, Gevirtz R, Arns M. Neuro-cardiac-guided TMS (NCG-TMS): probing DLPFC-sgACC-vagus nerve connectivity using heart rate - first results. Brain Stimulat. 2017;10(5):1006–8.
49. Makovac E, Thayer JF, Ottaviani C. A meta-analysis of non-invasive brain stimulation and autonomic functioning: Implications for brain-heart pathways to cardiovascular disease. Neurosci Biobehav Rev. 2017;74(Pt B):330–41.
50. Lefaucheur J-P, André-Obadia N, Antal A, Ayache SS, Baeken C, Benninger DH, et al. Evidence-based guidelines on the therapeutic use of repetitive transcranial magnetic stimulation (rTMS). Clin Neurophysiol. 2014;125(11):2150–206.
51. Sabesan P, Lankappa S, Khalifa N, Krishnan V, Gandhi R, Palaniyappan L. Transcranial magnetic stimulation for geriatric depression: promises and pitfalls. World J Psychiatry. 2015;5(2):170–81.
52. Croarkin PE, MacMaster FP. Transcranial magnetic stimulation for adolescent depression. Child Adolesc Psychiatr Clin N Am. 2019;28(1):33–43.
53. Felipe RM, Ferrão YA. Transcranial magnetic stimulation for treatment of major depression during pregnancy: a review. Trends Psychiatry Psychother. 2016;38(4):190–7.
54. Eryılmaz G, Sayar GH, Özten E, Gül IG, Yorbik Ö, Işiten N, et al. Follow-up study of children whose mothers were treated with transcranial magnetic stimulation during pregnancy: preliminary results. Neuromodulation. 2015;18(4):255–60.
55. Ganho-Ávila A, Poleszczyk A, Mohamed MMA, Osório A. Efficacy of rTMS in decreasing postnatal depression symptoms: a systematic review. Psychiatry Res. 2019;279:315–22.

TMS in Psychotic Disorders

Andre Aleman and Jozarni Dlabac-de Lange

7.1 Introduction

Most studies investigating the effect of Transcranial Magnetic Stimulation (TMS) in psychotic disorders have focused on patients with schizophrenia. Schizophrenia is one of the most debilitating mental disorders with a substantial burden of disease [1]. Schizophrenia typically begins in late adolescence or early adulthood and runs a life-long course characterised by relapses. Symptoms of schizophrenia are usually grouped into positive, negative and cognitive symptoms. Positive symptoms include psychotic symptoms such as hallucinations, delusions, disorganisation of thought and disorganised or catatonic behaviour. Positive symptoms of schizophrenia fluctuate and treatment with antipsychotic medication can often diminish positive symptoms of schizophrenia. However, non-response and non-remission percentages are notably high [2]. Negative symptoms include flattening of affect, alogia, avolition, apathy and social withdrawal. Negative symptoms are very invalidating and about 25% of the patients with schizophrenia suffer from severe and persistent negative symptoms [3]. Treatment options of these negative symptoms are limited and often not effective. Cognitive symptoms include impairments in attention, memory, executive functions and processing speed. These cognitive impairments persist throughout the course of the illness and may co-occur with negative symptoms. Negative and cognitive symptoms can be very debilitating and impair everyday life of patients with schizophrenia.

Due to the limitations of current treatment options for patients with schizophrenia, researchers have explored other treatment modalities, including neuromodulation. Neuromodulation strategies have been studied in various forms, however, in psychotic disorders, treatment with repetitive TMS (rTMS) is the most investigated application. Indeed, in the past two decades, a substantial amount of randomised,

A. Aleman (✉) · J. Dlabac-de Lange
University Medical Center Groningen, University of Groningen, Groningen, The Netherlands
e-mail: a.aleman@umcg.nl; jozarni@caiway.net

© Springer Nature Switzerland AG 2020
B. Dell'Osso, G. Di Lorenzo (eds.), *Non Invasive Brain Stimulation in Psychiatry and Clinical Neurosciences*,
https://doi.org/10.1007/978-3-030-43356-7_7

controlled trials have investigated the effect of rTMS to treat positive and negative symptoms. Regarding positive symptoms, most rTMS studies have focused on the treatment of auditory hallucinations. Several studies have combined their investigation with pre- and post-treatment assessments of cognitive functioning, in order to determine if treatment with rTMS affects cognition. This chapter reviews the literature with regard to the efficacy and safety of treatment with rTMS of positive and negative symptoms in psychotic disorders. In addition, it reviews the literature available on the effects of rTMS on cognition in psychotic disorders, although this was often not the primary research focus in most studies.

7.2   rTMS Treatment of Negative Symptoms

7.2.1   Introduction

Negative symptoms appear to be associated with reduced activation of the prefrontal cortex (PFC), in particular in the dorsolateral prefrontal cortex (DLPFC) [4]. High-frequency rTMS of the prefrontal cortex may treat negative symptoms by increasing local cortical excitability. Over the past decades, several studies have investigated the effect of rTMS on negative symptoms. Some of these studies found a significant improvement of negative symptoms after rTMS, but others failed to find a therapeutic effect. Since 2009, a total of 9 meta-analyses have been performed investigating the effect of rTMS for improving negative symptoms [5–13]. The latest and largest meta-analysis, involving 19 studies with a total $N = 825$, found a moderate treatment effect in favour of rTMS with a mean weighted effect size of 0.64 (0.32–0.96) [11]. Although these results are promising, it remains uncertain if this positive treatment effect is also clinically meaningful, and to which extent the therapeutic effects of rTMS are durable. One study found a positive treatment effect up to 3 months follow-up [14], but most studies did not have a follow-up or only had a short follow-up of up to 2 weeks.

This review aims to clarify the underlying mechanism of action and to investigate which moderators, including rTMS parameters and patient characteristics, increase treatment efficacy.

7.2.2   Mechanisms of Action of Prefrontal rTMS Treatment of Negative Symptoms

Negative symptoms of schizophrenia have been related to impaired functioning of the prefrontal cortex [15]. Prefrontal high-frequency rTMS may increase brain activity in the stimulated area, as well as in associated areas that are part of the same neural circuit, thereby reducing negative symptoms of schizophrenia. Studies have shown that rTMS can facilitate dopaminergic, GABAergic and glutaminergic neurotransmission [16–18], and in so doing may induce plasticity in the brain. In order to investigate the underlying working mechanism of prefrontal rTMS in schizophrenia, several neuroimaging studies have been performed. Two studies combined rTMS treatment with Single Photon Emission Computed Tomography (SPECT) scans, and both studies did not detect any changes in regional cerebral blood flow [19, 20]. One EEG study did find a significant cortical activation with the improvement of negative symptoms [21]. Two fMRI studies did not find statistically significant differences in neuronal activation during a working memory task between sham and active rTMS [22, 23]. One combined treatment and neuroimaging study that found a positive treatment effect [14] also found changes in brain activation between active and sham during an fMRI planning task [24] and a social-emotional evaluation fMRI task [25], accompanied by changes in brain metabolism during a ^{1}H-MRS study [26]. During the planning task, activity in the PFC increased and activity in the posterior brain decreased in the active group as compared to the sham group. During the social-emotional evaluation task, rTMS treatment resulted in reduced activation of striato-fronto-parietal brain areas. Furthermore, a ^{1}H-MRS study conducted among a subgroup of patients found increased glutamate and glutamine (Glx) concentration in the prefrontal cortex after bilateral rTMS in the active group as compared to the sham group. Although results are inconsistent, these neuroimaging studies provide evidence for the underlying rationale of prefrontal rTMS treatment for negative symptoms, namely that it can normalise prefrontal brain activity and metabolism. However, study sizes were small and further neuroimaging research is needed.

7.2.3 Potential Moderators of Effect

Non-invasive neurostimulation with rTMS can improve negative symptoms, but in order to optimise treatment parameters, it is important to investigate potential moderators of effect. These moderators of effect include rTMS treatment parameters, such as frequency of stimulation or duration of stimulation, as well as patient's characteristics such as duration of illness.

Studies on rTMS treatment of negative symptoms have all used different rTMS treatment parameters; see Table 7.1 for an overview of randomised controlled trials [14, 20, 27–47]. These studies varied in frequency of stimulation, location of stimulation (frontal, parietal, cerebellar vermis), percentage of motor threshold, duration of stimulation and number of TMS pulses administered. In general, a longer treatment duration of more than 2 weeks and a higher number of TMS pulses administered seem to be more effective [11]. Indeed, there is evidence for impaired cortical excitability, connectivity and plasticity in patients with schizophrenia in all stages of the disease [48]. To improve the efficacy of rTMS, it may be necessary to target neural plasticity, for example by applying a greater number of rTMS stimulations or by increasing treatment duration to enhance treatment response.

Regarding the frequency of stimulation, three studies have investigated low-frequency (1–3 Hz) stimulation of the prefrontal cortex [27, 29, 35] but failed to find an effect. Six studies investigated the effect of 20 Hz prefrontal rTMS [29, 30, 37, 39, 41, 42] but only one study found a significant improvement [41]. Most studies ($n = 16$) have examined the effect of 10 Hz rTMS, which seems the most promising,

Table 7.1 Overview of randomized placebo controlled rTMS studies for the treatment of negative symptoms of schizophrenia

Study	Study goal	N	Location	rTMS frequency (Hz)	rTMS intensity (% MT)	Total number of pulses	Treatment duration (days)	Results of the study (rTMS group versus sham group)
Klein et al. [27]	Examine effect on positive, negative or depressive symptoms	31	Right PFC	1	110	1200	10	No significant change
Hajak et al. [20]	Examine effect on negative and depressive symptoms	20	Left PFC	10	110	10,000	10	Significant decrease negative symptoms
Holi et al. [28]	Examine effect on cognition, positive and negative symptoms	22	Left PFC	10	100	10,000	10	No significant change
Jin et al. [29]	Examine effect of individual alpha TMS on negative symptoms	27	Bilateral PFC	3 rTMS groups: 3 Hz, 20 Hz, alpha TMS (8–13 Hz)	80	3 Hz: 1200 20 Hz: 8000 Alpha TMS: 3200–5200	10	Significant decrease negative symptoms in alpha TMS group
Novak et al. [30]	Examine effect on negative symptoms	16	Left PFC	20	90	20,000	10	No significant change
Mogg et al. [31]	Examine effect on negative symptoms	17	Left PFC	10	110	20,000	10	No significant change
Prikryl et al. [32]	Examine effect on negative symptoms	22	Left PFC	10	110	22,500	15	Significant decrease negative symptoms
Goyal et al. [33]	Examine effect on negative symptoms	10	Left PFC	10	110	9800	10	Significant decrease negative symptoms
Fitzgerald et al. [34]	Examine effect on negative symptoms	20	Bilateral PFC	10	90	60,000	15	No significant change
Schneider et al. [35]	Examine effect on negative symptoms	51	Left PFC	2 rTMS groups: 1 and 10 Hz	110	1 Hz: 2000 10 Hz: 20,000	20	Significant decrease negative symptoms in 10 Hz group

Study	Aim	N	Site	Frequency	Intensity	Total pulses	Sessions	Outcome
Cordes et al. [36]	Examine effect on clinical global impression, positive and negative symptoms	35	Left PFC	10	110	10,000	10	No significant change. Significant improvement in subgroup of patients with severe negative symptoms
Barr et al. [37]	Examine effect on negative symptoms	25	Bilateral PFC	20	90	30,000	20	No significant change
Jin et al. [38]	Examine effect on clinical symptoms of schizophrenia	78	2 groups: frontal and parietal	Individual EEG alpha (8–13 Hz)	80	Variable	10	No significant change in negative symptoms. Significant decrease positive symptoms in both frontal and parietal group
Zheng et al. [39]	To investigate the effect of different paradigms of rTMS on cognition, positive and negative symptoms	80	Left PFC	3 rTMS groups: 10 Hz, 20 Hz and theta burst stimulation (TBS)	80	6000	5	Significant decrease negative symptoms in 10 Hz and TBS group
Prikryl et al. [40]	Examine effect on negative symptoms	40	Left PFC	10	110	22,500	15	Significant decrease negative symptoms
Zhao et al. [41]	Examine the effectiveness of different rTMS stimulation protocols in the treatment of the negative symptoms	96	Left PFC	3 rTMS groups: 1 Hz, 20 Hz and theta burst stimulation (TBS) (5 and 50 Hz)	80	10 Hz: 30,000 20 Hz: 60,000 TBS: 48,000	20	Significant decrease negative symptoms in all 3 groups
Rabany et al. [42]	Examine effect on negative symptoms and cognition	30	Mainly left, weaker right PFC	20	120	33,600	20	No significant change

(continued)

Table 7.1 (continued)

Study	Study goal	N	Location	rTMS frequency (Hz)	rTMS intensity (% MT)	Total number of pulses	Treatment duration (days)	Results of the study (rTMS group versus sham group)
Dlabac-de Lange et al. [14, 24]	Examine effect on negative symptoms	32	Bilateral PFC	10	90	60,000 (30,000 per hemisphere)	15 (twice daily)	Significant decrease negative symptoms
Quan et al. [44]	Examine effect on negative symptoms	117	Left PFC	10	80	16,000	20	Significant decrease negative symptoms
Wobrock et al. [45]	Examine effect on negative symptoms	175	Left PFC	10	110	15,000	15	No significant change
Gan et al. [46]	Examine effect on negative symptoms	70	Left PFC	10	100	Not available	10 (twice daily)	Significant decrease negative symptoms
Li et al. [47]	Examine effect on negative symptoms	47	Left PFC	10	110	30,000	20	No significant change post-treatment, significant decrease negative symptoms at 4 weeks follow-up
Garg et al. [43]	Examine effect on clinical symptoms of schizophrenia	40	Cerebellar vermis	Theta patterned (trains of 5, 6 and 7 Hz followed each other sequentially)	100	6000	10	Significant decrease negative symptoms and depressive symptoms

rTMS repetitive Transcranial Magnetic Stimulation, *PFC* prefrontal cortex, *MT* motor threshold

as the majority of these studies ($n = 10$) found a significant improvement of negative symptoms in the rTMS group as compared to the sham group. A recent meta-analysis also found a greater effect size in studies applying 10 Hz prefrontal rTMS as compared to other frequencies [11]. Interesting developments include theta burst stimulation (TBS), which has been investigated by two trials, both of which found a significant treatment effect [39, 41].

The location of stimulation varies, but the majority of trials have investigated rTMS stimulation of the left or bilateral prefrontal cortex, and results were promising (see Table 7.1). Low-frequency stimulation of the right prefrontal cortex [27] and high-frequency rTMS of the parietal cortex [38] did not improve negative symptoms. Interestingly, one study ($n = 40$) investigating high-frequency rTMS of the cerebellar vermis did find a significant decrease in negative and depressive symptoms in the treatment group [43]. Authors hypothesised that high-frequency rTMS of the cerebellar vermis can, through neural network modulations, increase excitability in the frontal lobe.

Other treatment characteristics include type and dosage of medication. Patients with schizophrenia may use high dosages of medication, including antipsychotics, benzodiazepines and anticonvulsant medication. These medications may interfere with the putative mechanism of action of rTMS, namely increasing excitability and neurotransmitter (including dopamine) release in the prefrontal cortex. The vast majority of patients use antipsychotics to treat positive symptoms, but most antipsychotics have high affinity for dopamine (D2) receptors and thus block dopamine. Indeed, one exploratory study found active rTMS to improve antipsychotic-induced extrapyramidal symptoms (EPS), possibly by increasing dopamine release [49]. Clozapine is an atypical antipsychotic that was shown to be superior in the treatment of refractory schizophrenia. Clozapine, in contrast to most other antipsychotics, shows only weak antagonism to the dopamine D2 receptor. Patients with schizophrenia using clozapine may therefore more readily respond to rTMS treatment. Until now, only one exploratory study has been conducted in a cohort of patients on clozapine participating in the RESIS trial [50]. This study ($n = 26$) found a significant reduction of the PANSS positive subscale and the PANSS general subscale, but not on the PANSS negative subscale, in patients receiving active rTMS as compared to patients receiving sham rTMS. More research on the effect of type and dosage of medication on rTMS treatment response is warranted.

Besides investigating rTMS parameters as potential moderators of effect, it is also important to explore patient's characteristics as potential moderators. Exploratory analyses in an earlier meta-analysis found a higher effect in studies that included younger patients with a shorter duration of illness [11]. It may be easier to induce neuroplasticity in younger patients with a shorter duration of illness, and more rTMS studies conducted among patients with a first episode psychosis are required.

7.2.4 Conclusions

In conclusion, high-frequency prefrontal rTMS has been found to improve negative symptoms in patients with schizophrenia, and this improvement may last up to several months after rTMS treatment. Neuroimaging studies showed rTMS to potentially induce changes in brain activity in prefrontal and connected brain areas, thereby reducing negative symptoms. Although several studies have found a significant improvement of negative symptoms, it remains unclear if the results are clinically significant. Regarding rTMS treatment parameters, a treatment frequency of 10 Hz, a treatment location of the left or bilateral PFC, a longer treatment duration and a larger amount of total TMS pulses administered seem to enhance effectiveness. Regarding patient's characteristics, younger patients with a shorter duration of illness may respond better to rTMS treatment. Further research is needed to investigate the potential benefits of treatment with clozapine on rTMS treatment response. Future studies should also investigate the underlying neural working mechanism and further establish the most effective combination of rTMS parameters.

7.3 rTMS Treatment of Positive Symptoms

7.3.1 Introduction

Neuroimaging studies have shown hyperactivation of language areas of the brain to be involved in hallucinations. More specifically, increased activation of the superior temporal gyrus and of Broca's area (amongst others) have been consistently observed. Indeed, hyperexcitability of such language-related regions has been hypothesised to be associated with auditory hallucinations. The first attempt to use TMS to reduce the frequency and severity of hallucinations was made by Hoffman and colleagues in 1999 [51]. They investigated the effects of 1 Hz TMS over the temporoparietal cortex in patients with schizophrenia and chronic, medication-resistant auditory-verbal hallucinations (AVHs). After some preliminary and promising results, they conducted a RCT comparing two groups: one group of patients received active TMS, the other received sham TMS. A total of 132 minutes of rTMS was administered over 9 days at 90% of the motor threshold. The hallucination change score improved significantly more in the active as compared to the sham group. In particular, the frequency of hallucinations was reduced by the TMS.

Subsequent research confirmed this effect, although not all studies reported significant improvements due to TMS. Several meta-analyses reported medium effect sizes for active compared to sham TMS [52, 53]. The most recent meta-analysis [10] included 13 studies and showed a statistically significant effect size, albeit of smaller magnitude (standardised mean difference of 0.29). Of note, the authors reported that this result was not stable after sensitivity analysis, and publication bias had a substantial impact on the results. They therefore caution that, even though there may be a therapeutic effect for 1-Hz rTMS on auditory hallucinations in schizophrenia, this needs to be confirmed by large-scale RCTs before this finding can be recommended in clinical practice.

7.3.2 Mechanism of Action

Most studies that tried to improve hallucinations used 1 Hz stimulation, which was shown to reduce cortical excitability. This was based on neuroimaging studies that showed hyperactivation of superior temporal areas. Indeed, increased levels of excitability or spontaneous fluctuations in auditory (and related) cortex may be associated with hallucinatory activity [54].

Few studies have directly investigated the neural effects of 1 Hz rTMS over the temporoparietal junction (TPJ). Tracy et al. [55] tested the effects of a typical 1 Hz protocol (one session) on auditory brain activation in healthy volunteers. Stimulation with rTMS led to attenuation of the underlying auditory cortex response to the stimulus and a contralateral increase in cortical activity. This supports the underlying rationale for rTMS in hallucinations, i.e. to reduce activation of the auditory-verbal system. However, as the investigators rightly note, the lack of studies investigating immediate (and long-term) neural effects of the rTMS protocol highlights the insufficient knowledge of the effects of rTMS on normal physiology. They also suggest that this, combined with a lack of consensus on clinical trial parameters, may be contributing to the ambivalent data in therapeutic trials.

In a study of patients with schizophrenia and auditory-verbal hallucinations, Bais et al. [56] reported that, compared to sham rTMS, stimulation of the left TPJ resulted in a weaker network contribution of the left supramarginal gyrus to the bilateral fronto-temporal network. In addition, left-sided rTMS resulted in stronger network contributions of the right superior temporal gyrus to the auditory-sensorimotor network, right inferior gyrus to the left fronto-parietal network, and left middle frontal gyrus to the default mode network. The authors interpreted this as follows: the decreased contribution of the left supramarginal gyrus to the bilateral fronto-temporal network may reduce the likelihood of speech intrusions that have been shown to be associated with hallucinations. On the other hand, left rTMS appeared to increase the contribution of functionally connected regions involved in perception, cognitive control and self-referential processing, which may aid coping mechanisms. Although the findings hint to potential neural mechanisms underlying rTMS for hallucinations, the authors emphasise that they need corroboration in larger samples.

7.3.3 Potential Moderators of Effect

Several potential moderators of effects should be considered. Duration of treatment, number of sessions, location of stimulation, and use of sedatives (such as benzodiazepines) have all been suggested in the literature to possibly be of relevance. It seems logical to suppose that longer duration of treatment and the higher number of treatment sessions (or the total number of TMS pulses) will be as associated with better treatment outcomes. However, there is no strong evidence to support this, which may be due to our lack of studies with the proper comparisons. With regard to location of stimulation, the evidence supports the posterior superior temporal cortex as most effective target [57].

In recent years, three novel potential moderators of TMS treatment effect have been identified. First, TMS may be more effective in young and female participants [58]. Second, the distance between the scalp (where the TMS coil is held) and the cortex may matter [59]. That is, in people with a larger distance between the scalp and the cortex, TMS has less effect. The scalp to cortex distance can be measured using previously acquired MRI scans. Finally, a number of studies have shown that TMS response may be dependent, in part, on genetic variation. For example, variation in the BDNF gene has been associated with TMS effects in patients treated for depression [60, 61].

7.3.4 Conclusions

Meta-analysis shows a small but significant effect of rTMS on improving auditory-verbal hallucinations in schizophrenia. Delusions did not improve in those studies. No studies have targeted delusions and their underlying neural substrate specifically with rTMS; thus, this remains to be investigated. For hallucinations, it is imperative that larger effect sizes need to be observed in order to warrant clinical relevance. Further exploration of different parameters (e.g. intensity and frequency of stimulation, use of neuronavigation for coil placement, etc.) is needed.

7.4 Effect of rTMS on Cognition in Patients with a Psychotic Disorder

7.4.1 Introduction

Cognitive dysfunction is a core symptom of schizophrenia, and these cognitive deficits can be profound and disabling. Several studies investigating the effect of prefrontal rTMS on negative symptoms also investigated the effect of rTMS on cognitive function. For some studies, the primary focus of investigation was the effect of prefrontal rTMS on cognition in patients with schizophrenia. Initially, investigating the effect on cognition was important to rule out any adverse cognitive effects, as can be the case with ECT treatment, which can cause negative cognitive side effects. Fortunately, until now, no adverse cognitive side effects have been reported. Indeed, some studies have found prefrontal rTMS to improve certain domains of cognitive functioning. In the following section, the effect of prefrontal rTMS on different cognitive domains, including executive functioning, attention, working memory, verbal memory, processing speed, motor speed and social cognition, will be discussed.

7.4.2 Executive Functioning

Several studies have investigated the effect of rTMS on executive functioning [14, 22, 24, 31, 34, 39, 42, 45, 62–65]. Frequently used neuropsychological tests to assess executive functioning were verbal fluency tests, the Wisconsin Card Sorting Test (WCST) and the Trial Making Test (TMT). Executive functioning was also assessed with the Tower of London test, the Controlled Oral Word Association Test, the Stroop interference task, the Stockings of Cambridge (SOC) and a spatial working memory task of the Cambridge Neuropsychological Test Automated Battery (CANTAB). Interestingly, three out of the five studies that investigated changes in verbal fluency found a significant improvement of verbal fluency immediately post-treatment or at 2 weeks follow-up in the rTMS group as compared to sham [14, 34, 39, 62, 64]. One study found a trend for improvement as measured by the Stroop test ($t = 2.1$, df = 12, $p = 0.06$) [31]. There was no significant change as measured by the other neuropsychological tests. However, a recent meta-analysis [66] found rTMS to improve executive functioning at a trend level as compared to sham treatment ($p = 0.08$).

7.4.3 Attention

Three randomised controlled trials investigated the effect of rTMS on attention using the Tübinger Aufmerksamkeitsprüfung (TAP), the d2-attention task and the rapid visual information processing (RVP) task of the CANTAB [22, 42, 63]. None of them found any significant effects, nor did a recent meta-analysis [66].

7.4.4 Working Memory

Several studies assessed the effect of rTMS on working memory in patients with a psychotic disorder. The neuropsychological tests used were the n-back test, the digit span test, the pattern recognition memory (PRM) as measured by the CANTAB, the digit sequencing task of the Brief Assessment of Cognition in Schizophrenia (BACS) and a visuospatial working memory test [22, 23, 39, 42, 62, 64, 67, 68]. Most studies did not find any significant change in working memory performance between the sham and the real rTMS group. However, two studies applying high-frequency (20 Hz) rTMS found significant improvements in working memory. One study found that rTMS significantly improved 3-back accuracy to targets in the n-back test [68] and one study found a significant improvement in visuospatial working memory [39]. In addition, a meta-analysis on the effects of rTMS on cognition in schizophrenia found the effect of active rTMS to be significantly greater than that of sham rTMS in improving working memory [66].

7.4.5 Verbal Memory

Four RCTs investigated the effect of rTMS on verbal memory, using a parallel form of the Hopkins Verbal Learning Test, the BACS Verbal Memory test or the Rey Auditory Verbal Learning Test [14, 31, 62, 64]. Two studies did not find any significant changes between both groups [14, 62] and one found a significant change in BACS Verbal Memory scores, caused primarily by a decline of performance in the sham group rather than an improvement in the rTMS group [64]. Finally, one study found a significant improvement in the delayed recall of the verbal learning test in the rTMS group as compared to the sham group at 2 weeks follow-up [31]. The meta-analysis, including these four studies, did not find a significant difference of rTMS on verbal memory performance [66].

7.4.6 Processing Speed

One study used the BACS Symbol Coding to investigate the effect of rTMS on processing speed in patients in an early stage psychosis [64], and found a significant change in scores in the rTMS group at 2 weeks follow-up as compared to the sham group, caused by an improved performance in the rTMS group and a decreased performance in the sham group. Another study, conducted among patients with schizophrenia that used the Digit Symbol Substitution Test to measure processing speed, did not find any significant change [14].

7.4.7 Motor Speed

Motor speed was assessed in three studies using the Grooved Pegboard Test, the motor screening and reaction time of the CANTAB or the BACS Token Motor Total [31, 42, 64]. No significant changes in motor speed after rTMS were found as compared to sham treatment.

7.4.8 Social Cognition

Two studies have investigated the effect of rTMS on social cognition [24, 69]. One study found that facial affect recognition improved significantly in patients with schizophrenia after rTMS treatment as compared to sham treatment [69]. Another study investigated the effect of rTMS on brain activation during ambiguous social-emotional evaluation in patients with schizophrenia [24]. This study did not find differences in performance, but fMRI analysis showed that rTMS treatment resulted in reduced activation of striato-fronto-parietal brain areas, while sham treatment resulted in an increased activation as compared to baseline [24]. The authors speculate that rTMS therefore may normalise an increased brain response to ambiguous emotional stimuli. It is important to further investigate the effect of neuromodulation on social cognition, as many patients with schizophrenia are troubled by deficits in social cognition.

7.4.9 Conclusions

In conclusion, most studies that investigated the effect of rTMS on cognition in patients with a psychotic disorder did not find any significant change in cognition between the rTMS and sham group. Some studies found improvement in executive functioning and working memory in the rTMS group, and there is evidence that rTMS may help ameliorate deficits in social cognition. It is important to note that no adverse cognitive effects occurred. Future studies on prefrontal rTMS should include neuropsychological tests to further clarify the effect of rTMS on cognition.

7.5 Safety and Side Effects of rTMS Treatment in Patients with a Psychotic Disorder

Common reported side effects were facial muscle twitching during stimulation and transient headache after stimulation. It is important to note that the conducted studies on rTMS treatment in patients with a psychotic disorder did not report the occurrence of seizures or other life-threatening events. In general, the rTMS treatment was well tolerated.

7.6 Conclusions

In conclusion, in the past decades, several studies have investigated the effect of rTMS on auditory hallucinations, negative and cognitive symptoms in patients with a psychotic disorder, in particular schizophrenia. There is a growing body of evidence that rTMS can alleviate auditory hallucinations and reduce negative symptoms, although it should be noted that several studies failed to find effects. Furthermore, rTMS may improve cognitive functioning. However, the effect size of treatments with rTMS is not as yet clinically satisfactory, and more studies are needed to establish a durable and clinically meaningful improvement. More research is also needed concerning the neural effects of these non-invasive brain stimulation interventions.

References

1. Charlson FJ, Ferrari AJ, Santomauro DF, Diminic S, Stockings E, Scott JG, et al. Global epidemiology and burden of schizophrenia: findings from the global burden of disease study 2016. Schizophr Bull. 2018;44(6):1195–203.
2. Samara MT, Nikolakopoulou A, Salanti G, Leucht S. How many patients with schizophrenia do not respond to antipsychotic drugs in the short term? An analysis based on individual

patient data from randomized controlled trials. Schizophr Bull. 2018;45(3):ss639–46. https://doi.org/10.1093/schbul/sby095.

3. Buchanan RW. Persistent negative symptoms in schizophrenia: an overview. Schizophr Bull. 2007;33(4):1013–22.

4. Gruber O, Chadha Santuccione A, Aach H. Magnetic resonance imaging in studying schizophrenia, negative symptoms, and the glutamate system. Front Psychiatry. 2014;5:32.

5. Fusar-Poli P, Papanastasiou E, Stahl D, et al. Treatments of negative symptoms in schizophrenia: metaanalysis of 168 randomized placebo-controlled trials. Schizophr Bull. 2015;41(4):892–9.

6. Dlabac-de Lange JJ, Knegtering R, Aleman A. Repetitive transcranial magnetic stimulation for negative symptoms of schizophrenia: review and meta-analysis. J Clin Psychiatry. 2010;71(4):411–8.

7. Shi C, Yu X, Cheung EF, Shum DH, Chan RC. Revisiting the therapeutic effect of rTMS on negative symptoms in schizophrenia: a meta-analysis. Psychiatry Res. 2014;215(3):505–13.

8. Slotema CW, Blom JD, Hoek HW, Sommer IE. Should we expand the toolbox of psychiatric treatment methods to include repetitive transcranial magnetic stimulation (rTMS)? A meta-analysis of the efficacy of rTMS in psychiatric disorders. J Clin Psychiatry. 2010;71(7):873–84.

9. Freitas C, Fregni F, Pascual-Leone A. Meta-analysis of the effects of repetitive transcranial magnetic stimulation (rTMS) on negative and positive symptoms in schizophrenia. Schizophr Res. 2009;108(1–3):11–24.

10. He H, Lu J, Yang L, Zheng J, Gao F, Zhai Y, et al. Repetitive transcranial magnetic stimulation for treating the symptoms of schizophrenia: a PRISMA compliant meta-analysis. Clin Neurophysiol. 2017;128(5):716–24.

11. Aleman A, Enriquez-Geppert S, Knegtering H, Dlabac-de Lange JJ. Moderate effects of noninvasive brain stimulation of the frontal cortex for improving negative symptoms in schizophrenia: meta-analysis of controlled trials. Neurosci Biobehav Rev. 2018;89:111–8.

12. Kennedy NI, Lee WH, Frangou S. Efficacy of non-invasive brain stimulation on the symptom dimensions of schizophrenia: a meta-analysis of randomized controlled trials. Eur Psychiatry. 2018;49:69–77.

13. Osoegawa C, Gomes JS, Grigolon RB, Brietzke E, Gadelha A, Lacerda ALT, et al. Non-invasive brain stimulation for negative symptoms in schizophrenia: an updated systematic review and meta-analysis. Schizophr Res. 2018;197:34–44.

14. Dlabac-de Lange JJ, Bais L, van Es FD, et al. Efficacy of bilateral repetitive transcranial magnetic stimulation for negative symptoms of schizophrenia: results of a multicenter double-blind randomized controlled trial. Psychol Med. 2015;45(6):1263–75.

15. Hovington CL, Lepage M. Neurocognition and neuroimaging of persistent negative symptoms of schizophrenia. Expert Rev Neurother. 2012;12(1):53–69.

16. Strafella AP, Paus T, Barrett J, Dagher A. Repetitive transcranial magnetic stimulation of the human prefrontal cortex induces dopamine release in the caudate nucleus. J Neurosci. 2001;21(15):RC157.

17. Luborzewski A, Schubert F, Seifert F, et al. Metabolic alterations in the dorsolateral prefrontal cortex after treatment with high-frequency repetitive transcranial magnetic stimulation in patients with unipolar major depression. J Psychiatr Res. 2007;41(7):606–15.

18. Michael N, Gosling M, Reutemann M, et al. Metabolic changes after repetitive transcranial magnetic stimulation (rTMS) of the left prefrontal cortex: a sham-controlled proton magnetic resonance spectroscopy (1H MRS) study of healthy brain. Eur J Neurosci. 2003;17(11):2462–8.

19. Cohen E, Bernardo M, Masana J, et al. Repetitive transcranial magnetic stimulation in the treatment of chronic negative schizophrenia: a pilot study. J Neurol Neurosurg Psychiatry. 1999;67(1):129–30.

20. Hajak G, Marienhagen J, Langguth B, Werner S, Binder H, Eichhammer P. High-frequency repetitive transcranial magnetic stimulation in schizophrenia: a combined treatment and neuroimaging study. Psychol Med. 2004;34(7):1157–63.

21. Jandl M, Bittner R, Sack A, et al. Changes in negative symptoms and EEG in schizophrenic patients after repetitive transcranial magnetic stimulation (rTMS): an open-label pilot study. J Neural Transm. 2005;112(7):955–67.

22. Guse B, Falkai P, Gruber O, et al. The effect of long-term high frequency repetitive transcranial magnetic stimulation on working memory in schizophrenia and healthy controls--a randomized placebo-controlled, double-blind fMRI study. Behav Brain Res. 2013;237:300–7.
23. Prikryl R, Mikl M, Prikrylova Kucerova H, et al. Does repetitive transcranial magnetic stimulation have a positive effect on working memory and neuronal activation in treatment of negative symptoms of schizophrenia? Neuro Endocrinol Lett. 2012;33(1):90–7.
24. Dlabac-de Lange JJ, Liemburg EJ, Bais L, Renken RJ, Knegtering H, Aleman A. Effect of rTMS on brain activation in schizophrenia with negative symptoms: a proof-of-principle study. Schizophr Res. 2015;168(1–2):475–82.
25. Liemburg EJ, Dlabac-De Lange JJ, Bais L, Knegtering H, Aleman A. Effects of bilateral prefrontal rTMS on brain activation during social-emotional evaluation in schizophrenia: a double-blind, randomized, exploratory study. Schizophr Res. 2018;202:210–1.
26. Dlabac-de Lange JJ, Liemburg EJ, Bais L, van de Poel-Mustafayeva AT, de Lange-de Klerk ESM, Knegtering H, et al. Effect of bilateral prefrontal rTMS on left prefrontal NAA and Glx levels in schizophrenia patients with predominant negative symptoms: an exploratory study. Brain Stimul. 2017;10(1):59–64.
27. Klein E, Kolsky Y, Puyerovsky M, Koren D, Chistyakov A, Feinsod M. Right prefrontal slow repetitive transcranial magnetic stimulation in schizophrenia: a double-blind sham-controlled pilot study. Biol Psychiatry. 1999;46(10):1451–4.
28. Holi MM, Eronen M, Toivonen K, Toivonen P, Marttunen M, Naukkarinen H. Left prefrontal repetitive transcranial magnetic stimulation in schizophrenia. Schizophr Bull. 2004;30(2):429–34.
29. Jin Y, Potkin SG, Kemp AS, et al. Therapeutic effects of individualized alpha frequency transcranial magnetic stimulation (alphaTMS) on the negative symptoms of schizophrenia. Schizophr Bull. 2006;32(3):556–61.
30. Novak T, Horacek J, Mohr P, et al. The double-blind sham-controlled study of high-frequency rTMS (20 hz) for negative symptoms in schizophrenia: negative results. Neuro Endocrinol Lett. 2006;27(1–2):209–13.
31. Mogg A, Purvis R, Eranti S, et al. Repetitive transcranial magnetic stimulation for negative symptoms of schizophrenia: a randomized controlled pilot study. Schizophr Res. 2007;93(1–3):221–8.
32. Prikryl R, Kasparek T, Skotakova S, Ustohal L, Kucerova H, Ceskova E. Treatment of negative symptoms of schizophrenia using repetitive transcranial magnetic stimulation in a double-blind, randomized controlled study. Schizophr Res. 2007;95(1–3):151–7.
33. Goyal N, Nizamie SH, Desarkar P. Efficacy of adjuvant high frequency repetitive transcranial magnetic stimulation on negative and positive symptoms of schizophrenia: preliminary results of a double-blind sham-controlled study. J Neuropsychiatry Clin Neurosci. 2007;19(4):464–7.
34. Fitzgerald PB, Herring S, Hoy K, et al. A study of the effectiveness of bilateral transcranial magnetic stimulation in the treatment of the negative symptoms of schizophrenia. Brain Stimul. 2008;1(1):27–32.
35. Schneider AL, Schneider TL, Stark H. Repetitive transcranial magnetic stimulation (rTMS) as an augmentation treatment for the negative symptoms of schizophrenia: a 4-week randomized placebo controlled study. Brain Stimul. 2008;1(2):106–11.
36. Cordes J, Thunker J, Agelink MW, et al. Effects of 10 hz repetitive transcranial magnetic stimulation (rTMS) on clinical global impression in chronic schizophrenia. Psychiatry Res. 2010;177(1–2):32–6.
37. Barr MS, Farzan F, Tran LC, Fitzgerald PB, Daskalakis ZJ. A randomized controlled trial of sequentially bilateral prefrontal cortex repetitive transcranial magnetic stimulation in the treatment of negative symptoms in schizophrenia. Brain Stimul. 2012;5(3):337–46.
38. Jin Y, Kemp AS, Huang Y, et al. Alpha EEG guided TMS in schizophrenia. Brain Stimul. 2012;5(4):560–8.
39. Zheng L, Guo Q, Li H, Li C, Wang JJ. Effects of repetitive transcranial magnetic stimulation with different paradigms on the cognitive function and psychotic symptoms of schizophrenia patients. Beijing Da Xue Xue Bao. 2012;44:732–6.

40. Prikryl R, Ustohal L, Prikrylova Kucerova H, et al. A detailed analysis of the effect of repetitive transcranial magnetic stimulation on negative symptoms of schizophrenia: a double-blind trial. Schizophr Res. 2013;149(1–3):167–73.
41. Zhao S, Kong J, Li S, Tong Z, Yang C, Zhong H. Randomized controlled trial of four protocols of repetitive transcranial magnetic stimulation for treating the negative symptoms of schizophrenia. Shanghai Arch Psychiatry. 2014;26(1):15–21.
42. Rabany L, Deutsch L, Levkovitz Y. Double-blind, randomized sham controlled study of deep-TMS add-on treatment for negative symptoms and cognitive deficits in schizophrenia. J Psychopharmacol. 2014;28(7):686–90.
43. Garg S, Sinha VK, Tikka SK, Mishra P, Goyal N. The efficacy of cerebellar vermal deep high frequency (theta range) repetitive transcranial magnetic stimulation (rTMS) in schizophrenia: a randomized rater blind-sham controlled study. Psychiatry Res. 2016;243:413–20.
44. Quan WX, Zhu XL, Qiao H, Zhang WF, Tan SP, Zhou DF, et al. The effects of high-frequency repetitive transcranialmagnetic stimulation (rTMS) on negative symptoms of schizophrenia and the follow-up study. Neurosci Lett. 2015;584:197–201.
45. Wobrock T, Guse B, Cordes J, et al. Left prefrontal high-frequency repetitive transcranial magnetic stimulation for the treatment of schizophrenia with predominant negative symptoms: a sham-controlled, randomized multicenter trial. Biol Psychiatry. 2015;77(11):979–88.
46. Gan J, Duan H, Chen Z, Shi Z, Gao C, Zhu X, et al. Effectiveness and safety of high dose transcranial magnetic stimulation in schizophrenia with refractory negative symptoms: a randomized controlled study. Zhonghua Yi Xue Za Zhi. 2015;95(47):3808–12.
47. Li Z, Yin M, Lyu XL, Zhang LL, Du XD, Hung GCL. Delayed effect of repetitive transcranial magnetic stimulation (rTMS) on negative symptoms of schizophrenia: findings from a randomized controlled trial. Psychiatry Res. 2016;240:333–5.
48. Hasan A, Falkai P, Wobrock T. Transcranial brain stimulation in schizophrenia: targeting cortical excitability, connectivity and plasticity. Curr Med Chem. 2013;20(3):405–13.
49. Kamp D, Engelke C, Wobrock T, Wölwer W, Winterer G, Schmidt-Kraepelin C, et al. Left prefrontal high-frequency rTMS may improve movement disorder in schizophrenia patients with predominant negative symptoms—a secondary analysis of a sham-controlled, randomized multicenter trial. Schizophr Res. 2019;204:445–7.
50. Wagner E, Wobrock T, Kunze B, Langguth B, Landgrebe M, Eichhammer P, et al. Efficacy of high-frequency repetitive transcranial magnetic stimulation in schizophrenia patients with treatment-resistant negative symptoms treated with clozapine. Schizophr Res. 2019;208:370–6.
51. Hoffman RE, Boutros NN, Berman RM, Roessler E, Belger A, Krystal JH, Charney DS. Transcranial magnetic stimulation of left temporoparietal cortex in three patients reporting hallucinated "voices". Biol Psychiatry. 1999;46(1):130–2.
52. Aleman A, Sommer IE, Kahn RS. Efficacy of slow repetitive transcranial magnetic stimulation in the treatment of resistant auditory hallucinations in schizophrenia: a meta-analysis. J Clin Psychiatry. 2007 Mar;68(3):416–21.
53. Slotema CW, Aleman A, Daskalakis ZJ, Sommer IE. Meta-analysis of repetitive transcranial magnetic stimulation in the treatment of auditory verbal hallucinations: update and effects after one month. Schizophr Res. 2012;142(1–3):40–5.
54. Hunter MD, Eickhoff SB, Miller TW, Farrow TF, Wilkinson ID, Woodruff PW. Neural activity in speech-sensitive auditory cortex during silence. Proc Natl Acad Sci U S A. 2006;103(1):189–94.
55. Tracy DK, de Sousa de Abreu M, Nalesnik N, Mao L, Lage C, Shergill SS. Neuroimaging effects of 1 Hz right temporoparietal rTMS on normal auditory processing: implications for clinical hallucination treatment paradigms. J Clin Neurophysiol. 2014;31(6):541–6.
56. Bais L, Liemburg E, Vercammen A, Bruggeman R, Knegtering H, Aleman A. Effects of low frequency rTMS treatment on brain networks for inner speech in patients with schizophrenia and auditory verbal hallucinations. Prog Neuro-Psychopharmacol Biol Psychiatry. 2017;78:105–13.
57. Hoffman RE, Hampson M, Wu K, Anderson AW, Gore JC, Buchanan RJ, Constable RT, Hawkins KA, Sahay N, Krystal JH. Probing the pathophysiology of auditory/verbal hallucina-

tions by combining functional magnetic resonance imaging and transcranial magnetic stimulation. Cereb Cortex. 2007;17(11):2733–43.

58. Koops S, Slotema CW, Kos C, Bais L, Aleman A, Blom JD, Sommer IEC. Predicting response to rTMS for auditory hallucinations: younger patients and females do better. Schizophr Res. 2018;195:583–4.

59. Nathou C, Simon G, Dollfus S, Etard O. Cortical anatomical variations and efficacy of rTMS in the treatment of auditory hallucinations. Brain Stimul. 2015;8(6):1162–7.

60. Cheeran B, Talelli P, Mori F, Koch G, Suppa A, Edwards M, Houlden H, Bhatia K, Greenwood R, Rothwell JC. A common polymorphism in the brain-derived neurotrophic factor gene (BDNF) modulates human cortical plasticity and the response to rTMS. J Physiol. 2008;586(23):5717–25.

61. Bocchio-Chiavetto L, Miniussi C, Zanardini R, Gazzoli A, Bignotti S, Specchia C, Gennarelli M. 5-HTTLPR and BDNF Val66Met polymorphisms and response to rTMS treatment in drug resistant depression. Neurosci Lett. 2008;437(2):130–4.

62. Hasan A, Guse B, Cordes J, Wölwer W, Winterer G, Gaebel W, et al. Cognitive effects of high-frequency rTMS in schizophrenia patients with predominant negative symptoms: results from a multicenter randomized sham-controlled trial. Schizophr Bull. 2016;42(3):608–18.

63. Mittrach M, Thünker J, Winterer G, Agelink MW, Regenbrecht G, Arends M, et al. The tolerability of rTMS treatment in schizophrenia with respect to cognitive function. Pharmacopsychiatry. 2010;43(3):110–7.

64. Francis MM, Hummer TA, Vohs JL, Yung MG, Visco AC, Mehdiyoun NF, et al. Cognitive effects of bilateral high frequency repetitive transcranial magnetic stimulation in early phase psychosis: a pilot study. Brain Imaging Behav. 2019;13(3):852–61.

65. Rollnik JD, Huber TJ, Mogk H, Siggelkow S, Kropp S, Dengler R, et al. High frequency repetitive transcranial magnetic stimulation (rTMS) of the dorsolateral prefrontal cortex in schizophrenic patients. Neuroreport. 2000;11(18):4013–5.

66. Jiang Y, Guo Z, Xing G, He L, Peng H, Du F, et al. Effects of high-frequency transcranial magnetic stimulation for cognitive deficit in schizophrenia: a meta-analysis. Front Psych. 2019;10:135.

67. Barr MS, Farzan F, Arenovich T, Chen R, Fitzgerald PB, Daskalakis ZJ. The effect of repetitive transcranial magnetic stimulation on gamma oscillatory activity in schizophrenia. PLoS One. 2011;6(7):e22627.

68. Barr MS, Farzan F, Rajji TK, Voineskos AN, Blumberger DM, Arenovich T, et al. Can repetitive magnetic stimulation improve cognition in schizophrenia? Pilot data from a randomized controlled trial. Biol Psychiatry. 2013;73(6):510–7.

69. Wölwer W, Lowe A, Brinkmeyer J, Streit M, Habakuck M, Agelink MW, et al. Repetitive transcranial magnetic stimulation (rTMS) improves facial affect recognition in schizophrenia. Brain Stimul. 2014;7(4):559–63.

Transcranial Magnetic Stimulation in OCD

8

Lior Carmi

Transcranial Magnetic Stimulation (TMS) is a noninvasive technique, initially introduced by Barker and colleagues [1]. It consists of pulses that are administered by passing alternating high currents through an electromagnetic coil placed upon the scalp, which, in turn, generates a briefly pulsed magnetic field (1.5–2.0 T) and induces electrical currents in the underlying cortical tissue [2]. These electrical currents may lead to local and remote effects on cortical and subcortical neuronal circuitry, metabolism, monoamine neurotransmitter release, alteration in noradrenergic and serotonergic receptors as well as induction of gene expression [3–5].

TMS may include several protocols (e.g., single pulse, paired pulse); however, when applied in clinical settings, it is often used in a repetitive pulse mode, known as repetitive TMS (rTMS). Usually, trains of pulses delivered at high-frequency stimulation (HF; >5 Hz) lead to a facilitatory effect and induce increased neuronal excitability (long-term potentiation; LTP-like effect), while low-frequency stimulation (LF; ~1 Hz) reduces neuronal excitability (long-term depression; LTD-like effect) [6, 7]. Nevertheless, cumulative evidence suggests that the notion of excitatory HF vs. inhibitory LF stimulation is oversimplified [8], and that additional factors may contribute to the effect of TMS. These factors include the type of coil used, the frequency and intensity of stimulation, and the state of the relevant neuronal circuit. Specifically, the effects of TMS seem to be most pronounced when the targeted circuit is active [9, 10].

L. Carmi (✉)
The Post Trauma Center, Chaim Sheba Medical Center, Ramat Gan, Israel

The Data Science institution, The Interdisciplinary Center, Herzliya, Israel
e-mail: Lior.Carmi@sheba.health.gov.il

© Springer Nature Switzerland AG 2020
B. Dell'Osso, G. Di Lorenzo (eds.), *Non Invasive Brain Stimulation in Psychiatry and Clinical Neurosciences*,
https://doi.org/10.1007/978-3-030-43356-7_8

8.1   TMS in OCD

Although the combination of cognitive behavioral therapy (CBT) and serotonin reuptake inhibitors (SRIs) stands as a first-line treatment for OCD [11], the clinical challenge still remains. This is due to the complexity and heterogeneity of the disorder [12], the high percentage of patients that are drug resistant or that cannot tolerate the drug-related side effects [13, 14], and the relative low percentage of patients that receive CBT [15].

Converging evidence highlights the involvement of the Cortico-Striatal-Thalamic Circuitry (CSTC) in the etiology of OCD [16]. Indeed, impaired function of the CSTC circuit as a whole [16–18], or of its elements [19, 20], has been detected in OCD patients (Fig. 8.1) and hence became potential therapeutic targets for TMS.

These areas include the dorsolateral prefrontal cortex (DLPFC), orbitofrontal cortex (OFC), medial prefrontal cortices (mPFC), anterior cingulate cortex (ACC), and supplementary motor area (SMA). However, although TMS was found to be clinically and statistically superior to sham [22], a consensus intervention protocol has yet to emerge.

8.2   Trials of rTMS of the Dorsolateral Prefrontal Cortex

Greenberg and colleagues [23] made the first attempt to treat OCD with rTMS by stimulating the DLPFC as a starting point to induce remote stimulation in the CSTC. Twelve patients were given high-frequency rTMS (80% MT, 20 Hz/2 seconds per minute for 20 minutes) to the right and left lateral prefrontal, and to the midoccipital site as control, on separate days (randomized). In this study, right

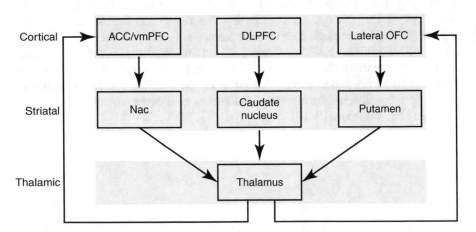

Fig. 8.1 Schematic illustration of the components of the cortico-striato-thalamo-cortical (CSTC) pathway. This pathway is commonly implicated in the psychopathology of obsessive-compulsive disorder (OCD). *ACC* anterior cingulate cortex, *vmPFC* ventromedial prefrontal cortex, *DLPFC* dorsolateral prefrontal cortex, *OFC* orbitofrontal cortex, *Nac* nucleus accumbens. (Adapted from [21])

lateral prefrontal stimulation caused compulsive urges to decrease significantly for 8 hours, and mood improvement during and 30 minutes after stimulation; left lateral prefrontal stimulation caused a shorter-lasting (30 minutes), modest, and nonsignificant reduction in compulsive urges, and midoccipital stimulation causes nonsignificant increases in compulsive urges.

During the following years, other researchers have tried to stimulate the circuitry, targeting the DLPFC on OCD: however, conflicting findings emerged. Alonso and co-workers [24] targeted the right DLPFC with low-frequency rTMS for 18 sessions (1 Hz, 110% MT for 20 minutes) and detected no significant changes in symptom severity.

Prasko and colleagues [25] targeted the left DLPFC with low-frequency rTMS (1 Hz, 110% MT, 10 sessions; $n = 30$), and found that both real and sham groups improved during the study period but with no treatment effect.

Sachdev and co-authors [26] found no significant difference between the active ($n = 10$) and sham ($n = 8$) stimulation of high-frequency rTMS to the left DLPFC (10 Hz at 110% of MT, 10 sessions). At the end of the blind trial, 3/10 in the active and 2/8 in the sham groups were responders. When analysis included an additional 10 sessions of open trial, there was a significant overall reduction in total YBOCS scores, which was due to a fall in YBOCS obsession but not compulsion subscale. However, correcting for depression using MADRS made these results nonsignificant.

Along these lines, Sarkhel and colleagues [27] found that both active ($n = 21$) and sham ($n = 21$) high-frequency stimulation of the right DLPFC evinced significant improvement in obsessions and compulsions (10 Hz at 110% of MT, 10 sessions—4 seconds per train, 20 trains per session). However, active rTMS treatment was not superior to sham in reducing YBOCS scores.

On the other hand, positive results were found in two recent studies, which reported a reduction in YBOCS score in the active group compared to sham via bilateral stimulation of the DLPFC [28, 29]. Thus, despite long years of attempts, a consensus on the efficacy of rTMS of the dorsolateral PFC for OCD is still lacking.

8.3   Trials of rTMS Over the Supplementary Motor Area (SMA)

The SMA is involved in motor planning and response inhibition along with emotional and cognitive processes [30–32]. Findings from recent years have demonstrated high level of cortical excitability of motor areas in OCD patients [33] and were the basis for clinical trials that have chosen the SMA as a target for LF-rTMS.

In an open trial with a relatively small sample, Mantovani and colleagues [34] reported a clinical improvement in OCD symptoms as early as the first week of low-frequency rTMS to the SMA bilaterally (1 Hz at 100% of MT, 10 sessions, 1200 stimuli/day). In a follow-up of this study with a sham-controlled design, Mantovani and colleagues [35] reported that low-frequency rTMS delivered to the SMA (1 Hz at 100% of MT, 20 sessions) resulted in more clinical responders among those patients who completed 4-week active treatment (67%, $n = 9$), compared to those who received sham treatment (22%, $n = 9$).

The utility of low-frequency stimulation came from several other studies. Gomes and co-authors. reported a significant improvement of YBOCS scores in a double-blind study following pre-SMA stimulation (1 Hz, 100% MT stimulation, 10 sessions). In this study, YBOCS scores in the active group reached a 35% reduction as compared to only 6.2% in the sham group [36]. Mantovani and co-workers also found an average reduction of 25% in the YBOCS score in the active group as compared with 12% in the sham group (1 Hz, 100% MT, for 4 weeks) [37].

In another study, bilateral rTMS over the SMA (1 Hz, 15 sessions) was compared with antipsychotics intervention in SRIs-refractory OCD patients [38]. An overall 66% of the TMS group responded positively as compared to 25% in the antipsychotic group, suggesting the superiority of rTMS targeting SMA over the treatment with antipsychotics in OCD refractory patients. TMS over the SMA as an augmentation for treatment-resistant OCD patients was also studied by Lee and colleagues from South Korea. They reported a significant reduction in YBOCS (mainly compulsions) score at the fourth week of treatment (open label) in patients with treatment-resistant OCD [39].

An interesting study conducted by Kang and colleagues [40] investigated the effect of combined low-frequency stimulation of the right DLPFC and SMA in a double-blind design (1 Hz, 110% MT, 10 sessions). In each session, stimulation of the RDLPFC was followed by bilateral stimulation of the SMA (1 Hz, 100% MT). However, at treatment endpoint (week 2), and at follow-up assessment (week 4), YBOCS severity scores were significantly reduced in both active and sham groups without any statistically significant differences.

8.4 Trials of rTMS Over the Orbitofrontal Cortex

The OFC is part of the CSTC and it has been found to be hyperactivated in OCD and linked to the development of compulsive-like behaviors [41]. However, despite its involvement in the pathophysiology of the disorder, this region has attracted less attention as a stimulation target for TMS.

This may be due to practical problems in stimulating the OFC with rTMS, such as access—the OFC is rather deeply buried beneath the scalp—and side effects (e.g., excessive twitching of eye muscles) [42].

The first exploratory treatment of stimulating the OFC was carried out by Ruffini and co-authors in 2009 [43]. In a single-blind study, 23 drug-resistant OCD patients were given rTMS (80% motor threshold, 1 Hz, 10 min every day for 15 days) to the left OFC parallel to the scalp (16 active and 7 sham). They found a significant reduction in YBOCS scores, comparing active versus sham treatment for 10 weeks after the end of rTMS treatment, for active TMS; however, this significance was lost after 12 weeks, suggesting only a time-limited improvement.

Another study [44] targeted the right OFC (1 Hz, 120% MT, twice daily (1200 pulses/session) using a double-cone coil (which allows deeper stimulation compared to figure-of-eight coil [45]). This was a double-blind, crossover study, with two treatment phases of 1 week each, separated by 1-month washout period. In addition, PET scans were conducted on some of the patients and were correlated to the clinical outcome. Both active and sham groups showed a significant reduction in the YBOCS score, with significantly larger reduction in the active group. However, this signal was lost a month after the second period of stimulation. In addition, the clinical effect was correlated with the decrease in metabolic activity of the right OFC.

8.5 Deep TMS

Deep TMS (dTMS) is a relatively new form of TMS that enables direct stimulation of deep neuronal pathways [46]. It operates according to the same basic principles as the superficial Figure-8 coil for rTMS, by which a rapidly pulsed magnetic field induces an electric field within the cortex. However, the two coils differ with regard to the spatial distribution of the electric field [47–50]. For example, when stimulating at standard intensities for depression treatment (a condition for which both coils are FDA approved), the Figure-8 coil induces suprathreshold fields that stimulate 3 cm^3 of brain volume up to 0.7 cm from the brain surface, while the H-coil induces suprathreshold fields that stimulate 17 cm^3 of brain volume up to 1.8 cm beneath the cortical surface [51]. This increased stimulation depth is achieved due to the multiple windings in multiple planes inside the H-coil helmet, which in effect improves the depth penetration of the electromagnetic field without necessitating increased electric intensity [52].

8.6 Deep TMS in OCD

Carmi and colleagues conducted two studies using Deep TMS, and both targeted the Medial Prefrontal Cortex (mPFC) and the Anterior Cingulate Cortex (ACC). In the first study [9], treatment-resistant OCD participants were treated with either high-frequency (HF; 20 Hz), low-frequency (LF; 1 Hz), or sham dTMS for 5 weeks, in a double-blinded manner. Interim analysis revealed that YBOCS scores were significantly improved following HF ($n = 7$), but not LF stimulation ($n = 8$), compared to sham ($n = 8$), and thus recruitment for the LF group was terminated. Following completion of the study, the response rate in the HF group ($n = 18$) was significantly higher than that of the sham group ($n = 15$) for at least 1 month following the end of the treatment. Notably, the clinical response in the HF group correlated with increased Error-Related Negativity (ERN) in the Stroop task, an electrophysiological component that is attributed to ACC activity. Following this study, Carmi and colleagues conducted a randomized double-blind multicenter study [53]. At 11 centers, 99 OCD patients were randomly allocated to treatment with either high-frequency (20 Hz) or sham dTMS and received daily treatments following individualized symptom provocation, for 6 weeks. The reduction in YBOCS score among patients who received active dTMS treatment was significantly greater than among patients who received sham treatment (reductions of 6.0 points and 3.3 points, respectively), with response rates of 38.1% and 11.1%, respectively. At the 1-month follow-up, the response rates were 45.2% in the active treatment group and 17.8% in the sham treatment group. Significant differences between the groups were maintained at follow-up. Based on this study, the treatment of dTMS targeting the mPFC and the ACC was recently approved by the FDA for treatment of OCD.

8.7   Summary

Although the combination of CBT and SRIs stands as a first-line treatment for OCD, the clinical challenge remains. The knowledge of the neurological circuitry involved in OCD, along with the technology to stimulate it noninvasively, has harnessed researchers to employ TMS as an important tool for intervention. Accordingly, several areas were targeted via TMS and dTMS: the DLPFC, SMA, OFC, and the mPFC-ACC.

The DLPFC was widely investigated with most studies yielding negative results. However, as recent studies have produced positive results, stimulation of DLPFC may still be a relevant region for TMS stimulation in OCD. Targeting of pre-SMA and SMA with rTMS has produced a number of positive results and may be considered a promising era for intervention. As for the stimulation of the OFC, due to practical problems, only a few studies have stimulated this area: however, both have shown improvement in OCD symptoms. Deep TMS (dTMS) is a relatively new form of TMS that enables direct stimulation of deep neuronal pathways. Two studies targeted the mPFC and the ACC via dTMS, and both yielded positive results upon which a new therapeutic indication (dTMS over the Mpfc in OCD patients) was approved.

References

1. Barker AT, Jalinous R, Freeston IL. Non-invasive magnetic stimulation of human motor cortex. Lancet. 1985;1:1106–7.
2. Peterchev AV, Wagner TA, Miranda PC, Nitsche MA, Paulus W, Lisanby SH, et al. Fundamentals of transcranial electric and magnetic stimulation dose: definition, selection, and reporting practices. Brain Stimul. 2012;5(4):435–53.
3. Jaafari N, Rachid F, Rotge JY, Polosan M, El-Hage W, Belin D, et al. Safety and efficacy of repetitive transcranial magnetic stimulation in the treatment of obsessive-compulsive disorder: a review. World J Biol Psychiatry. 2012;13(3):164–77.
4. Strafella AP, Paus T, Fraraccio M, Dagher A. Striatal dopamine release induced by repetitive transcranial magnetic stimulation of the human motor cortex. Brain. 2003;126:2609–15.
5. Szuba MP, O'Reardon JP, Rai AS, Snyder-Kastenberg J, Amsterdam JD, Gettes DR, et al. Acute mood and thyroid stimulating hormone effects of transcranial magnetic stimulation in major depression. Biol Psychiatry. 2001;50:22–7.
6. Pell GS, Roth Y, Zangen A. Modulation of cortical excitability induced by repetitive transcranial magnetic stimulation: influence of timing and geometrical parameters and underlying mechanisms. Prog Neurobiol. 2011;93(1):59–98.

7. Voineskos D, Daskalakis ZJ. A primer on the treatment of schizophrenia through repetitive transcranial magnetic stimulation. Expert Rev Neurother. 2013;13(10):1079.
8. Lefaucheur J-P, et al. Evidence-based guidelines on the therapeutic use of repetitive transcranial magnetic stimulation (rTMS). Clin Neurophysiol. 2014;125(11):2150–206.
9. Carmi L, Alyagon U, Barnea-Ygael N, Zohar J, Dar R, Zangen A. Clinical and electrophysiological outcomes of deep TMS over the medial prefrontal and anterior cingulate cortices in OCD patients. Brain Stimul. 2018;11(1):158–65.
10. Isserles M, Shalev AY, Roth Y, Peri T, Kutz I, Zlotnick E, Zangen A. Effectiveness of deep transcranial magnetic stimulation combined with a brief exposure procedure in post-traumatic stress disorder–a pilot study. Brain Stimul. 2013;6(3):377–83.
11. Öst L-G, Havnen A, Hansen B, Kvale G. Cognitive behavioral treatments of obsessive–compulsive disorder. A systematic review and meta-analysis of studies published 1993–2014. Clin Psychol Rev. 2015;40:156–69.
12. Hollander E. Obsessive-compulsive disorder: the hidden epidemic. J Clin Psychiatry. 1997;58:3–6.
13. Leckman JF, Denys D, Simpson HB, Mataix-Cols D, Hollander E, Saxena S, et al. Obsessive–compulsive disorder: a review of the diagnostic criteria and possible subtypes and dimensional specifiers for DSM-V. Depress Anxiety. 2010;27(6):507.
14. Mataix-Cols D, do Rosario-Campos MC, Leckman JF. A multidimensional model of obsessive-compulsive disorder. Am J Psychiatry. 2005;162(2):228–38.
15. O'Neill J, Feusner JD. Cognitive-behavioral therapy for obsessive–compulsive disorder: access to treatment, prediction of long-term outcome with neuroimaging. Psychol Res Behav Manag. 2015;8:211.
16. Bear RE, et al. Neurosurgery for obsessive-compulsive disorder: contemporary approaches. J Clin Neurosci. 2010;17(1):1–5.
17. Coles ME, et al. Not just right experiences and obsessive–compulsive features: experimental and self-monitoring perspectives. Behav Res Ther. 2005;43(2):153–67.
18. Speer AM, et al. Opposite effects of high and low frequency rTMS on regional brain activity in depressed patients. Biol Psychiatry. 2000;48(12):1133–41.
19. Yin HH, Knowlton BJ. The role of the basal ganglia in habit formation. Nat Rev Neurosci. 2006;7(6):464–76.
20. Lehéricy S, et al. Diffusion tensor fiber tracking shows distinct corticostriatal circuits in humans. Ann Neurol. 2004;55(4):522–9.
21. Del Casale A, et al. Functional neuroimaging in obsessive-compulsive disorder. Neuropsychobiology. 2011;64(2):61–85.
22. Trevizol AP, Shiozawa P, Cook IA, Sato IA, Kaku CB, Guimarães FB, et al. Transcranial magnetic stimulation for obsessive-compulsive disorder: an updated systematic review and meta-analysis. J ECT. 2016;32(4):262–6.
23. Greenberg BD, et al. Effect of prefrontal repetitive transcranial magnetic stimulation in obsessive-compulsive disorder: a preliminary study. Am J Psychiatry. 1997;154(6):867–9.
24. Alonso P, et al. Right prefrontal repetitive transcranial magnetic stimulation in obsessive-compulsive disorder: a double-blind, placebo-controlled study. Am J Psychiatry. 2001;158(7):1143–5.
25. Prasko J, et al. The effect of repetitive transcranial magnetic stimulation (rTMS) on symptoms in obsessive compulsive disorder. A randomized, double blind, sham controlled study. Neuro Endocrinol Lett. 2006;27(3):327–32.
26. Sachdev PS, et al. Repetitive transcranial magnetic stimulation for the treatment of obsessive compulsive disorder: a double-blind controlled investigation. Psychol Med. 2007;37(11):1645–9.
27. Sarkhel S, Sinha VK, Praharaj SK. Adjunctive high-frequency right prefrontal repetitive transcranial magnetic stimulation (rTMS) was not effective in obsessive-compulsive disorder but improved secondary depression. J Anxiety Disord. 2010;24(5):535–9.

28. Xiaoyan M, Yueqin H, Liwei L, Yi J. A randomized double-blinded sham-controlled trial of electroencelogram-guided transcranial magnetic stimulation for obsessive compulsive disorder. Chin Med J. 2014;127:601–6.
29. Elbeh KAM, Elserogy YMB, Khalifa HE, Ahmed MA, Hafez MH, Khedr EM. Repetitive transcranial magnetic stimulation in the treatment of obsessive-compulsive disorders: double blind randomized clinical trial. Psychiatry Res. 2016;238:264–9.
30. Mostosfsky SH, Simmonds DJ. Response inhibition and response selection: two sides of the same coin. J Cogn Neurosci. 2008;20(5):751–61.
31. Picard N, Strick PL. Activation of the supplementary motor area (SMA) during performance of visually guided movements. Cereb Cortex. 2003;13:977–86.
32. Oliveri M, Babiloni C, Filippi MM, Caltagirone C, Babiloni F, Cicinelli P, et al. Influence of the supplementary motor area on primary motor cortex excitability during movements triggered by neutral or emotionally unpleasant visual cues. Exp Brain Res. 2003;149:1214–21.
33. Rossi S, Bartalini S, Ulivelli M, Mantovani A, Di Muro A, Goracci A, et al. Hypofunctioning of sensory gating mechanisms in patients with obsessive-compulsive disorder. Biol Psychiatry. 2005;57:16–20.
34. Mantovani A, et al. Repetitive transcranial magnetic stimulation (rTMS) in the treatment of obsessive-compulsive disorder (OCD) and Tourette's syndrome (TS). Int J Neuropsychopharmacol. 2006;9(1):95–100.
35. Mantovani A, et al. Randomized sham-controlled trial of repetitive transcranial magnetic stimulation in treatment-resistant obsessive-compulsive disorder. Int J Neuropsychopharmacol. 2010;13(2):217–27.
36. Gomes PVO, Brasil-Neto JP, Allam N, de Souza ER. A randomized, double blind trial of repetitive transcranial magnetic stimulation in obsessive-compulsive disorder with three months follow-up. J Neuropsychiatry Clin Neurosci. 2012;24(4):437–43.
37. Montovani A, Rossi S, Bassi BD, Simpson HB, Fallon BA, Lisanby SH. Modulation of motor-cortex excitability in obsessive-compulsive disorders: an exploratory study on the relations of neurophysiology measures with clinical outcome. Psychiatry Res. 2013;210(3):1026–32.
38. Pallanti S, Marras A, Salerno L, Makris N, Hollander E. Better than treated as usual: transcranial magnetic stimulation augmentation in selective serotonin reuptake inhibitor-refractory obsessive-compulsive disorder, minireview and pilot open-label trial. J Psychopharmacol. 2016;30:568–78.
39. Lee YJ, Koo BH, Seo WS, Kim HG, Kim JY, Cheon EJ. Repetitive transcranial magnetic stimulation of the supplementary motor area in treatment-resistant obsessive-compulsive disorder: an open-label pilot study. J Clin Neurosci. 2017;44:264–8 . pii: S0967-5868(17)30538-6. https://doi.org/10.1016/j.jocn.2017.06.057.
40. Kang JI, Kim CH, Namkoong K, Lee C, Kim SJ. A randomized controlled study of sequentially applied repetitive transcranial magnetic stimulation in obsessive-compulsive disorder. J Clin Psychiatry. 2009;70:1645–51.
41. Evans DW, Lewis MD, Iobst E. The role of the orbitofrontal cortex in normally developing compulsivelike behaviors and obsessive-compulsive disorder. Brain Cogn. 2004;55:220–34.
42. Zaman R, Robbins TW. Is there potential for Repetitive Transcranial Magnetic Stimulation (RTMS) as a treatment of OCD. Psychiatr Danub. 2017;29(Suppl 3):672–8.
43. Ruffini C, Locatelli M, Luca A, Benedetti F, Insacco C, Smeraldi E. Augmentation effect of repetitive transcranial magnetic stimulation over the orbitofrontal cortex in drugresistant obsessive-compulsive disorder patients: a controlled investigation. Prim Care Comp J Clin Psychiatry. 2009;11(5):226–30.
44. Nauczyciel C, Le Jeune F, Naudet F, Douabin S, Esquevin A, Verin M, Dondaine T, Robert G, Drapier D, Millet B. Repetitive transcranial magnetic stimulation over the orbitofrontal cortex for obsessive-compulsive disorder: a double-blind, crossover study. Transl Psychiatry. 2014;4:e436.
45. Deng ZD, Lisanby SH, Peterchev AV. Electric field depth focality trade off in transcranial magnetic stimulation: simulation comparison of 50 coil designs. Brain Stimul. 2013;6:1–13.

46. Roth Y, Zangen A. Reaching deep brain structures: the H-coils. Neuromethods. 2014;89:57–65.
47. Deng Z-D, Lisanby SH, Peterchev AV. Electric field depth–focality tradeoff in transcranial magnetic stimulation: simulation comparison of 50 coil designs. Brain Stimul. 2013;6(1):1–13.
48. Rosenberg O, et al. Deep TMS in a resistant major depressive disorder: a brief report. Depress Anxiety. 2010;27(5):465–9.
49. Roth Y, et al. Three-dimensional distribution of the electric field induced in the brain by transcranial magnetic stimulation using figure-8 and deep H-coils. J Clin Neurophysiol. 2007;24(1):31–8.
50. Roth Y, Zangen A. Reaching deep brain structures: the H-coils. In: Neuromethods: transcranial magnetic stimulation. New York: Humana Press/Springer; 2014. p. 57–69.
51. Ginou A, Roth Y, Zangen A. Comparison of superficial TMS and deep TMS for major depression. Brain Stimul. 2014;5(7):e19.
52. Tendler A, et al. Deep transcranial magnetic stimulation (dTMS)–beyond depression. Expert Rev Med Devices. 2016;13(10):987–1000.
53. Carmi L, et al. Efficacy and safety of deep transcranial magnetic stimulation for obsessive-compulsive disorder: a prospective multicenter randomized double-blind placebo-controlled trail. Am J Psychiatry. 2019 Nov 1;176(11):931–8.

Neuromodulation in Attention-Deficit/Hyperactivity Disorder: Toward a Precision Psychiatry Approach

9

Luana Salerno, Sonia Gaur, Giacomo Grassi, and Stefano Pallanti

9.1 Introduction

Attention-deficit/hyperactivity disorder (ADHD) is a neurodevelopmental disorder with a childhood onset, characterized by developmentally inadequate levels of inattention, hyperactivity, and impulsivity [1]. Epidemiological studies show a prevalence rate of ADHD in children of 5–6% [2, 3] and of 2.8% in adults [4]. ADHD persists in most cases from childhood to adulthood, and even if ADHD is considered "in partial remission," it still causes interference with the individual functioning and psychosocial impairment [5–7]. Apart from the widely recognized impairment associated with untreated ADHD, including academic failure, self-esteem problems, and interpersonal relationship difficulties, people with ADHD have an increased risk for being involved in criminal situations, for facing unplanned pregnancies, for suffering from sexually transmitted diseases and several health problems due to their maladaptive lifestyle habits, such as excessive cigarette consumption, impulsive and dysregulated eating leading to obesity, hypertension, and type 2 diabetes mellitus [8]. Also, a high prevalence of fibromyalgia syndrome (FMS) has been reported in patients with ADHD [9].

A hallmark of ADHD is its high heterogeneity, which can manifest not only between individuals who received the diagnosis but also within the same individuals across the lifespan. The classification of ADHD in the three presentations of predominantly hyperactive-impulsive, predominantly inattentive, or combined ADHD

L. Salerno · S. Pallanti (✉)
INS Istituto di Neuroscienze, Firenze, Italy
e-mail: stefanopallanti@yahoo.it

S. Gaur
Stanford University School of Medicine, Stanford, CA, USA

G. Grassi
Florence, Italy

© Springer Nature Switzerland AG 2020
B. Dell'Osso, G. Di Lorenzo (eds.), *Non Invasive Brain Stimulation in Psychiatry and Clinical Neurosciences*,
https://doi.org/10.1007/978-3-030-43356-7_9

is only an attempt to deal with its heterogeneity, but even in this way two subjects with the same ADHD clinical presentation share no more than three symptoms [10]. Moreover, the ADHD presentation is not stable during the lifespan, as a child who received a diagnosis of predominantly inattentive ADHD can become an adult with a combined ADHD. The ADHD heterogeneity affects not only symptom profiles, but even neuropsychological impairments. In fact, although the evidence indicating that people with ADHD, as a group, are more impaired in some neuropsychological domains compared to healthy controls, and particularly in executive functioning and motivational processes [11–15], not all individuals with ADHD present this kind of deficits [11, 16, 17]. Furthmore, 50–75% of adults with ADHD have at least one comorbid learning, neurodevelopmental, or psychiatric disorder [18–22] complicating the current clinical presentation, and it is possible that some comorbid conditions, such as anxiety or depression, are not simple coexistent disorders, but rather the direct consequence of the lifelong impairment caused by untreated ADHD.

At present, the diagnosis of ADHD does not take into account etiological sources or biological markers, but it is established on the presence of a certain number of symptoms, presenting in more than one context and with an onset before age 12. However, even though the current manuals for diagnosing psychiatric disorders have been of value in facilitating communication between clinicians and researchers, they did not keep the promise of a heightened focus on neurobiological markers and on the use of a dimensional system, and failed in establishing the validity of their diagnostic categories beyond the clinical level. The relationship between ADHD clinical definition and its neurobiological substrates constitutes an important issue, as its etiological heterogeneity can be the result of diverse neural correlates, which in turn can explain the treatment response to different therapeutic agents, to different doses, and to a combination of them. In this context, the approach proposed by the National Institute of Mental Health (NIMH) called Research Domain Criteria (RDoC) emerged as a useful framework, as a project aiming to transform diagnosis by incorporating genetics, imaging, cognitive science, and other information levels in order to establish the starting point for a new classification system [23]. It assumes that mental disorders are biological conditions involving brain circuits that implicate specific domains of cognition, emotion, and behavior, and therefore symptoms cannot be constrained by the categories of current diagnostic manuals. Its ultimate goal is "precision medicine" for psychiatry, and therefore a diagnostic refinement based on a deeper understanding of the circuitries and networks of psychiatric disorders considered to be responsible for brain diseases [24].

Even though the treatment with psychostimulants is a mainstay of ADHD treatment, it is still challenged by stigma and fear regarding potential side effects. Moreover, it is estimated that at least 30% of individuals do not appropriately respond to, or are not able to tolerate them [25]. Last but not least, there are some concerns about the risk for stimulant misuse and diversion in ADHD patients [26]. Noninvasive brain stimulation (NIBS) techniques, such as repetitive transcranial magnetic stimulation (rTMS) and transcranial direct current stimulation (tDCS), have been increasingly used in different contexts to improve cognitive performance and ameliorate depressive symptoms [27]. Their use can be of value also for the treatment of the dysfunctional networks underpinning the clinical manifestation of ADHD.

9.2   The Rationale for the Use of NIBS in ADHD: Main Dysfunctional Networks

ADHD in children and adults is associated with several cognitive deficits and brain alterations. Studies on children with ADHD found impairments related to inhibitory control, sustained attention, visuospatial and verbal working memory, timing, vigilance, planning, and reward processing [11, 28–30]. Recently, great attention was focused on the finding regarding the association of ADHD with reaction time variability (RTV), which is thought to represent attentional lapses [28, 31, 32]. Similar impairments have been found in adults with ADHD [31–35]. There is consistent evidence indicating a disruption in several brain networks explaining the variety of cognitive deficits and behavioral symptoms characterizing people with ADHD. Impairments in the anterior cingulate cortico-striato-thalamo-cortical (ACCSTC) circuit, known as the selective attention circuit [36], are considered responsible for the lack of attention to details and distractibility characterizing people with ADHD. Deficient response inhibition appears related to impaired circuitry, including inferior frontal gyrus, anterior insula cortex, dorsomedial frontal cortex with the presupplementary motor area or pre-SMA and caudate [37–40]. Timing-related dysfunction is associated with functional hypo-activation of inferior frontal cortex, dorsolateral prefrontal cortex, supplementary motor area, anterior cingulate cortex, basal ganglia, parietal regions, and cerebellum [41, 42]. Impulsive decision making has been associated with disrupted connectivity between the nucleus accumbens and the anterior prefrontal cortex (PFC) and ventromedial PFC [43], ventro–striatal hypo-responsiveness during reward anticipation [44] and hyper-responsiveness in the ventral striatum/nucleus accumbens upon receipt of reward [45]. Alterations in the cortico-striatal network have been considered as underlying the deficits in motor control characterizing ADHD, causing excessive moving or talking in subjects affected by the disorder [46, 47]. Moreover, hypofunctionality in basal ganglia showed to predict poor movement preparations as well as cognitive planning deficits [48]. Emotional dysregulation seemed to be associated with an impaired emotion regulation network, including circuitry implicated in the emotional impulsivity (EI) and therefore mesolimbic circuitry, involving the orbitofrontal cortex, the amygdala, and the ventral striatum [49–51] as well as that of deficient emotional self-control (DESR) mediated by the ventrolateral prefrontal cortex, the medial prefrontal cortex, and the anterior cingulate cortical region [52–55]. Finally, ADHD is associated with reduced activation in neuroanatomical regions involved in working memory such as occipital, inferior parietal cortex, caudate nucleus, cerebellar regions [56] during working memory tasks, and in left and right prefrontal brain regions in both children and adults [57, 58].

Besides the rationale provided by the brain circuits alterations reported here, important insights for the use of NIBS for the treatment of ADHD symptomatology derive from studies indicating that the most used pharmacological agents for treating ADHD work by altering cortical excitability [59]. Indeed, methylphenidate influences motor cortex excitability in both inhibitory and excitatory neuronal circuitry in healthy subjects [59, 60].

On the basis of such evidence, NIBS techniques represent potential alternative tools with respect to ADHD medications for influencing cortical excitability. NIBS techniques offer the opportunity to develop a tailored intervention targeting a specific cognitive domain or other symptomatological dimension and, therefore, to the specific disrupted brain networks. Up until now, the NIBS brain targets in ADHD have been the dorsolateral prefrontal cortex (DLPFC) for inhibitory deficits, and the orbitofrontal cortex (OFC), which is more closely involved in motivational dysfunction [61].

The most used NIBS in ADHD are Transcranial Magnetic Stimulation or TMS and transcranial Direct Current Stimulation or tDCS. Both TMS and tDCS permit to modulate cortical and brain regions through electromagnetic fields or direct electrical currents over the scalp, which can either increase or decrease cortical excitability in relatively focal areas according to different stimulation parameters [62].

rTMS consists of repetitive trains of magnetic pulses, inducing temporary electrical currents in localized cortical tissue. Recently, two new rTMS protocols have been introduced, using theta burst stimulation or TBS. TBS consists of bursts of three pulses of stimulation with a frequency of 50 Hz repeated every 200 ms, provided through an intermittent bursting frequency (iTBS) with a facilitatory effect, or through a continuous bursting frequency (cTBS) with an inhibitory effect, inducing transient long-term depression of behavior [63, 64].

tDCS uses low-intensity direct current (up to 2.0 mA) through two or more electrodes placed on the scalp and modulates the resting membrane potential according to the type of electrode application.

9.3   TMS as a Therapeutic Tool: rTMS Studies in ADHD

To date, there are still few rTMS studies in people with ADHD, and the vast majority has been performed in children and adolescents. Helfrich and colleagues [65], in a randomized, sham-controlled study, investigated the effects of inhibitory rTMS in modifying the inhibitory/excitatory (I/E) unbalance in the motor system of children with ADHD ($N = 25$), by using as neurophysiological measures the TMS-evoked potentials (TEPs) and the motor-evoked potentials (MEPs). TEPs and MEPs in response to single-pulse TMS (110% resting motor threshold, RMT) were measured before and after active 1-Hz rTMS (900 pulses, 80% RMT) or sham stimulation (achieved through a deactivated coil) over the left M1, with the stimulation conditions delivered in counterbalanced order 30 minutes apart. rTMS showed to be safe and well tolerated, but the study results showed a decrease in N100 after inhibitory low frequency-rTMS (LF-rTMS) rather than an increase [66], not supporting the use of rTMS to increase intracortical inhibition in ADHD [61]. However, findings from this study indicated that the N100 amplitude may be useful as an indicator to maximize the functional effects of rTMS on the cortex [65].

In a randomized, sham-controlled crossover study, nine adolescents and young adults with ADHD received either active or sham high frequency-rTMS (HF-rTMS) over the right DLPFC. The protocol was implemented in a counterbalanced order in two phases, each lasting 2 weeks, with 1-week interval of no treatment between phases. Ten-Hertz rTMS was delivered at 100% of the MT (2000 pulses per session, 5 sessions per week), with informant ratings regarding functional impairment and ADHD symptoms obtained at baseline, midpoint, and end of the study. Results by the comparison of rating scales scores showed that, despite a significant improvement in ADHD symptoms and impairment, there were no differences between active and sham rTMS [67]. Instead, a tolerability and safety pilot study performed by the group of Gómez and colleagues [68] using LF-rTMS in ten children with ADHD classified as nonresponders to conventional treatment showed interesting results. This study investigated the effects of 5 consecutive daily sessions of 1-Hz rTMS (90% RMT) over the left DLPFC, with a total of 1500 stimuli per session, by comparing informant reports (parents and teachers) collected before and 1 week after completing the rTMS sessions. For what concerns tolerability, all children completed treatment, reporting a slight headache or local discomfort in 70% of cases, neck pain in 20%, and one patient reporting brief dizziness (only in two sessions). Results from informant ratings showed a significant improvement in inattentive symptoms at school and hyperactive/impulsive behavior at home. However, several limitations of the study, such as the open-label design, the small sample, and the lack of a sham arm, could not allow testing its clinical efficacy [61].

Studies on the effectiveness of rTMS in adults with ADHD are very scarce. Bloch and co-workers [69], in their crossover double-blind, randomized, sham-controlled pilot study, investigated the effect of either a single session of HF-rTMS directed to the right prefrontal cortex (active rTMS) or a single session of sham rTMS on adults with an ADHD diagnosis according to DSM-IV ($N = 13$). The stimulation protocol consisted of a 20-Hz stimulation over the right DLPFC at a 100% MT for a total of 1680 stimuli per session. They found a specific beneficial effect on attention 10 minutes after active rTMS, with a subsequent improvement in attention, according to Positive and Negative Affect Schedule (PANAS) scores. Any significant effect on measures of mood and anxiety was detected and the sham rTMS showed no effect at all.

Niederhofer [70] reported improved ADHD symptoms in a case study that consisted of motor cortex stimulation using 1 Hz rTMS at 1200 pulses per day for 5 days.

Even though there are no published large, randomized, sham-controlled trials of therapeutic rTMS in ADHD so far, several clinical trials are ongoing, as documented on the website https://clinicaltrials.gov/.

Recently, also a trial with deep-TMS (dTMS), which uses special coils for reaching up to 4 cm beneath the surface of the skull, and that has been recently approved for both treatment-resistant major depressive disorder and treatment-resistant obsessive-compulsive disorder, has been performed in subjects with ADHD. Specifically, 26 adults with ADHD were included in a double-blind sham-controlled study exploring the safety and effectiveness of bilateral prefrontal deep rTMS [71]. Subjects underwent 20 daily sessions targeting the prefrontal cortex with a bilateral coil at 120% of MT at high frequency, and behavioral and cognitive ADHD symptoms were evaluated through an ADHD-rating scale and a continuous performance test. At the end of the trial, results showed no differences in clinical outcomes between the active dTMS and sham groups, providing no support to the utility of such a bilateral prefrontal stimulation to treat adult ADHD.

Despite mixed results, the potential application of rTMS as an alternative or add-on treatment in ADHD seems supported by evidence emerging from positron emission tomography (PET) studies of rTMS, which revealed changes in striatal dopamine receptor occupancy following rTMS, being the changes localized to the specific region of the striatum serving the cortical target (dorsomedial prefrontal cortex, DMPFC, and dorsolateral prefrontal cortex, DLPFC) of stimulation [72, 73]. Moreover, dopamine agonists and antagonists appeared to potentiate or block the effects of rTMS [74]. Furthermore, there is growing evidence indicating the utility of rTMS in enhancing cognitive control, such as the excitatory dorsomedial rTMS protocol, which resulted effective in reducing impulsivity on a delay-discounting task [75, 76]. In relation to tolerability, TMS treatment is generally well tolerated, and among adverse reactions, the most frequently reported are mild and self-limited headache, scalp pain at the stimulation site, and potential transient hearing alterations caused by the clicking sound of the machine. The most serious adverse event is the seizure induction, which, however, is rare [77].

9.4   TMS as an Investigative Tool in ADHD

Since it permits us to evaluate motor pathways excitability, TMS represents a very useful investigative tool helping us to improve our understanding of the neurobiology of ADHD. TMS pulses are delivered to the primary motor cortex, and single- and paired-pulse TMS can capture the neurophysiological correlates of behavioral symptoms of ADHD in the motor cortex. For example, evidence from TMS studies as an investigative tool showed an inverse correlation between the Short-Interval Cortical Inhibition (SICI) and hyperactivity. As low levels of intracortical inhibition appeared associated with greater hyperactivity, and these abnormalities normalized after methylphenidate (MPH) administration [78], it has been suggested that SICI may represent a putative biomarker of ADHD symptom severity [78–82]. Interestingly, another TMS study, investigating motor cortex excitability and its modulation by attention in healthy adults, showed that SICI decreases under task conditions requiring attentional focus on an internal or external locus, compared to a resting condition [83]. Authors suggested that altered SICI characterizing other conditions, such as Tourette's syndrome [84] and ADHD [82, 85], may not be only the reflections of impaired intracortical GABA circuits per se, but the result of disorder-specific (and therefore different) attentional states [83].

Other TMS studies showed impaired transcallosal-mediated inhibition in ADHD [86–88], and that both latency and duration of the ipsilateral silent period (iSP) are prolonged in children with ADHD [86–88], with the duration being correlated with hyperactivity and restlessness [89]. Instead, adults with ADHD showed a shortened iSP but a normal latency [89]. The increased iSP latencies in children with ADHD have been explained as a defective myelination of fast-conducting fibers in corpus callosum [86], indicating a callosal maturation deficit in ADHD approximating normality with increased age [86, 87]. Therefore, it is likely that the different iSP latencies found between children and adults with ADHD are due to developmental differences in the inhibitory intracortical pathways [90].

TMS can be a useful tool for guiding ADHD pharmacotherapy. ADHD children under medication with methylphenidate showed a significant prolongation of iSP duration and a latency shortening [88], indicating that methylphenidate, as an indirect dopamine agonist, might improve the imbalance between excitatory and inhibitory interneuronal activities of this neuronal network, via dopaminergic modulatory effects on the striato-thalamo-cortical loop [89]. As TMS studies showed SICI to be correlated with hyperactivity, and MPH administration showed a normalizing effect on SICI and hyperactivity, SICI has been suggested as an objective and quantitative proxy of the therapeutic effectiveness of MPH [81]. By identifying ADHD individuals showing a greater SICI change after MPH administration, it would be possible to identify potential responders from nonresponders. Moreover, by monitoring SICI changes, clinicians could optimize drug titration [81]. However, these hypotheses require more research and may benefit from the advances of TMS-evoked potentials. The combination of TMS with electroencephalography (TMS-EEG) appears as a powerful technology for characterizing and modulating brain networks. Indeed, TMS-EEG allows us to assess in vivo neural excitation, inhibition, connectivity as well as plasticity across brain regions providing useful information regarding brain function-behavior relationship in health and disease [91]. In this context, future research should take into account findings related to the utility of TEP monitoring, together with clinical EEG, for assessing the immediate online effects of rTMS on cortical excitability (N100 amplitude changed during 1 Hz stimulation) that may serve as a safety measure and to maximize the functional effects of rTMS on the cortex [65]. Moreover, TMS-EEG use may allow the assessment of neurophysiological responses to medications outside of the motor cortex [81, 92].

9.5 tDCS Studies in ADHD

In respect to the evidence of TMS as a therapeutic tool for both behavioral and cognitive symptoms in ADHD, which requires more research for establishing its efficacy, promising results come from the studies investigating the tDCS use on people with the disorder. Studies performed in children and adolescents with ADHD investigated the acute effects of a single session of tDCS on working memory dysfunction and inhibitory control deficits. A double-blind, sham-controlled experimental design investigated the effect of a single session of anodal active electrode (1 mA) over the left DLPFC and cathodal active electrode over the Cz during an N-back working memory (WM) task. Interestingly, tDCS demonstrated to improve significantly WM performance, but also the activation and connectivity of the WM network. Compared to sham condition, tDCS led to a greater activation of the left

DLPFC, left premotor cortex, left supplementary motor cortex, and precuneus, and its effect was long lasting. In fact, tDCS influenced the resting-state functional connectivity even 20 minutes after the stimulation [93].

In a sham-controlled experiment performed on 25 children with ADHD, anodal stimulation over the left DLPFC and cathodal stimulation over the right DLPFC showed a significant effect of tDCS on WM and interference inhibition. By changing parameters, using therefore cathodal stimulation of the left DLPFC and anodal stimulation of the right orbitofrontal cortex (OFC), a positive tDCS effect on response inhibition and improvement of attentional shifting have been also found [94].

Both anodal and cathodal tDCS on the left DLPFC improved performance accuracy during a Go/NoGo task in a sham-controlled trial performed on students with ADHD, indicating that both types of stimulation could improve executive functions in people with the disorder [95].

As the right inferior frontal gyrus has been recognized as an important region in the inhibitory control network, the effects of tDCS applied over this area in 21 male adolescents with ADHD and matched controls were explored. Subjects underwent three separate sessions of tDCS (anodal, cathodal, and sham) while completing a Flanker task. The overall analysis did not show a significant effect of tDCS, but in consideration of the learning effect from the first to the second session, the performance in the first session was therefore separately analyzed. This second analysis revealed that while ADHD patients receiving sham stimulation in the first session showed impaired interference control compared to controls, ADHD subjects who received anodal stimulation showed comparable performance levels (commission errors, reaction time variability) to the control group. According to these results, the authors concluded that anodal tDCS over the right inferior frontal gyrus could improve interference control in patients with ADHD [96].

A study exploring the effect of repeated sessions of tDCS (30 minutes for 5 days) with 2 mA anodal stimulation of the left DLPFC and cathode positioned over the right supraorbital area in a small group of children and adolescents with ADHD ($N = 9$) showed that tDCS induced a more efficient processing speed, improved detection of stimuli, and improved ability in switching between an ongoing activity and a new one [97].

In a randomized, double-blinded, sham-controlled crossover study performed on adolescents with ADHD ($N = 15$), 1 session a day for 5 consecutive days of anodal tDCS (active stimulation: 1 mA) over the left DLPC and cathodal active electrode over the Cz (vertex), during which patients performed a working memory task, anodal tDCS showed to significantly reduce clinical symptoms of inattention and impulsivity compared to sham stimulation. Noteworthy, tDCS effects appeared more pronounced 7 days after the end of stimulation, supporting the putative long-lasting clinical and neuropsychological changes of tDCS [98].

For what concerns adults with ADHD, tDCS studies performed on this kind of population showed promising results. A recent double-blind sham-controlled study investigated the effects of tDCS (2 mA) daily sessions of 20 minutes for 5 days with the anode over the right DLPFC and cathode over the left DLPFC in adults with ADHD ($N = 17$), through self-report measures for both ADHD symptoms and impairment (Adult ADHD Report Scale and Sheehan Disability Scale). Results showed that subjects treated with active vs. sham tDCS with ADHD displayed a symptom reduction and a decreased impairment. Follow-up data analysis revealed a positive interaction between time and treatment in both self-rated inattention, impairment, and total ADHD score [99]. As the study of Cachoeira et al. [99] showed a clinical positive effect on ADHD symptomatology, which was driven primarily by attentional improvement rather than impulsivity/hyperactivity reduction, another group of researchers explored the effectiveness of 2 mA anodal stimulation (tDCS) applied over the left DLPFC versus sham stimulation in improving impulse control. Overall, 37 adults with ADHD completed two periods of three tDCS (or sham) sessions 2 weeks apart in a within-subject, double-blind, counterbalanced order and performed a fractal N-back training task concurrent with tDCS (or sham) stimulation. For this aim, participants also performed the Conners Continuous Performance Test (CPT) and the Stop Signal Task (SST), and the CPT and the SST reaction time (SSRT) were analyzed. A comparison between the CPT and SST scores performed at baseline, at the end of the treatment, and at a 3-day post-stimulation follow-up showed no significant change in SSRT but rather a decrease in CPT false-positive errors from baseline to end of treatment in the tDCS group, reflecting a reduction in impulsive response. Such positive effect did not persist at the follow-up conducted 3 days after the final stimulation session, but authors concluded that repeated tDCS may be a novel treatment for impulsivity in ADHD, although additional research was necessary to determine whether an optimized treatment approach could induce persistent effects [100].

A parallel, randomized, double-blind, sham-controlled trial performed on 30 adults with ADHD explored the efficacy of a single session of tDCS (1 mA anode over the left DLPFC and cathode over the right DLPFC) on the modulation of inhibitory control, as measured by a go/no-go task before and after the active/sham stimulation [101]. Results did not show any significant differences between active and sham tDCS, and it is not clear whether this lack of effect was due to the use of 1 mA current stimulation rather than 2 mA (the most used tDCS intensity in psychiatric disorders), or to the fact that, unlike many tDCS trials, in this study people were not required to simultaneously perform a cognitive task (online tDCS). The latter hypothesis has been considered as very likely, as the application of tDCS when subjects are actively involved in a cognitive task may activate more specific brain networks, resulting in better performance than when they are at rest. This is in line with evidence from studies coupling tDCS with cognitive training showing greater effects compared to tDCS intervention at rest [102, 103]. Furthermore, evidence from neuroimaging studies showed that people with ADHD are characterized by reduced brain activation in the prefrontal regions, and therefore one single session of tDCS may not be strong enough to improve their cognitive performance, even though it may enhance cortical excitability [104].

In consideration of the high frequency of comorbid disorders in people with ADHD, such as sleep-wake disorders, the recent findings from a study performed by Munz et al. [105] using slow-oscillating tDCS (so-tDCS) on children with ADHD ($N = 14$), aged 10–14 years, are noteworthy. They used so-tDCS, 0.75 Hz, over the right and left DLPFC during non-REM sleep and evaluated its effect on inhibition using a Go/no-go Task. They found an enhancement of endogenous oscillatory activity as a result of their intervention, with an improvement of behavioral inhibition performance, which is typically impaired in ADHD. Previously, so-tDCS applied to 12 children with ADHD over the bilateral DLPFC in a double-blind crossover design showed an enhancement of declarative memory [106]. Therefore, Slow Oscillation (SO) has been considered as a promising somatic marker in the pathophysiology of ADHD [106–108] and a future potential therapeutic target [105].

In conclusion, tDCS is a low-cost, easily accessible, and pain-free stimulation method that is generally well tolerated, having limited side effects, such as itchiness or scalp irritation. It is easily applicable to children as well as adults with ADHD, notwithstanding the presence of a high level of hyperactivity. tDCS has been successfully used in the treatment of several neurological and psychiatric disorders, including Parkinson's disease and major depression [109]. Even though its mechanism of action is not fully understood, tDCS demonstrated the potential to induce some neurochemical modifications in targeted brain tissues, which last longer than the period of active stimulation [110], therefore allowing maintenance of results.

9.6   Summary of NIBS in ADHD

Collectively, evidence up to date provides support to the use of NIBS as a treatment tool for neurodevelopmental disorders such as ADHD, as these interventions showed to produce positive effects and particularly when combined with functional cognitive training. However, the studies conducted hitherto are characterized by some methodological issues, such as small sample sizes and lack or inconsistent use of sham protocols. Moreover, despite the high heterogeneity characterizing the ADHD phenotype, the vast majority of studies have focused mainly on the DLPFC stimulation. It should be underscored that, in spite of being NIBS protocols divided into excitatory and inhibitory, many subjects show opposite effects or even no effect at all. In fact, about 50% of subjects who receive 1-Hz rTMS show a pattern of excitation instead of inhibition, and similarly, a consistent proportion of people who receive 10-Hz rTMS display an inhibitory rather than excitatory pattern [76]. Variability appeared to characterize also 1-Hz parietal rTMS on resting-state functional connectivity, according to findings from fMRI studies [111]. As for TMS, also in studies using tDCS it has been reported that only the 36% show an excitatory effect after anodal stimulation and inhibitory effect after cathodal stimulation, while the opposite has been reported in 21% of cases [112].

In conclusion, NIBS techniques offer a promising new approach to reduce some ADHD dimensions of pathology. Although research in the use of NIBS in ADHD is still in its infancy, data deriving from protocols for strengthening cognitive control [76] may help to personalize the treatment plan of people with this neurodevelopmental disorder, and may be particularly well suited for comorbid cases. The use of combined TMS-EEG appears as particularly useful for the goal of "precision medicine" for psychiatry, as interindividual differences in TMS-EEG markers of brain health seem to have a genetic basis [113]. Finally, the utility of Transcranial Near-Infrared Light Therapy, a noninvasive intervention in which near-infrared light (830 nm) is applied to forebrain, should be explored in ADHD, considering the recent evidence indicating some positive effects on core symptoms of autism spectrum disorders [114].

References

1. American Psychiatric Association. Diagnostic and statistical manual of mental disorders, 5th Edition (DSM-5). Diagnostic and statistical manual of mental disorder, 4th Ed. TR. 280; 2013.
2. Polanczyk G, de Lima MS, Horta BL, Biederman J, Rohde LA. The worldwide prevalence of ADHD: a systematic review and metaregression analysis. Am J Psychiatry. 2007;164(6): 942–8.
3. Willcutt EG. The prevalence of DSM-IV attention-deficit/hyperactivity disorder: a meta-analytic review. Neurotherapeutics. 2012;9(3):490–9.
4. Fayyad J, Sampson NA, Hwang I, Adamowski T, Aguilar-Gaxiola S, Al-Hamzawi A, et al. The descriptive epidemiology of DSM-IV adult ADHD in the world health organization world mental health surveys. Atten Defic Hyperact Disord. 2017;9(1):47–65.
5. Barkley RA, Fischer M, Smallish L, Fletcher K. The persistence of attention- deficit/hyperactivity disorder into young adulthood as a function of reporting source and definition of disorder. J Abnorm Psychol. 2002;111(2):279–89.
6. Mannuzza S, Klein RG, Moulton JL 3rd. Persistence of attention-deficit/hyperactivity disorder into adulthood: what have we learned from the prospective follow-up studies? J Atten Disord. 2003;7(2):93–100.
7. Kooij JJS, Bijlenga D, Salerno L, Jacschke R, Bitter I, Balázs J, et al. Updated European Consensus Statement on diagnosis and treatment of adult ADHD. Eur Psychiatry. 2019;56:14–34.
8. Pallanti S, Salerno L. The burden of adult ADHD in comorbid psychiatric and neurological disorders. 1st ed. 2020, XVII, 402 p. Basel: Springer; 2020.
9. van Rensburg R, Meyer HP, Hitchcock SA, Schuler CE. Screening for adult ADHD in patients with fibromyalgia syndrome. Pain Med. 2018;19(9):1825–31. https://doi.org/10.1093/pm/pnx275.
10. Dias TGC, Kieling C, Graeff-Martins AS, Moriyama TS, Rohde LA, Polanczyk GV. Developments and challenges in the diagnosis and treatment of ADHD. Rev Bras Psiquiatr. 2013;35(Suppl 1):S40–50.
11. Willcutt EG, Doyle AE, Nigg JT, Faraone SV, Pennington BF. Validity of the executive function theory of attention-deficit/hyperactivity disorder: a meta-analytic review. Biol Psychiatry. 2005;57(11):1336–46.
12. Luman M, Oosterlaan J, Sergeant JA. The impact of reinforcement contingencies on AD/HD: a review and theoretical appraisal. Clin Psychol Rev. 2005;25:183–213.
13. Nikolas MA, Nigg JT. Neuropsychological performance and attention-deficit hyperactivity disorder subtypes and symptom dimensions. Neuropsychology. 2013;27:107–20.
14. Rapport MD, Bolden J, Kofler MJ, Sarver DE, Raiker JS, Alderson RM. Hyperactivity in boys with attention-deficit/hyperactivity disorder (ADHD): a ubiquitous core symptom or manifestation of working memory deficits? J Abnorm Child Psychol. 2009;37:521–34.
15. Doyle AE. Executive functions in attention-deficit/hyperactivity disorder. J Clin Psychiatry. 2006;67:21–6.
16. Nigg JT, Willcutt EG, Doyle AE, Sonuga-Barke EJ. Causal heterogeneity in attention-deficit/hyperactivity disorder: do we need neuropsychologically impaired subtypes? Biol Psychiatry. 2005;57:1224–30.

17. Luo Y, Weibman D, Halperin JM, Li X. A review of heterogeneity in attention deficit/hyperactivity disorder (ADHD). Front Hum Neurosci. 2019;13:42. Retrieved from https://www.frontiersin.org/article/10.3389/fnhum.2019.00042.
18. Barkley RA. Attention-deficit hyperactivity disorder: a hand- book for diagnosis and treatment, vol. 1. New York: Guilford Press; 2005.
19. Biederman J, Newcorn J, Sprich S. Comorbidity of attention deficit hyperactivity disorder. Am J Psychiatry. 1991;148(5):564–77.
20. Jensen PS, Martin D, Cantwell DP. Comorbidity in ADHD: implications for research, practice, and DSM-V. J Am Acad Child Adolesc Psychiatry. 1997;36(8):1065–79.
21. Patel N, Patel M, Patel H. ADHD and comorbid conditions. Atten Deficit Hyperact Disord. 2012;1:978–9.
22. Pliszka SR, Carlson CL, Swanson JM. ADHD with comorbid disorders: clinical assessment and management. New York: Guilford Press; 1999.
23. Insel T, Cuthbert B. Research Domain Criteria (RDoC): toward a new classification framework for research on mental disorders. Am J Psychiatry. 2010;167:748–51.
24. Insel TR. The NIMH Research Domain Criteria (RDoC) Project: precision medicine for psychiatry. Am J Psychiatry. 2014;171:395–7.
25. Davidson MA. ADHD in adults: a review of the literature. J Atten Disord. 2008;11:628.
26. Chang Z, Lichtenstein P, Halldner L, et al. Stimulant ADHD medication and risk for substance abuse. J Child Psychol Psychiatry. 2014;55(8):878–85. https://doi.org/10.1111/jcpp.12164.
27. Tortella G, Selingardi PM, Moreno ML, Veronezi BP, Brunoni AR. Does non-invasive brain stimulation improve cognition in major depressive disorder? A systematic review. CNS Neurol Disord Drug Targets. 2014;13(10):1759–69.
28. Karalunas SL, Geurts HM, Konrad K, Bender S, Nigg JT. Annual research review: reaction time variability in ADHD and autism spectrum disorders: measurement and mechanisms of a proposed trans-diagnostic phenotype. J Child Psychol Psychiatry. 2014;55(6):685–710.
29. van Lieshout M, Luman M, Buitelaar J, Rommelse NN, Oosterlaan J. Does neurocognitive functioning predict future or persistence of ADHD? A systematic review. Clin Psychol Rev. 2013;33:539–60. https://doi.org/10.1016/j.cpr.2013.02.003.
30. Huang-Pollock CL, Karalunas SL, Tam H, Moore AN. Evaluating vigilance deficits in ADHD: a meta- analysis of CPT performance. J Abnorm Psychol. 2012;121(2):360–71.
31. Frazier-Wood AC, Bralten J, Arias-Vasquez A, Luman M, Ooterlaan J, Sergeant J, Faraone SV, Buitelaar J, Franke B, Kuntsi J, Rommelse NN. Neuropsychological intra-individual variability explains unique genetic variance of ADHD and shows suggestive linkage to chromosomes 12, 13, and 17. Am J Med Genet B Neuropsychiatr Genet. 2012;159b(2):131–40.
32. Kuntsi J, Wood AC, Rijsdijk F, Johnson KA, Andreou P, Albrecht B, Arias-Vasquez A, Buitelaar JK, McLoughlin G, Rommelse NN, Sergeant JA, Sonuga-Barke EJ, Uebel H, van der Meere JJ, Banaschewski T, Gill M, Manor I, Miranda A, Mulas F, Oades RD, Roeyers H, Rothenberger A, Steinhausen HC, Faraone SV, Asherson P. Separation of cognitive impairments in attention- deficit/hyperactivity disorder into 2 familial factors. Arch Gen Psychiatry. 2010;67(11):1159–67.
33. Mostert JC, Onnink AM, Klein M, Dammers J, Harneit A, Schulten T, van Hulzen KJ, Kan CC, Slaats-Willemse D, Buitelaar JK, Franke B, Hoogman M. Cognitive heterogeneity in adult attention deficit/hyperactivity disorder: a systematic analysis of neuropsychological measurements. Eur Neuropsychopharmacol. 2015;25(11):2062–74.
34. Mowinckel AM, Pedersen ML, Eilertsen E, Biele G. A meta-analysis of decision-making and attention in adults with ADHD. J Atten Disord. 2015;19(5):355–67.
35. Sonuga-Barke E, Bitsakou P, Thompson M. Beyond the dual pathway model: evidence for the dissociation of timing, inhibitory, and delay-related impairments in attention-deficit/hyperactivity disorder. J Am Acad Child Adolesc Psychiatry. 2010;49(4):345–55.
36. Zhu Y, Yang D, Ji W, et al., The relationship between neurocircuitry dysfunctions and attention deficit hyperactivity disorder: a review. BioMed Res Int. 2016, Article ID 3821579, 7 pages.

37. Aron AR, Cai W, Badre D, Robbins TW. Evidence supports specific braking function for inferior PFC. Trends Cogn Sci. 2015;19(12):711–2.
38. Aron AR, Poldrack RA. The cognitive neuroscience of response inhibition: relevance for genetic research in attention-deficit/hyperactivity disorder. Biol Psychiatry. 2005;57(11):1285–92.
39. Chambers CD, Garavan H, Bellgrove MA. Insights into the neural basis of response inhibition from cognitive and clinical neuroscience. Neurosci Biobehav Rev. 2009;33(5):631–46.
40. Hwang S, Me H, Parsley I, Tyler PM, Erway AK, Botkin ML, et al. Segregating sustained attention from response inhibition in ADHD: an fMRI study. NeuroImage Clin. 2019;21:101677.
41. Noreika V, Falter CM, Rubia K. Timing deficits in attention-deficit/hyperactivity disorder (ADHD): evidence from neurocognitive and neuroimaging studies. Neuropsychologia. 2013;51:235–66.
42. Hart H, Radua J, Mataix-Cols D, Rubia K. Meta-analysis of fMRI studies of timing in attention-deficit hyperactivity disorder (ADHD). Neurosci Biobehav Rev. 2012;36:2248–56.
43. Costa Dias TG, Wilson VB, Bathula DR, Iyer S, Mills KL, Thurlow BL, et al. Reward circuit connectivity relates to delay discounting in children with attention-deficit/hyperactivity disorder. Eur Neuropsychopharmacol. 2012;23:33–45.
44. Plichta MM, Scheres A. Ventral-striatal responsiveness during reward anticipation in ADHD and its relation to trait impulsivity in the healthy population: a meta-analytic review of the fMRI literature. Neurosci Biobehav Rev. 2014;38:125–34.
45. Furukawa E, Bado P, Tripp G, Mattos P, Wickens JR, Bramati IE, et al. Abnormal striatal BOLD responses to reward anticipation and reward delivery in ADHD. PLoS One. 2014;9:e89129.
46. Makris N, Biederman J, Monuteaux MC, Seidman LJ. Towards conceptualizing a neural systems-based anatomy of attention-deficit/hyperactivity disorder. Dev Neurosci. 2009;31(1–2):36–49.
47. Salerno L, Makris N, Pallanti S. Sleep disorders in adult ADHD: a key feature. J Psychopathol. 2016;22(2):135–40.
48. Bradshaw JL, Mattingley JB. Clinical neuropsychology: behavioral and brain science. Amsterdam: Elsevier; 2013.
49. Shaw P, Stringaris A, Nigg J, Leibenluft E. Emotion dysregulation in attention deficit hyperactivity disorder. Am J Psychiatry. 2014;171:276–93.
50. Koob GF. Negative reinforcement in drug addiction: the darkness within. Curr Opin Neurobiol. 2013;23(4):559–63.
51. Seeman P. Parkinson's disease treatment may cause impulse control disorder via dopamine D3 receptors. Synapse. 2015;69(4):183–9.
52. Phillips ML, Ladouceur CD, Drevets WC. A neural model of voluntary and automatic emotion regulation: implications for understanding the pathophysiology and neurodevelopment of bipolar disorder. Mol Psychiatry. 2008;13(9):829, 833–57.
53. Volkow ND, Fowler JS. Addiction, a disease of compulsion and drive: involvement of the orbitofrontal cortex. Cereb Cortex. 2000;10(3):318–25.
54. Cortese S, Kelly C, Chabernaud C, et al. Toward systems neuroscience of ADHD: a meta-analysis of 55 fMRI studies. Am J Psychiatry. 2012;169(10):1038–55.
55. Hart H, Radua J, Nakao T, et al. Meta-analysis of functional magnetic resonance imaging studies of inhibition and attention in attention-deficit/hyperactivity disorder: exploring task-specific, stimulant medication, and age effects. JAMA Psychiat. 2013;70(2):185–98.
56. Massat I, Slama H, Kavec M, Linotte S, Mary A, Baleriaux D, et al. Working memory-related functional brain patterns in never medicated children with ADHD. PLoS One. 2012;7:e49392.
57. Fassbender C, Schweitzer JB, Cortes CR, Tagamets MA, Windsor TA, Reeves GM, et al. Working memory in attention deficit/hyperactivity disorder is characterized by a lack of specialization of brain function. PLoS One. 2011;6:e27240.
58. Bollmann S, Ghisleni C, Poil SS, Martin E, Ball J, Eich-Höchli D, et al. Age-dependent and-independent changes in attention-deficit/hyperactivity disorder (ADHD) during spatial working memory performance. World J Biol Psychiatry. 2017;18(4):279–90.

59. Gilbert DL, Ridel KR, Sallee FR, Zhang J, Lipps TD, Wassermann EM. Comparison of the inhibitory and excitatory effects of ADHD medications methylphenidate and atomoxetine on motor cortex. Neuropsychopharmacology. 2006;31(2):442–9.

60. Kratz O, Diruf MS, Studer P, Gierow W, Buchmann J, Moll GH, Heinrich H. Effects of methylphenidate on motor system excitability in a response inhibition task. Behav Brain Funct. 2009;5:12. https://doi.org/10.1186/1744-9081-5-12.

61. Finisguerra A, Borgatti R, Urgesi C. Non-invasive brain stimulation for the rehabilitation of children and adolescents with neurodevelopmental disorders: a systematic review. Front Psychol. 2019;10:135. https://doi.org/10.3389/fpsyg.2019.00135. eCollection 2019.

62. Pallanti S, Grassi G, Marras A, Hollander E. Can we modulate obsessive-compulsive networks with neuromodulation? Neuromodulazione dei network ossessivo-compulsivi: è possibile? J Psychopathol. 2015;21:262–5.

63. Huang YZ, Edwards MJ, Rounis E, et al. Theta burst stimulation of the human motor cortex. Neuron. 2005;45:201–6.

64. Hanlon CA, Dowdle LT, Austelle CW, et al. What goes up, can come down: novel brain stimulation paradigms may attenuate craving and craving-related neural circuitry in substance dependent individuals. Brain Res. 2015;1628:199–209.

65. Helfrich C, Pierau SS, Freitag CM, Roeper J, Ziemann U, Bender S. Monitoring cortical excitability during repetitive transcranial magnetic stimulation in children with ADHD: a single-blind, sham-controlled TMS-EEG study. PLoS One. 2012;7:e50073.

66. Casula EP, Tarantino V, Basso D, Arcara G, Marino G, Toffolo GM, et al. Low-frequency rTMS inhibitory effects in the primary motor cortex: insights from TMS-evoked potentials. NeuroImage. 2014;98:225–32.

67. Weaver L, Rostain AL, Mace W, Akhtar U, Moss E, O'Reardon JP. Transcranial magnetic stimulation (TMS) in the treatment of attention-deficit/hyperactivity disorder in adolescents and young adults: a pilot study. J ECT. 2012;28(2):98–103.

68. Gómez L, Vidal B, Morales L, Báez M, Maragoto C, Galvizu R, et al. Low frequency repetitive transcranial magnetic stimulation in children with attention deficit/hyperactivity disorder. preliminary results. Brain Stimul. 2014;7:760–2.

69. Bloch Y, Harel EV, Aviram S, et al. Positive effects of repetitive transcranial magnetic stimulation on attention in ADHD Subjects: a randomized controlled pilot study. World J Biol Psychiatry. 2010;11:755–8.

70. Niederhofer H. Effectiveness of the repetitive Transcranical Magnetic Stimulation (rTMS) of 1 Hz for Attention-Deficit Hyperactivity Disorder (ADHD). Psychiatr Danub. 2008;20(1):91–2.

71. Zangen A, Roth AY, Voller B, et al. Transcranial magnetic stimulation of deep brain regions: evidence for efficacy of the H-coil. Clin Neurophysiol. 2005;116(4):775–9.

72. Pogarell O, Koch W, Pöpperl G, et al. Acute prefrontal rTMS increases striatal dopamine to a similar degree as d-amphetamine. Psychiatry Res. 2007;156:251–5.

73. Pogarell O, Koch W, Pöpperl G, et al. Striatal dopamine release after prefrontal repetitive transcranial magnetic stimulation in major depression: preliminary results of a dynamic [123I] IBZM SPECT study. J Psychiatr Res. 2006;40:307–14.

74. Monte-Silva K, Ruge D, Teo JT, et al. D2 receptor block abolishes θ burst stimulation-induced neuroplasticity in the human motor cortex. Neuropsychopharmacology. 2011;36:2097–102.

75. Cho SS, Kosimori Y, Aminian K, et al. Investing in the future: stimulation of the medial prefrontal cortex reduces discounting of delayed rewards. Neuropsychopharmacology. 2015;40:546–53.

76. Dunlop K, Hanlon CA, Downar J. Noninvasive brain stimulation treatments for addiction and major depression. Ann N Y Acad Sci. 2017;1394(1):31–54.

77. Benatti B, Cremaschi L, Oldani L, De Cagna F, Vismara M, Dell'Osso B. Past, present and future of transcranial magnetic stimulation (TMS) in the treatment of psychiatric disorders. Evid Based Psychiatr Care. 2016;2:77–85.

78. Buchmann J, Gierow W, Weber S, et al. Restoration of disturbed intracortical motor inhibition and facilitation in attention deficit hyperactivity disorder children by methylphenidate. Biol Psychiatry. 2007;62(9):963–9.

79. Gilbert DL, Bansal AS, Sethuraman G, et al. Association of cortical disinhibition with TIC, ADHD, and OCD severity in Tourette syndrome. Mov Disord. 2004;19(4):416–25.
80. Gilbert DL, Sallee FR, Zhang J, Lipps TD, Wassermann EM. Transcranial magnetic stimulation-evoked cortical inhibition: a consistent marker of attention-deficit/hyperactivity disorder scores in Tourette syndrome. Biol Psychiatry. 2005;57(12):1597–600.
81. Rubio B, Boes AD, Laganiere S, Rotenberg A, Jeurissen D, Pascual-Leone A. Noninvasive brain stimulation in pediatric attention-deficit hyperactivity disorder (ADHD): a review. J Child Neurol. 2016;31(6):784–96.
82. Gilbert DL, Isaacs KM, Augusta M, Macneil LK, Mostofsky SH. Motor cortex inhibition: a marker of ADHD behavior and motor development in children. Neurology. 2011;76(7):615–21.
83. Ruge D, Muggleton N, Hoad D, Caronni A, Rothwell JC. An unavoidable modulation? Sensory attention and human primary motor cortex excitability. Eur J Neurosci. 2014;40(5): 2850–8.
84. Orth M, Rothwell JC. Motor cortex excitability and co-morbidity in Gilles de la Tourette syndrome. J Neurol Neurosurg Psychiatry. 2009;80(1):29–34.
85. Moll GH, Heinrich H, Trott G, Wirth S, Rothenberger A. Deficient intracortical inhibition in drug-naive children with attention-deficit hyperactivity disorder is enhanced by methylphenidate. Neurosci Lett. 2000;284(1–2):121–5.
86. Buchmann J, Wolters A, Haessler F, Bohne S, Nordbeck R, Kunesch E. Disturbed transcallosally mediated motor inhibition in children with attention deficit hyperactivity disorder (ADHD). Clin Neurophysiol. 2003;114:2036–42.
87. Garvey MA, Barker CA, Bartko JJ, Denckla MB, Wassermann EM, Castellanos FX, Dell ML, et al. The ipsilateral silent period in boys with attention-deficit/hyperactivity disorder. Clin Neurophysiol. 2005;116:1889–96.
88. Buchmann J, Gierow W, Weber S, et al. Modulation of transcallosally mediated motor inhibition in children with attention deficit hyperactivity disorder (ADHD) by medication with methylphenidate (MPH). Neurosci Lett. 2006;405(1–2):14–8. https://doi.org/10.1016/j.neulet.2006.06.026.
89. Hoeppner J, Wandschneider R, Neumeyer M, et al. Impaired transcallosally mediated motor inhibition in adults with attention-deficit/hyperactivity disorder is modulated by methylphenidate. J Neural Transm. 2008;115(5):777–85. https://doi.org/10.1007/s00702-007-0008-1.
90. Walther M, Berweck S, Schessl J, et al. Maturation of inhibitory and excitatory motor cortex pathways in children. Brain Dev. 2009;31(7):562–7. https://doi.org/10.1016/j.braindev.2009.02.007.
91. Farzan F, Vernet M, Shafi MMD, Rotenberg A, Daskalakis ZJ, Pascual-Leone A. Characterizing and modulating brain circuitry through transcranial magnetic stimulation combined with electroencephalography. Front Neural Circuits. 2016;10:73.
92. Bortoletto M, Veniero D, Thut G, Miniussi C. The contribution of TMS-EEG coregistration in the exploration of the human cortical connectome. Neurosci Biobehav Rev. 2014;49C:114–24. https://doi.org/10.1016/j.neubiorev.2014.12.014.
93. Sotnikova A, Soff C, Tagliazucchi E, et al. Transcranial direct current stimulation modulates neuronal networks in attention deficit hyperactivity disorder. Brain Topogr. 2017;30(5):656–72.
94. Nejati V, Salehinejad MA, Nitsche MA, et al. Transcranial direct current stimulation improves executive dysfunctions in ADHD: implications for inhibitory control, interference control, working memory, and cognitive flexibility. J Atten Disord. 2017;1:1087054717730611.
95. Soltaninejad Z, Nejati V, Ekhtiari H. Effect of anodal and cathodal transcranial direct current stimulation on DLPFC on modulation of inhibitory control in ADHD. J Atten Disord. 2015;23(4):325–32.
96. Breitling C, Zaehle T, Dannhauer M, et al. Improving interference control in ADHD patients with transcranial direct current stimulation (tDCS). Front Cell Neurosci. 2016;10:72.
97. Bandeira ID, Guimarães RS, Jagersbacher JG, et al. Transcranial direct current stimulation in children and adolescents with attention-deficit/hyperactivity disorder (ADHD): a pilot study. J Child Neurol. 2016;31(7):918–24.

98. Soff C, Sotnikova A, Christiansen H, Becker K. Transcranial direct current stimulation improves clinical symptoms in adolescents with attention deficit hyperactivity disorder. J Neural Transm. 2017;124(1):133–44.
99. Cachoeira CT, Leffa DT, Mittelstadt SD, et al. Positive effects of transcranial direct current stimulation in adult patients with attention-deficit/hyperactivity disorder—a pilot randomized controlled study. Psychiatry Res. 2017;247:28–32.
100. Allenby C, Falcone M, Bernardo L, et al. Transcranial direct current brain stimulation decreases impulsivity in ADHD. Brain Stimul. 2018;11(5):974–81.
101. Cosmo C, Baptista AF, de Araújo AN, et al. A randomized, double-blind, sham-controlled trial of transcranial direct current stimulation in attention-deficit/hyperactivity disorder. PLoS One. 2015;12:10(8).
102. Elmasry J, Loo C, Martin D. A systematic review of transcranial electrical stimulation combined with cognitive training. Restor Neurol Neurosci. 2015;33(3):263–78.
103. Martin DM, Liu R, Alonzo A, et al. Use of transcranial direct current stimulation (tDCS) to enhance cognitive training: effect of timing of stimulation. Exp Brain Res. 2014;232(10):3345–51.
104. Oliveira JF, Zanão TA, Valiengo L, et al. Acute working memory improvement after tDCS in antidepressant-free patients with major depressive disorder. Neurosci Lett. 2013;537:60–4.
105. Munz MT, Prehn-Kristensen A, Thielking F, et al. Slow oscillating transcranial direct current stimulation during non-rapid eye movement sleep improves behavioral inhibition in attention-deficit/hyperactivity disorder. Front Cell Neurosci. 2015;9:307.
106. Prehn-Kristensen A, Munz M, Goder R, Wilhelm I, Korr K, Vahl W, et al. Transcranial oscillatory direct current stimulation during sleep improves declarative memory consolidation in children with attention-deficit/hyperactivity disorder to a level comparable to healthy controls. Brain Stimul. 2014;7:793–9.
107. Prehn-Kristensen A, Munz M, Molzow I, Wilhelm I, Wiesner CD, Baving L, et al. Sleep promotes consolidation of emotional memory in healthy children but not in children with attention-deficit hyperactivity disorder. PLoS One. 2013;8:e65098.
108. Ringli M, Souissi S, Kurth S, et al. Topography of sleep slow wave activity in children with attention-deficit/hyperactivity disorder. Cortex. 2013;49(1):340–7.
109. Woods AJ, Antal A, Bikson M, et al. A technical guide to tDCS, and related non-invasive brain stimulation tools. Clin Neurophysiol. 2016;127:1031–48.
110. Utz KS, Dimova V, Oppenlander K, et al. Electrified minds: transcranial direct current stimulation (tDCS) and galvanic vestibular stimulation (GVS) as methods of non-invasive brain stimulation in neuropsychology—a review of current data and future implications. Neuropsychologia. 2010;48:2789–810.
111. Eldaief MC, Halko MA, Buckner RL, Pascual-Leone A. Transcranial magnetic stimulation modulates the brain's intrinsic activity in a frequency-dependent manner. Proc Natl Acad Sci U S A. 2011;108:21229–34.
112. Wiethoff S, Hamada M, Rothwell JC. Variability in response to transcranial direct current stimulation of the motor cortex. Brain Stimul. 2014;7:468–75.
113. Lett TA, Kennedy JL, Radhu N, Dominguez LG, Chakravarty MM, Nazeri A, et al. Prefrontal white matter structure mediates the influence of GAD1 on working memory. Neuropsychopharmacology. 2016;41:2224–31.
114. Ceranoglu T, Hoskova B, Cassano P, Biederman J, Joshi G. Efficacy of transcranial near-infrared light treatment in ASD: interim analysis of an open-label proof of concept study of a novel approach. Biol Psychiatry. 2019;85(10 Suppl):S153–4.

Application of Repetitive Transcranial Magnetic Stimulation in Tourette Syndrome

10

Antonio Mantovani

Tic disorders have been the subject of etiological speculation for at least the past 300 years. Over the past 35 years, Tourette syndrome (TS) has come to be recognized as a model of neurodevelopmental disorder representing the nexus between neurology and psychiatry [1, 2]. The identification of abnormalities involving the basal ganglia in postmortem [3] and neuroimaging studies [4], the possibility of a post-infectious etiology for some cases of the disorder [5, 6], and the increasing appreciation of the interaction of genetic [7] and environmental factors [8] in disease expression, have all contributed to making TS a model for understanding developmental psychopathology more broadly. The reality for patients is that TS can be a devastating condition, which alone, or in combination with other closely associated forms of psychopathology, causes patients and their families considerable suffering [9, 10].

TS is a childhood-onset neuropsychiatric disorder characterized by chronic motor and vocal tics that are often preceded by premonitory urges [11]. Although tic symptoms in the majority of children with TS improve during adolescence, adults with persistent illness can experience chronic and severe tics [12].

Randomized controlled trials (RCTs) have documented the efficacy of several behavioral and pharmacological treatments for TS [13, 14]. However, approximately one-third of individuals with TS do not benefit from first-line treatments, and several of the most effective medications used to treat tics have significant side effects [15, 16].

Considering that the basal ganglia and the thalamocortical systems play an important role in habit formation and are implicated in the pathophysiology of TS [17], the experimental use of deep brain stimulation (DBS), targeting the thalamus,

A. Mantovani (✉)
Department of Cellular, Molecular and Biomedical Sciences, CUNY School of Medicine, City University of New York, New York, NY, USA

Department of Medicine and Health Sciences "V. Tiberio", Molise University, Campobasso, Italy
e-mail: AMantovani@med.cuny.edu

the posteroventrolateral part and the anteromedial part of the globus pallidus internus, the anterior limb of the internal capsule and the nucleus accumbens, has been shown to produce positive results for a proportion of children, adolescents, and adults with severe TS [18–20].

However, to date, the largest RCT failed to prove the efficacy of DBS in TS [21], and the optimal site for electrode placement has yet to be determined [22, 23]. In addition, DBS can be associated with serious adverse effects, including an increased risk of infection [24, 25]. In this context, novel, less-invasive treatments to reduce tic severity are urgently needed, especially for patients with severe TS.

Transcranial magnetic stimulation (TMS) is a noninvasive tool of stimulating targeted cortical regions in TS [26]. Initial repetitive TMS (rTMS) studies targeting motor and premotor cortical sites with either low-frequency (1-Hz) or high-frequency (15-Hz) protocols have had limited or no success in treating individuals with severe TS [27–29]. More recently, several open-label studies have reported that 1-Hz rTMS targeting the supplementary motor area (SMA) can decrease the frequency and intensity of tics [30–35].

Based on the importance of sensory signals and their integration with subsequent motor acts [36–38], the SMA seems to be a promising target for rTMS. As early as the 1980s, Eccles [39] speculated that the SMA was involved in the intentional preparation of movements [40]. More recently, event-related functional Magnetic Resonance Imaging (fMRI) and Positron Emission Tomography (PET) techniques have implicated the SMA in the preparation and organization of voluntary movements [41, 42]. Not only does stimulation of this region produce both movements and urges to move (reminiscent of the premonitory urges of TS) but also the nature of the movements or corresponding urges ranges from simple motor acts to complex movements, paralleling the range of simple to complex tics experienced in TS [43]. Neuroimaging studies examining patterns of brain activation in individuals with TS have consistently identified the SMA as one of the structures that is active simultaneously with tics as well as in the seconds preceding tics [44–48].

Hampson et al. [49] compared the temporal patterns of brain activity during tics in 16 TS patients to those during intentional "tic-like" movements in control subjects. Rather than relying on a subjective judgment of when tics occurred, a novel method was employed that first identified that part of the motor cortex specific to each patient's tic movement, and then cross-correlated activity in that region with activity in other brain areas during tics. Regions implicated in sensory urges, particularly the SMA and somatosensory cortex, were hypothesized to show differential time courses in patients and controls. A nearly identical sequence of brain activity was observed across groups. However, only the SMA showed a significantly different profile with cross-correlations to motor cortex extending over a significantly broader time window in the patients relative to controls. The SMA was active both earlier and later in the patients, implying that it is involved in both tics and intentional movements. These findings highlight the potential importance of the SMA in tic generation and point toward novel focal brain stimulation intervention strategies for TS.

An RCT with 1-Hz rTMS targeting the SMA failed to find a statistical difference in clinical improvement between the active and the sham (placebo) groups after 3 weeks. However, in the 3-week open-label continuation phase of the study, patients who received a total of 6 weeks of rTMS showed on average 30% decrease in the Yale Global Tic Severity Score (YGTSS) with a sizable proportion of the TS subjects who received active rTMS for 6 weeks judged to be responders (57.1%) [50].

rTMS was administered with the Magstim super-rapid stimulator (Magstim Company Ltd, UK) using a vacuum-cooled 70-mm figure-of-eight coil. Stimulation parameters were 1-Hz, 30-min train (1800 pulses/day) at 110% of resting motor threshold-MT (using the lowest value of right or left hemisphere), once a day, 5 days/week, for 3 (in the double-blind phase) to 6 weeks (in the continuation open-label phase). The coil was positioned over pre-SMA using the International 10–20 EEG System coordinates. Pre-SMA was defined at 15% of the distance between inion and nasion anterior to Cz (vertex) on the sagittal midline [33]. Brainsight TMS navigation system was used to locate and monitor online the stability of coil placement during each rTMS session. The coil was placed with the handle along the sagittal midline, pointing toward the occiput to stimulate bilaterally and simultaneously the pre-SMA.

Sham rTMS was administered using the Magstim sham coil, which contains a mu-metal shield that diverts the majority of the magnetic flux so that a minimal (<3%) magnetic field is delivered to the cortex [51]. To maintain the blind, raters were blinded to treatment condition with a separation between the clinical team and rTMS treating physician(s). Moreover, patients who had received TMS treatments in the past were excluded.

Before and after each session, patients were asked a series of questions in a structured form to rate rTMS side-effects. In addition, subjects were asked to complete the Systematic Assessment for Treatment Emergent Effects (SAFTEE) [52].

Twenty patients entered and 18 completed phase 1 (3-week double-blind phase). Regarding the 20 patients who met criteria for TS, a 33% (3/9) response rate was observed in those randomized to active rTMS and 18% (2/11) with sham rTMS (Fisher's exact test, $p = 0.62$). Analysis of 18 completers showed a response rate of 37.5% (3/8) with active and 20% (2/10) with sham rTMS (Fisher's exact test, $p = 0.61$) at the end of the double-blind phase.

Seventeen patients entered and 16 completed the open-label phase (seven initially randomized to active and nine to sham). Nine patients initially randomized to sham had no significant change in their YGTSS total tic scores after 3 weeks of active rTMS (from 32.9 ± 8.4 to 31.8 ± 8.5; $F = 0.64$, df = 2,16, $p = 0.54$). Seven patients initially randomized to active rTMS, who received an additional 3-week active rTMS, showed further improvements from weeks 3 to 6 on the YGTSS total tic scores (from 31.1 ± 9.5 to 25.3 ± 6.7, $F = 0.58$, df = 2,12, $p = 0.57$). The mean improvement in the total tic severity score from baseline to 6 weeks [mean reduction of YGTSS score = 10.7 points (29.7%)] for the 7 patients who completed the 6 weeks of active treatment was statistically significant ($t = 2.6$, df = 6, $p = 0.04$).

No major side effects were noted during the course of treatment. Specifically, there were no seizures, neurological complications, or complaints about memory or concentration difficulties. Headache, neck pain, and muscle sprain were the only side effects reported as "severe" in active treatment. Only in one instance was there a "severe" side effect, i.e., a severe headache, judged to be treatment related.

A major limitation of this study is the relatively small sample size and short blinded phase. A larger sample and longer blinded phase will be needed to definitively evaluate whether 6 weeks of low-frequency rTMS targeting the SMA is clinically efficacious in reducing tic severity. This is an important consideration given that optimal antidepressant effects result from the application of rTMS for 4–6 weeks [53].

In fact, recently, three patients with severe, medication-refractory TS, and comorbid obsessive-compulsive disorder (OCD) in two of them, received rTMS at 1-Hz to the SMA for 4-week duration. The first two cases of TS-OCD showed, on average, 57% improvement in the YGTSS scores and 45% improvement in Yale-Brown Obsessive–Compulsive Scale (Y-BOCS) scores; the third case of pure-TS showed marginal improvement of 10% only. The improvement in TS-OCD patients with rTMS treatment was maintained at the end of 3-month follow-up, with an average reduction of about 49% and 36% observed in YGTSS and Y-BOCS scores, respectively [54].

rTMS to the SMA has been successfully tested in treatment-resistant OCD in RCTs [55–57] and as an augmentation to pharmacotherapy [58–60]. A recent meta-analysis showed that low-frequency rTMS of the SMA yielded the greatest reductions in Y-BOCS scores relative to other cortical targets in the short- and long-term follow-ups [61]. Specifically, the clinical effect of 1-Hz rTMS to the SMA correlated with changes in cortical excitability measures, consistent with an inhibitory action of rTMS on dysfunctional premotor and motor circuits in OCD [62]. The SMA target was selected, based on the results of a deficient sensory gating and enhanced precentral somatosensory-evoked potentials in OCD, which might reflect the inability to modulate sensory information due to a tonic high level of cortical excitability of motor and related areas [63].

Recently, optogenetic stimulation revealed that secondary motor area (M2) postsynaptic responses in central striatum were significantly increased in strength and reliability in *Sapap3* knockout mouse model of compulsive behaviors, suggesting that increased M2-striatal drive may contribute to both striatal hyperactivity and compulsive behaviors. Because M2 is thought to be homologous to pre-SMA/SMA in humans, regions considered important for movement preparation and behavioral sequencing, these results are consistent with a model in which increased drive from M2 leads to the excessive selection of sequenced motor patterns and support a potential role for pre-SMA/SMA in the pathology and treatment of compulsive behavior disorders, like OCD and Tourette syndrome [64].

Considering the overlap in the pathophysiology of OCD and TS [65], with OCD symptoms reported in 50–90% of patients with TS [66], with studies suggesting an involvement of the basal ganglia circuit, especially disruption of the indirect pathway resulting in repetitive behaviors and thoughts in comorbid OCD and TS [67], and considering that single and paired-pulse TMS found a deficit in intracortical inhibition in both OCD and TS [68], it is plausible to think that the application of low-frequency rTMS to the SMA might be particularly helpful in patients with comorbid TS-OCD.

Studies using motor-evoked potential (MEP) and phosphene threshold have shown that 1-Hz rTMS to motor and occipital cortex, respectively, reduces cortical excitability [69, 70]. One-Hertz rTMS to prefrontal cortex reduces blood flow [71, 72]. Studies have demonstrated that suppressive effects of rTMS to one region can be propagated to other cortical regions via functional connections. For example, 1-Hz rTMS to motor cortex reduces MEP induction in the contralateral motor cortex [73] and reduces the Bereitschaftspotential, a slow negative EEG potential arising from the SMA [74].

The mechanism of action of 1-Hz rTMS is thought to be analogous to long-term depression induced by direct electrical stimulation. One-Hertz rTMS may produce neuroplastic effects similar to that produced by direct 1-Hz electrical stimulation of gray matter in animal studies, which often produces a phenomenon known as long-term depression (LTD). LTD in the hippocampus and cerebral cortex has been widely replicated [75–77]. Like 1-Hz rTMS, LTD requires 15–30 minutes of continuous 1-Hz stimulation, has cumulative effects if stimulation is repeated over many days, and propagates trans-synaptically to other functionally connected brain regions [78]. LTD can last for many weeks, indeed as long as the experimental animal can be maintained [79]. If 1-Hz rTMS produces LTD-like effects, rTMS-induced alterations in brain function may produce clinically significant effects lasting beyond the period of stimulation.

Our pioneering open-label study, which targeted the SMA, demonstrated that 1-Hz rTMS produced a significant clinical improvement (67% reduction in tic severity) in patients with comorbid OCD and TS [33]. We demonstrated in two other cases affected with TS and comorbid OCD a 52% clinical improvement that matches or exceeds approved behavioral or pharmacological interventions for TS [80].

The clinical efficacy of rTMS in patients with TS and OCD was reported in a recent meta-analysis. The authors included eight studies, with a sample of 113 subjects, and showed that rTMS significantly improved tic ($g = -0.61$; CI: -0.94 to -0.29) and OCD ($g = -0.48$; CI: -0.83 to -0.14) symptoms in TS patients. Stimulation of the SMA was more effective in tic symptoms than the stimulation of other areas ($g = -0.70$; CI: -1.11 to -0.30 vs. $g = -0.36$; CI: -0.84 to 0.14), and younger age was associated with a better treatment effect (coefficient = 0.03, $p = 0.027$) [81].

Wu et al. [82] suggested using a patient-specific targeting procedure and a novel rTMS paradigm, named continuous theta burst stimulation (cTBS). In their RCT, mean YGTSS scores decreased in both active (27.5 ± 7.4 to 23.2 ± 9.8) and sham (26.8 ± 4.8 to 21.7 ± 7.7) groups. No significant difference in video-based tic severity rating was detected between the two groups. However, the two-day post-treatment fMRI activation during finger tapping decreased significantly with active rTMS and not with sham in the SMA ($p = 0.02$), left M1 ($p = 0.0004$), and right M1 ($p < 0.0001$). Therefore, active fMRI-navigated cTBS administered over 2 days to the SMA induced significant inhibition in the motor network (SMA, bilateral M1), but larger sample size and protocol modifications (i.e., higher number of rTMS sessions) may be needed to produce clinically significant tic reduction.

Since cTBS provides more potent inhibitory neuromodulatory effects [83], the efficacy of fMRI targeted cTBS should be evaluated over a longer period of time in TS patients before any definite conclusions can be made concerning its clinical efficacy. In addition, based on our laterality findings in TS and OCD patients' right hemisphere cortical excitability measures after active rTMS but not sham [33, 50, 56, 57, 62], and the recent work of Obeso et al. [84], a case can potentially be made to target preferentially the right pre-SMA with cTBS. Specifically, combining cTBS with oxygen 15-labeled water ($H_2^{15}O$) PET scans acquired during a stop signal task, Obeso and colleagues found that cTBS-induced changes in the excitability of the right pre-SMA (as compared to sham cTBS) enhanced response inhibition. They also found that cTBS over the right pre-SMA was associated with increased blood flow in the left pre-SMA, the left inferior frontal gyrus, as well as the right premotor and right inferior parietal cortex. If cTBS over the right pre-SMA can enhance response inhibition, then it might also have a beneficial effect on tics. In a recent RCT, including 27 treatment-refractory OCD patients, fMRI-guided rTMS to the pre-SMA improved significantly symptoms, and such improvement correlated with measures of cortical excitability (i.e., % of reduction on self-reported YBOCS correlated with increased MT) [85]. In another study, bilateral stimulation of the pre-SMA induced a clinical improvement in OCD symptoms and increased functional connectivity between the rTMS target and the right inferior frontal gyrus and orbito-frontal cortex (Mantovani et al. unpublished data).

Therefore, based on the preliminary evidence of a clinical and neurophysiological effect of rTMS applied to the SMA in patients with TS and OCD, the application of low-frequency rTMS protocols holds promise in the treatment of refractory cases and might be tried in the future with improved target selection and stimulation procedures before the application of more invasive interventions, such as electroconvulsive therapy [86], DBS [20], and gamma knife capsulotomy [87].

References

1. Leckman JF. Tourette syndrome. Lancet. 2002;360:1577–86.
2. Leckman JF, Vaccarino FM, Kalanithi PS, Rothenberger A. Annotation: Tourette syndrome: a relentless drumbeat driven by misguided brain oscillations. J Child Psychol Psychiatry. 2006;47:537–50.
3. Kalanithi PS, Zheng W, DiFiglia M, DiFiglia M, Grantz H, Saper CB, et al. Altered parvalbumin-positive neuron distribution in basal ganglia of individuals with Tourette syndrome. Proc Natl Acad Sci U S A. 2005;102:13307–12.
4. Albin RL, Mink JW. Recent advances in Tourette syndrome research. Trends Neurosci. 2006;29:175–82.
5. Mell LK, Davis RL, Owens D. Association between streptococcal infection and obsessive-compulsive disorder, Tourette's syndrome, and tic disorder. Pediatrics. 2005;116:56–60.
6. Swedo SE, Leonard HL, Garvey M, Mittleman B, Allen AJ, Perlmutter S, et al. Pediatric autoimmune neuropsychiatric disorders associated with streptococcal infections: clinical description of the first 50 cases. Am J Psychiatry. 1998;155:264–71.

7. Abelson JF, Kwan KY, O'Roak BJ, Baek DY, Stillman AA, Morgan TM, et al. Mutations in *SLITRK1* are associated with Tourette syndrome. Science. 2005;310:317–20.
8. Lin H, Katsovich L, Ghebremichael M, Findley DB, Grantz H, Lombroso PJ, et al. Psychosocial stress predicts future symptom severities in children and adolescents with Tourette syndrome and/or obsessive-compulsive disorder. J Child Psychol Psychiatry. 2007;48:157–66.
9. Davis KK, Davis JS, Dowler L. In motion, out of place: the public space(s) of Tourette syndrome. Soc Sci Med. 2004;59:103–12.
10. Elstner K, Selai CE, Trimble MR, Robertson MM. Quality of Life (QOL) of patients with Gilles de la Tourette's syndrome. Acta Psychiatr Scand. 2001;103:52–9.
11. Leckman JF, Bloch MH, Sukhodolsky DG. Phenomenology of tics and sensory urges: the self under siege. In: Martino D, Leckman JF, editors. Tourette syndrome. New York: Oxford University Press; 2013. p. 3–25.
12. Bloch MH, Peterson BS, Scahill L, Otka J, Katsovich L, Zhang H, et al. Adulthood outcome of tic and obsessive-compulsive symptom severity in children with Tourette syndrome. Arch Pediatr Adolesc Med. 2006;160:65–9.
13. McGuire JF, Piacentini J, Brennan EA, Lewin AB, Murphy TK, Small BJ, et al. A meta-analysis of behavior therapy for Tourette syndrome. J Psychiatr Res. 2014;50:106–12.
14. Roessner V, Rothenberger A, Rickards H, Ludolph AG, Rizzo R, Skov L, et al. European clinical guidelines for Tourette syndrome and other tic disorders. Eur Child Adolesc Psychiatry. 2011;20:153–4.
15. Robertson MM, Stern JS. Gilles de la Tourette syndrome: symptomatic treatment based on evidence. Eur Child Adolesc Psychiatry. 2000;9:60–75.
16. Roessner V, Rothenberger A. Pharmacological treatment of tics. In: Martino D, Leckman JF, editors. Tourette syndrome. New York: Oxford University Press; 2013. p. 454–62.
17. Groenewegen HJ, van den Heuvel OA, Cath DC, Voorn P, Veltman DJ. Does an imbalance between the dorsal and ventral striatopallidal systems play a role in Tourette's syndrome? A neuronal circuit approach. Brain Dev. 2003;25(Suppl 1):S3–S14.
18. Baldermann JC, Schüller T, Huys D, Becker I, Timmermann L, Jessen F, et al. Deep brain stimulation for Tourette syndrome: a systematic review and meta-analysis. Brain Stimul. 2016;9:296–304. https://doi.org/10.1016/j.brs.2015.11.005.
19. Coulombe MA, Elkaim LM, Alotaibi NM, Gorman DA, Weil AG, Fallah A, et al. Deep brain stimulation for Gilles de la Tourette syndrome in children and youth: a meta-analysis with individual participant data. J Neurosurg Pediatr. 2018;23:236–46. https://doi.org/10.3171/201 8.7.PEDS18300.
20. Martinez-Ramirez D, Jimenez-Shahed J, Leckman JF, Porta M, Servello D, Meng FG, et al. Efficacy and safety of deep brain stimulation in Tourette syndrome: the international Tourette syndrome deep brain stimulation public database and registry. JAMA Neurol. 2018;75:353–9.
21. Welter ML, Houeto JL, Thobois S, Bataille B, Guenot M, Worbe Y, et al. STIC study group. Anterior pallidal deep brain stimulation for Tourette's syndrome: a randomised, double-blind, controlled trial. Lancet Neurol. 2017;16:610–19.
22. Johnson KA, Fletcher PT, Servello D, Bona A, Porta M, Ostrem JL, et al. Image-based analysis and long-term clinical outcomes of deep brain stimulation for Tourette syndrome: a multisite study. J Neurol Neurosurg Psychiatry. 2019;90(10):1078–90. pii: jnnp-2019-320379. https://doi.org/10.1136/jnnp-2019-320379.
23. Kakusa B, Saluja S, Tate WJ, Espil FM, Halpern CH, Williams NR. Robust clinical benefit of multi-target deep brain stimulation for treatment of Gilles de la Tourette syndrome and its comorbidities. Brain Stimul. 2019;12:816–8.
24. Buhmann C, Huckhagel T, Engel K, Gulberti A, Hidding U, Poetter-Nerger M, et al. Adverse events in deep brain stimulation: a retrospective long-term analysis of neurological, psychiatric and other occurrences. PLoS One. 2017;12:e0178984. https://doi.org/10.1371/journal.pone.0178984.
25. Servello D, Sassi M, Gaeta M, Ricci C, Porta M. Tourette syndrome bears a higher rate of inflammatory complications at the implanted hardware in deep brain stimulation. Acta Neurochir (Wien). 2011;153:629–32.

26. Orth M. Transcranial magnetic stimulation in Gilles de la Tourette syndrome. J Psychosom Res. 2009;67:591–8.
27. Chae JH, Nahas Z, Wassermann E, Li X, Sethuraman G, Gilbert D, et al. A pilot safety study of repetitive transcranial magnetic stimulation in Tourette's syndrome. Cogn Behav Neurol. 2004;17:109–17.
28. Munchau A, Bloem BR, Thilo KV, Trimble MR, Rothwell JC, Robertson MM. Repetitive transcranial magnetic stimulation for Tourette syndrome. Neurology. 2002;59:1789–91.
29. Orth M, Kirby R, Richardson MP, Rothwell JC, Trimble MR, Robertson MM, et al. Subthreshold rTMS over pre-motor cortex has no effect on tics in patients with Gilles de la Tourette syndrome. Clin Neurophysiol. 2005;116:764–8.
30. Bloch Y, Arad S, Levkovitz Y. Deep TMS add-on treatment for intractable Tourette syndrome: a feasibility study. World J Biol Psychiatry. 2016;17:557–61. https://doi.org/10.3109/1562297 5.2014.964767.
31. Kwon HJ, Lim WS, Lim MH, Lee SJ, Hyun JK, Chae JH, et al. 1-Hz low frequency repetitive transcranial magnetic stimulation in children with Tourette's syndrome. Neurosci Lett. 2011;492:1–4.
32. Le K, Liu L, Sun MHL, Xiao N. Transcranial magnetic stimulation at 1 Hertz improves clinical symptoms in children with Tourette syndrome for at least 6 months. J Clin Neurosci. 2013;20:257–62.
33. Mantovani A, Lisanby SH, Pieraccini F, Ulivelli M, Castrogiovanni P, Rossi S. Repetitive transcranial magnetic stimulation in the treatment of obsessive-compulsive disorder and Tourette's syndrome. Int J Neuropsychopharmacol. 2006;9:95–100.
34. Mantovani A, Leckman JF, Grantz H, King RA, Sporn AL, Lisanby SH. Repetitive transcranial magnetic stimulation of the supplementary motor area in the treatment of Tourette syndrome: report of two cases. Clin Neurophysiol. 2007;118:2314–5.
35. Salatino A, Momo E, Nobili M, Berti A, Ricci R. Awareness of symptoms amelioration following low-frequency repetitive transcranial magnetic stimulation in a patient with Tourette syndrome and comorbid obsessive-compulsive disorder. Brain Stimul. 2014;7:341–3.
36. Alexander G, Crutcher M, DeLong M. Basal ganglia-thalamocortical circuits: parallel substrates for motor, oculomotor, "prefrontal", and "limbic" functions. Prog Brain Res. 1990;85:119–46.
37. Graybiel AM. The basal ganglia: learning new tricks and loving it. Curr Opin Neurobiol. 2005;15:638–44.
38. Haber SN. The primate basal ganglia: parallel and integrative networks. J Chem Neuroanat. 2003;26:317–30.
39. Eccles JC. The initiation of voluntary movements by the supplementary motor area. Arch Psychiatr Nervenkr. 1982;231:423–41.
40. Wiesendanger M. Eccles' perspective of the forebrain, its role in skilled movements, and the mind-brain problem. Prog Neurobiol. 2006;78:304–21.
41. Cunnington R, Windischberger C, Moser E. Premovement activity of the pre-supplementary motor area and the readiness for action: studies of time-resolved event-related functional MRI. Hum Mov Sci. 2005;24:644–56.
42. Lerner A, Bagic A, Hanakawa T, Boudreau EA, Pagan F, Mari Z, et al. Involvement of insula and cingulate cortices in control and suppression of natural urges. Cereb Cortex. 2009;19:218–23.
43. Fried I, Katz A, McCarthy G, Sass KJ, Williamson P, Spencer SS, et al. Functional organization of human supplementary motor cortex studied by electrical stimulation. J Neurosci. 1991;11:3656–66.
44. Bohlhalter S, Goldfine A, Matteson S, Garraux G, Hanakawa T, Kansaku K, et al. Neural correlates of tic generation in Tourette syndrome: an event-related functional MRI study. Brain. 2006;129:2029–37.
45. Braun AR, Stoetter B, Randolph C, Hsiao JK, Vladar K, Gernert J, et al. The functional neuroanatomy of Tourette's syndrome: an FDG-PET study. Regional changes in cerebral glucose metabolism differentiating patients and controls. Neuropychopharmacology. 1993;9:277–91.

46. Chase TN, Geoffrey V, Gillespie M, Burrows GH. Structural and functional studies of Gilles de la Tourette syndrome. Rev Neurol. 1986;142:851–5.
47. Eidelberg D, Moeller JR, Antonini A, Kazumata K, Dhawan V, Budman C, et al. The metabolic anatomy of Tourette's syndrome. Neurology. 1997;48:927–34.
48. Stern E, Silbersweig DA, Chee KY, Holmes A, Robertson MM, Trimble M, et al. A functional neuroanatomy of tics in Tourette Syndrome. Arch Gen Psychiatry. 2000;57:741–8.
49. Hampson M, Tokoglu F, King RA, Constable RT, Leckman JF. Brain areas coactivating with motor cortex during chronic motor tics and intentional movements. Biol Psychiatry. 2009;65:594–9. https://doi.org/10.1016/j.biopsych.2008.11.012.
50. Landeros-Weisenberger A, Mantovani A, Motlagh MG, de Alvarenga PG, Katsovich L, Leckman JF, et al. Randomized sham controlled double-blind trial of repetitive transcranial magnetic stimulation for adults with severe Tourette syndrome. Brain Stimul. 2015;8:574–81. https://doi.org/10.1016/j.brs.2014.11.015.
51. Rossi S, Ferro M, Cincotta M, Ulivelli M, Bartalini S, Miniussi C, et al. A real electromagnetic placebo device for sham transcranial magnetic stimulation. Clin Neurophysiol. 2007;118:709–16.
52. Levine J, Schooler NR. SAFETEE: a technique for the systematic assessment of side effects in clinical trials. Psychopharmacol Bull. 1986;22:343–81.
53. O'Reardon JP, Solvason HB, Janicak PG, Sampson S, Isenberg KE, Nahas Z, et al. Efficacy and safety of transcranial magnetic stimulation in the acute treatment of major depression: a multisite randomized controlled trial. Biol Psychiatry. 2007;62:1208–16.
54. Singh S, Kumar S, Kumar N, Verma R. Low-frequency repetitive transcranial magnetic stimulation for treatment of Tourette syndrome: a naturalistic study with 3 months of follow-up. Indian J Psychol Med. 2018;40:482–6.
55. Hawken ER, Dilkov D, Kaludiev E, Simek S, Zhang F, Milev R. Transcranial magnetic stimulation of the supplementary motor area in the treatment of obsessive-compulsive disorder: a multi-site study. Int J Mol Sci. 2016;17:420. https://doi.org/10.3390/ijms17030420.
56. Mantovani A, Simpson HB, Fallon BA, Rossi S, Lisanby SH. Randomized sham-controlled trial of repetitive transcranial magnetic stimulation in treatment-resistant obsessive-compulsive disorder. Int J Neuropsychopharmacol. 2010;13:217–27. https://doi.org/10.1017/S1461145709990435.
57. Mantovani A, Westin G, Hirsch J, Lisanby SH. Functional magnetic resonance imaging guided transcranial magnetic stimulation in obsessive-compulsive disorder. Biol Psychiatry. 2010;67.e39–40. https://doi.org/10.1016/j.biopsych.2009.08.009
58. Kumar N, Chadda RK. Augmentation effect of repetitive transcranial magnetic stimulation over the supplementary motor cortex in treatment refractory patients with obsessive compulsive disorder. Indian J Psychiatry. 2011;53:340–2. https://doi.org/10.4103/0019-5545.91909.
59. Lee YJ, Koo BH, Seo WS, Kim HG, Kim JY, Cheon EJ. Repetitive transcranial magnetic stimulation of the supplementary motor area in treatment-resistant obsessive-compulsive disorder: an open-label pilot study. J Clin Neurosci. 2017;44:264–8. https://doi.org/10.1016/j.jocn.2017.06.057.
60. Pallanti S, Marras A, Salerno L, Makris N, Hollander E. Better than treated as usual: transcranial magnetic stimulation augmentation in selective serotonin reuptake inhibitor-refractory obsessive-compulsive disorder, mini-review and pilot open-label trial. J Psychopharmacol. 2016;30:568–78. https://doi.org/10.1177/0269881116628427.
61. Rehn S, Eslick GD, Brakoulias V. A meta-analysis of the effectiveness of different cortical targets used in repetitive transcranial magnetic stimulation (rTMS) for the treatment of obsessive-compulsive disorder (OCD). Psychiatry Q. 2018;89:645–65. https://doi.org/10.1007/s11126-018-9566-7.
62. Mantovani A, Rossi S, Bassi BD, Simpson HB, Fallon BA, Lisanby SH. Modulation of motor cortex excitability in obsessive-compulsive disorder: an exploratory study on the relations of neurophysiology measures with clinical outcome. Psychiatry Res. 2013;210:1026–32. https://doi.org/10.1016/j.psychres.2013.08.054.

63. Rossi S, Bartalini S, Ulivelli M, Mantovani A, Di Muro A, Goracci A. Hypofunctioning of sensory gating mechanisms in patients with obsessive-compulsive disorder. Biol Psychiatry. 2005;57:16–20.

64. Corbit VL, Manning EE, Gittis AH, Ahmari SE. Strengthened inputs from secondary motor cortex to striatum in a mouse model of compulsive behavior. J Neurosci. 2019;39:2965–75. https://doi.org/10.1523/JNEUROSCI.1728-18.2018.

65. Hirschtritt ME, Darrow SM, Illmann C, Osiecki L, Grados M, Sandor P, et al. Genetic and phenotypic overlap of specific obsessive-compulsive and attention-deficit/hyperactive sub-types with Tourette syndrome. Psychol Med. 2018;48:279–93. https://doi.org/10.1017/S0033291717001672.

66. Gaze C, Kepley HO, Walkup JT. Co-occurring psychiatric disorders in children and adolescents with Tourette syndrome. J Child Neurol. 2006;21:657–64.

67. Nambu A, Tokuno H, Takada M. Functional significance of the cortico-subthalamo-pallidal 'hyperdirect' pathway. Neurosci Res. 2002;43:111–7.

68. Bunse T, Wobrock T, Strube W, Padberg F, Palm U, Falkai P, et al. Motor cortical excitability assessed by transcranial magnetic stimulation in psychiatric disorders: a systematic review. Brain Stimul. 2014;7:158–69.

69. Boroojerdi B, Prager A, Muelibacher W, Cohen LG. Reduction of human visual cortex excitability using 1-Hz transcranial magnetic stimulation. Neurology. 2000;11:1529–31.

70. Chen R, Classen J, Gerloff C, Celnik P, Wassermann EM, Hallett M, et al. Depression of motor cortex excitability by low-frequency transcranial magnetic stimulation. Neurology. 1997;48:1398–403.

71. Speer AM, Kimbrell TA, Wassermann EM, Repella J, Willis MW, Herscovitch P, et al. Opposite effects of high and low frequency rTMS on regional brain activity in depressed patients. Biol Psychiatry. 2000;48:133–41.

72. Speer AM, Willis MW, Herscovitch P, Daube-Witherspoon M, Shelton JR, Benson BE, et al. Intensity-dependent regional cerebral blood flow during 1-Hz repetitive transcranial magnetic stimulation (rTMS) in healthy volunteers studied with H215O positron emission tomography: II. Effects of prefrontal cortex rTMS. Biol Psychiatry. 2003;54:826–32.

73. Wassermann EM, Wedegaertner FR, Ziemann UI, George MS, Chen R. Crossed reduction of human motor cortex excitability by 1-Hz transcranial magnetic stimulation. Neurosci Lett. 1998;250:141–4.

74. Rossi S, Pasqualetti P, Rossini PM, Feige B, Ulivelli M, Glocker FX, et al. Effects of repetitive transcranial magnetic stimulation on movement-related cortical activity in humans. Cereb Cortex. 2000;10:802–8.

75. Artola A, Brocher S, Singer W. Different voltage-dependent thresholds for inducing long-term depression and long-term potentiation in slices of rat visual cortex. Nature. 1990;347:69–72.

76. Kirkwood A, Dudek S, Gold JT, Aizenman CD, Bear MF. Common forms of synaptic plasticity in the hippocampus and neocortex in vitro. Science. 1993;260:1518–21.

77. Stanton PK, Sejnowsky TJ. Associative long-term depression in the hippocampus induced by hebbian covariance. Nature. 1989;339:215–8.

78. Hoffman RE, Cavus I. Slow transcranial magnetic stimulation, long-term depotentiation, and brain hyperexcitability disorders. Am J Psychiatry. 2002;159:1093–102.

79. Bliss TVP, Gardner-Medwin AR. Long-lasting potentiation of the synaptic transimission in the detate area of the unanesthatized rabbit following stimulation of the perforant path. J Physiol. 1973;232:357–75.

80. Scahill L, Leckman JF, Schultz RT, Katsovich L, Peterson BS. A placebo-controlled trial of risperidone in Tourette syndrome. Neurology. 2003;60:1130–5.

81. Hsu CW, Wang LJ, Lin PY. Efficacy of repetitive transcranial magnetic stimulation for Tourette syndrome: a systematic review and meta-analysis. Brain Stimul. 2018;11:1110–8.

82. Wu SW, Maloney T, Gilbert DL, Dixon SG, Horn PS, Huddleston DA, et al. Functional MRI-navigated repetitive transcranial magnetic stimulation over supplementary motor area in chronic tic disorders. Brain Stimul. 2014;7:212–8.

83. Di Lazzaro V, Dileone M, Pilato F, Capone F, Musumeci G, Ranieri F, et al. Modulation of motor cortex neuronal networks by rTMS: comparison of local and remote effects of six different protocols of stimulation. J Neurophysiol. 2011;105:2150–6. https://doi.org/10.1152/jn.00781.2010.

84. Obeso I, Cho SS, Antonelli F, Houle S, Jahanshahi M, Ko JH, et al. Stimulation of the pre-SMA influences cerebral blood flow in frontal areas involved with inhibitory control of action. Brain Stimul. 2013;6:769–76.

85. Mantovani A, personal communication. Transcranial magnetic stimulation in obsessive-compulsive disorder: clinical, neurophysiolOGY and neuroimaging outcomes. In: Italian Society of Psychiatry National Meeting, June 23-26, 2019.

86. Dos Santos-Ribeiro S, de Salles Andrade JB, Quintas JN, Quintas JN, Baptista KB, Moreira-de-Oliveira ME, et al. A systematic review of the utility of electroconvulsive therapy in broadly defined obsessive-compulsive-related disorders. Prim Care Companion CNS Disord. 2018;18:20.

87. Zhang C, Deng Z, Pan Y, Zhang J, Zeljic K, Jin H, et al. Pallidal deep brain stimulation combined with capsulotomy for Tourette's syndrome with psychiatric comorbidity. J Neurosurg. 2019;4:1–9. https://doi.org/10.3171/2018.8.JNS181339.

Repetitive Transcranial Magnetic Stimulation in Addiction

11

Giovanni Martinotti, Mauro Pettorruso,
Chiara Montemitro, Hamed Ekhtiari, Colleen A. Hanlon,
Primavera A. Spagnolo, Elliot Stein,
and Massimo Di Giannantonio

G. Martinotti (✉)
Department of Neuroscience, Imaging and Clinical Sciences,
"G. D'Annunzio" University, Chieti, Italy

Department of Pharmacy, Pharmacology and Clinical Sciences,
University of Hertfordshire, Herts, UK

SRP "Villa Maria Pia", Rome, Italy
e-mail: giovanni.martinotti@gmail.com

M. Pettorruso · M. Di Giannantonio
Department of Neuroscience, Imaging and Clinical Sciences,
"G. D'Annunzio" University, Chieti, Italy

C. Montemitro
Department of Neuroscience, Imaging and Clinical Sciences,
"G. D'Annunzio" University, Chieti, Italy

Neuroimaging Research Branch, National Institute on Drug Abuse,
Intramural Research Program, National Institutes of Health, Baltimore, MD, USA

H. Ekhtiari
Laureate Institute for Brain Research, Tulsa, OK, USA

C. A. Hanlon
Medical University of South Carolina (MUSC), Charleston, SC, USA

P. A. Spagnolo
National Institute on Neurological Disorders and Stroke, National Institute of Health,
Bethesda, MD, USA

E. Stein
Neuroimaging Research Branch, National Institute on Drug Abuse, Intramural Research
Program, National Institutes of Health, Baltimore, MD, USA

© Springer Nature Switzerland AG 2020
B. Dell'Osso, G. Di Lorenzo (eds.), *Non Invasive Brain Stimulation
in Psychiatry and Clinical Neurosciences*,
https://doi.org/10.1007/978-3-030-43356-7_11

11.1 The Addicted Brain: From Neurotransmitters to Neural Circuits

Drug addiction, currently included in the field of Substance-Use Disorders (SUDs), can be defined as a chronically relapsing disorder, characterized by compulsive drug seeking and taking, loss of control over drug use, behavioral inflexibility, and emergence of negative emotional states (e.g., dysphoria, anxiety, irritability, anhedonia) [1]. Preclinical investigations, human neuroimaging and clinical studies have provided extensive evidence that these manifestations result from long-lasting neuroadaptations in several brain circuits, including basal ganglia, extended amygdala, and prefrontal cortex circuits [1].

Specifically, a central feature in the framework of causation of SUDs and other addictive disorders is represented by neuroadaptations in the reward neural circuitry (i.e., mesocorticolimbic dopamine (DA) system) and in the glutamatergic corticolimbic circuitry, in which the dopamine projections are embedded [2–5]. Although having diverse primary neurocircuitry and neurotransmitters targets, all addictive agents initially act by enhancing reward via increased dopamine release in the nucleus accumbens (NAc) [6] and other areas of the limbic forebrain, including the amygdala and prefrontal cortex [7]. According to the incentive-sensitization theory proposed by Robinson and Berridge [4], a sensitization of the mesolimbic dopaminergic system is critically implicated in the development of drug addiction and in the emergence of craving. Craving is a multifaceted construct, known is shown to be one of the most important contributors to relapse, thus representing an important treatment target [1].

The repeated stimulation of DA pathways, induced by exposure to addictive agents, evokes plastic changes in the reward neural circuitry, which leads to hypersensitivity to drugs, as well as to drug-associated cues [4]. Indeed, preclinical studies have shown that with repeated drug exposure neutral stimuli paired with the drug (conditioned stimuli) start to increase dopamine by themselves [8–12]. Brain imaging studies confirm that drug-associated cues induce dopamine increases, particularly in the dorsal striatum (region implicated in habit learning and action initiation). Thus, cue-induced conditioning plays a critical role in strengthening habitual responding in drug-seeking behavior, which reflects a transition from prefrontal cortical to striatal control over responding, and a transition from ventral striatal to more dorsal striatal subregions ([13, 14]). Indeed, studies using positron emission tomography (PET) reported reduced ventral striatal D2 receptors and diminished dopamine release in patients with substance dependence [15].

The changes in striatal dopamine function are accompanied by decreased activity in several prefrontal and associated regions. Alterations and dysfunction in prefrontal circuits have been shown to underlie the loss of inhibitory control, behavioral inflexibility, and impairment in executive functioning commonly observed in individuals with SUDs. The dorsal prefrontal cortex (PFC) network, including the dorsolateral prefrontal cortex (DLPFC) and the dorsal anterior cingulate cortex (dACC), controls executive functioning, including decision making and self-control, while the ventral PFC network, including the medial prefrontal cortex (MPFC), orbitofrontal cortex (OFC), and ventral anterior cingulate cortex (vACC), governs limbic arousal and emotion processing [16]. An imbalance of these two systems, specifically a hyperactive emotional processing and hypoactive executive functioning system, has been hypothesized as one of the main factors contributing to the transition to compulsive drug seeking and taking [17]. Indeed, hyperactivation of the ventral PFC network has been associated with craving [18], resulting in substance use [19], whereas hypoactivity of the left [20], as well as the right DLPFC [21], has been described in drug addicts while performing cognitive tasks, indicating impairments in executive functioning, which is modulated by the DLPFC network.

In addition to the alterations in reward neural circuitry and prefrontal circuits, SUDs are also characterized by neuroadaptations in the circuitry of the extended amygdala (central nucleus of the amygdala, bed nucleus of the stria terminalis, and NAc shell) and also in the lateral habenula. These changes are associated with abnormalities in neurotransmitter systems involved in stress response (e.g., corticotropin-releasing factor, CRF; neuropeptide 1, NK1; norepinephrine; and dynorphin). Engagement of these circuits and neurotransmitters leads to the emergence of negative affective states, which are manifest when the drug is removed during acute withdrawal but also during protracted abstinence [22]. Thus, negative states may powerfully motivate drug seeking via negative reinforcement and may trigger relapse even after prolonged periods of abstinence.

Taken together, these findings demonstrate that SUDs, as well as other addictive disorders rather than being expressions of a single brain region or neurotransmitter system, are mediated and maintained by alterations in multiple, integrated neural circuits, and allostatic alterations in the expression of their related neurotransmitters and molecular mediators. Therefore, effective treatments should be ideally able to address such complexity, by targeting and remodeling impaired circuits. In this perspective, an integrated, multidisciplinary approach based on combining pharmacotherapies, behavioral and cognitive interventions, and neurocircuitry-based interventions, such as transcranial magnetic stimulation and transcranial direct current stimulation, may represent a safe, effective, and feasible therapeutic option for patients with SUDs. As a neuroscientific, transdiagnostic-based approach has been proposed also for addictive disorders, including behavioral addictions [23–25], intermediate phenotypes of addiction, and their underlying neurobiological underpinnings, are being characterized. This can further fuel the development and use of interventions targeting these common underlying mechanisms.

11.2   The Rationale for Repetitive Transcranial Magnetic Stimulation (rTMS) for Addictive Disorders

Although in the last two decades important advances have been made in understanding the neurobiological underpinnings of ADs, this knowledge has not yet been translated into effective treatments for these disorders. Psychosocial interventions and currently FDA-approved pharmacotherapies for alcohol- and substance-use disorders (AUD and SUDs) have been shown to improve clinical outcomes. However, not all patients respond to these treatments, and relapse rates remain high. For example, SUDs present with disturbingly high recidivism rates, estimated between 40–60%, but in some instances exceeding 90%, depending on the primary substance being abused and how one measures the time frame of the treatment outcome (www. drugabuse.gov). This has prompted the investigation of novel pharmacotherapeutic targets, mostly with unsuccessful results [26–29]. Despite all these efforts, still there are no FDA-approved pharmacotherapies for cocaine- or amphetamine-use disorders, whose treatment relies mainly on behavioral and cognitive interventions, with variable success rates [30]. Furthermore, it is important to consider that pharmacotherapies such as methadone and buprenorphine, for opioid-use disorders, and naltrexone, for alcohol-use disorders, have been shown to modulate neural circuits implicated in ADs, but they lack spatial and temporal specificity of action.

Recent findings have indicated that brain stimulation techniques can be effective in reducing craving and consumption across different substances, and may also be efficacious for behavioral addictions, given their ability to induce neuroplasticity and modulate brain activity and connectivity. The rationale for the application of rTMS in the treatment of SUDs and other behavioral addictions lies in preclinical investigations. In a seminal optogenetic study, in vivo stimulation of prelimbic cortex (PLC) reversed cocaine-induced prefrontal hypofunction, and blocked drug-seeking behaviors [31, 32] in compulsive cocaine-seeking rats. The PLC in rats is the closest functional homologue of the DLPFC and the anterior cingulate cortex (ACC) in humans [33–35]. Consensus on this matter is still missing, due to the relevant large anatomical diversity between the rodent and the human frontal/anterior cortices, but both DLPFC and ACC play a major role in top-down inhibitory control and reward mechanisms. Thus, the aforementioned preclinical findings may be translated in humans by noninvasive stimulation of homologous areas (e.g., the DLPFC) [31] to test whether this intervention may reduce cocaine craving and consumption. This hypothesis has been preliminarly tested using transcranial magnetic stimulation (TMS).

The rationale of targeting the DLPFC is based also on the key role that this brain region plays in decision-making processes [36]. Addiction is associated with increased impulsivity and impaired risky decision making [37]. These decision-making processes in addiction can be modulated by rTMS on the DLPFC-enhancing inhibitory control, which may lead to a reduction in the use of substances. Therefore, the stimulation of the DLPFC by high-frequency pulses should increase its activity and its inhibitory control function. In particular, with drug-addicted subjects, this treatment should increase DLPFC function implementing the possibility to control craving and to cope with it.

The complex trajectory of addiction development from impulsive to compulsive substance use is thought to be reflected in changes in various cognitive constructs and their underlying networks, including reward processing [38], salience detection [39], executive control [39], and internal ruminations [40], with cycling phases, including binge/intoxication (i.e., reward seeking), withdrawal (negative affect) and drug-craving brain circuits and networks [1, 41]. The hypothesis of an imbalance between drive state and reward processing (so-called "Go-circuits") and executive control ("Stop-circuits") processes [16, 42–46] is a manifestation of such dysregulation. As reported by Hanlon et al. [47]) in their recent studies, two neurobehavioral systems may be targeted by TMS in order to treat substance-use disorders: an executive control system, namely, the *dorsal-lateral* frontal-striatal, likely involved in resisting drug use, and an impulsive system, namely, the *ventral-medial* frontal-striatal, likely involved in craving and use. Under this framework, a *Stop* system would inhibit the *Go*-craving system and stress system. It may therefore be useful to either increase activity in the DLPFC-dorsal striatal circuit or to decrease the activity in the ventral medial prefrontal cortex-caudate circuit using an inhibitory rTMS (1 Hz or continuous Theta Burst Stimulation, cTBS) [47]. It is therefore a possibility that the stimulation of the DLPFC could be less associated with a direct anticraving effect, probably exerting its action in terms of relapse prevention, increasing the possibility to control craving and to cope with it through a top-down mechanism.

A further aspect to consider is that targeting prefrontal areas via TMS also affects dopaminergic neurotransmission. Strafella and colleagues [48] found that high-frequency rTMS on the prefrontal cortex in humans induces subcortical release of dopamine in caudate nucleus, whereas Cho and Strafella [49] showed that rTMS over the left DLPFC modulates the release of dopamine in anterior cingulated cortex and orbitofrontal cortex in the same hemisphere. These findings have been recently confirmed in a longitudinal study investigating alcohol intake and dopamine transporter (DAT) availability in the striatum before and after deep rTMS. With respect to sham stimulation, active stimulation significantly reduced both alcohol craving and intake and DAT availability, suggesting a modulatory effect on dopaminergic terminals [50].

Also in the long-term perspective, in addicted brain where a repeated exposure to drugs has determined long-term neural adaptations, rTMS can exert its effect reverting the process of neuroadaptation. These neuroadaptations are partly associated with altered dopamine activity in the mesocorticolimbic circuitry [51] and lead to an alteration of cortical excitability [52], which have been implicated in the persistence of drug-seeking behaviors and in an increased likelihood of relapse. Repeated applications of rTMS can affect cortical excitability and increase the release of dopamine in the mesolimbic dopaminergic system, affecting neuroadaptation induced by the chronic use of substances [48, 53].

In addition to dopaminergic signaling, some of the TMS-induced effects depend on glutamatergic transmission [31, 54]. Different preclinical studies have clearly demonstrated that rTMS induced-LTP/LTD are strictly dependent on NMDA and AMPA receptor signaling [55, 56] within glutamatergic synapses within addiction-related brain areas [56, 57]. Additionally, rTMS has been shown to enhance GABA neurotransmission [58] through increased cortical inhibitory activity [59]. GABA neurotransmission is relevant in SUDs, and its modulation showed to have some potentials in terms of treatment outcomes [60–62].

Finally, rTMS could also exert its effects modulating the expression of neurotrophic factors, such as BDNF, an active regulator of synaptic plasticity, within cortical and subcortical areas [55]. More recently, nonsynaptic events have been suggested as mediators of rTMS long-term effects, including plasticity-related gene expression and neurogenesis [63, 64]. The role of BDNF should be also better explored, given its role in ADs [65, 66]. Whether these mechanisms are involved in rTMS-mediated effects in SUDs remains to be explored.

11.3   rTMS as a Therapeutic Tool in the Treatment of Addictive Disorders (ADs)

Repetitive transcranial magnetic stimulation (rTMS), including theta burst stimulation (TBS) and deep TMS (dTMS), has emerged as a potential treatment for ADs due to its promising results in terms of craving reduction [56, 67]. Most studies target the DLPFC by means of excitatory stimulation in order to strengthen executive functions and cognitive control [68].

A recent meta-analysis, including data from 748 patients with SUDs, showed that left DLPFC stimulation had a significant anticraving effect with medium effect size compared with sham stimulation [67]. However, this effect was limited in duration, as indicated by a nonsignificant treatment effect at follow-up. Meta-regression indicated an association between stimulation dosage (i.e., total number of stimulation pulses) and anticraving effect, whereas the number of sessions, pulse per session, frequency, and intensity was not significant [67]. This analysis yielded a large effect size for illicit drug dependence (including cocaine, opiates, methamphetamine, and cannabis), followed by a medium effect size for nicotine dependence and a small effect size for alcohol dependence [67]. Conversely, meta-analysis, including all studies for right DLPFC stimulation, showed no significant anticraving effect compared to sham stimulation [67]. Inhibitory stimulation protocols as well as dTMS had no significant effects on craving. Deep TMS is performed using a group of coils, called H coils, whose geometry and configuration allow to reach deeper brain regions [69], at the expense of focality. With regard to drug consumption, the analysis revealed that both excitatory rTMS of the left DLPFC and excitatory dTMS of the bilateral DLPFC and insula resulted in a significant reduction of substance consumption, compared with sham stimulation. Recently, other brain targets have been tested. For example, Hanlon and colleagues used continuous theta burst stimulation to attenuate MPFC activity during cue exposure [70, 71]. However, results were not supportive of an anticraving effect using this protocol.

The following sections describe trials exploring the experimental evidence for rTMS in SUD and other addictive behaviors.

11.3.1 rTMS in Nicotine-Use Disorder

There are three FDA-approved medications for smoking cessation, all of which promote abstinence: nicotine replacement therapies, bupropion, and varenicline. However, the outcomes are still far from satisfactory and there is ground for developments in the area of noninvasive brain stimulation (NIBS).

The first to investigate the efficacy of rTMS for smoking addiction were Johann and colleagues [72], who examined whether rTMS of the DLPFC could modulate tobacco craving. Following a 12-hour period of abstinence, 11 treatment-seeking smokers received either one active or one sham session of 20 Hz rTMS over the left DLPFC at 90% of MT. The session consisted of 20 trains of stimuli of 2.5 seconds. The levels of tobacco craving were assessed using a 100-point visual analogue scale (VAS) both 30 minutes prior to and following the rTMS treatment. rTMS significantly reduced the level of tobacco craving at 30 minutes post-treatment [72]. These findings, therefore, motivated further investigation on the efficacy of rTMS as a potential treatment in nicotine addiction, with the aim to test also whether this intervention could reduce cigarette consumption. Following this pilot study, the same research group [73] investigated the effects of two sessions of active and sham rTMS at the same parameters with a double-blind crossover design study. The second study demonstrated reduced smoking consumption following rTMS session, thus contributing to the preliminary evidence of the utility of rTMS treatment in nicotine dependence [74]. Based on these findings, the authors proposed that high-frequency rTMS could have potential therapeutic value in the treatment of nicotine dependence by reducing the levels of craving [72] and its consumption [73].

Amiaz and colleagues were also interested in evaluating the effects of high-frequency rTMS of the left DLPFC, combined with either smoking or neutral cues exposure, on cigarette consumption, dependence, and craving. Thus, there were four experimental groups: active TMS with smoking pictures, active TMS with neutral pictures, sham TMS with smoking pictures, and sham TMS with neutral pictures. The authors assessed the effects of 10 days of treatment with either active or sham 10 Hz rTMS treatment applied to the left DLPFC. Stimulation included 20 trains/day at 100% of MT and each train consisted of 50 pulses at 10 Hz. rTMS, independent of exposure to smoking pictures, reduced subjective and objective measures of cigarette consumption and nicotine dependence. However, these effects reduced gradually after completing the rTMS sessions and the reduction in cigarette use was not significant 6 months after treatment termination, although in the group of smokers who received active rTMS-smoking picture cigarette consumption was lower at 6-month follow-up compared to the other treatment groups. Overall, results from this study suggested that high-frequency rTMS over the DLPFC could reduce cigarette consumption and nicotine dependence [75].

Consistent with findings in nonpsychiatric smokers, some studies [72, 76] showed that treatment with rTMS significantly reduced craving in treatment-seeking individuals with schizophrenia, a population of smokers who are typically highly nicotine dependent. While there was a robust increase in craving following the rTMS session in the sham group (due to abstinence from smoking), post-treatment craving levels in the active group were the same or lower than the pretreatment assessment. Despite attenuation of tobacco craving, rTMS did not increase abstinence rates, thus suggesting that the number of rTMS sessions could be a critical factor modulating rTMS efficacy [76]. Rose et al. [77], instead, tested whether either excitatory and inhibitory stimulation of superior frontal gyrus (SFG) had anti-craving effects, with promising results. In one of the largest studies carried out to date, Dinur-Klein et al. [78] enrolled 115 smokers to either receive, in a randomized order, 13 sessions of high-frequency, low-frequency, or sham stimulation to the lateral PFC and insula bilaterally. This stimulation was done using an H-coil for deep TMS designed to target the DLPFC and insula, crucially involved in cigarette craving [79]. High-frequency deep TMS (10 Hz), in association with smoking cues during the stimulation procedure, was found to significantly reduce cigarette consumption, as well as nicotine dependence.

While other types of brain stimulation techniques (transcranial direct current stimulation, cranial electrostimulation, and deep brain stimulation) have been evaluated in the treatment of nicotine addiction, there is more evidence to support rTMS' potential to treat nicotine dependence. According to the criteria suggested by Brainin et al. [80], research on the therapeutic use of rTMS for nicotine dependence has one study in class II, three studies in class III, and one study in class IV that showed reduction in craving, consumption, and dependence [68]. Thus, according to the available evidence, rTMS falls within the level B recommendation as probably effective in the treatment of nicotine addiction [68].

11.3.2 rTMS in Alcohol-Use Disorder (AUD)

There are currently four FDA-approved pharmacotherapies for alcohol-use disorder: disulfiram, oral naltrexone, extended-release injectable naltrexone, and acamprosate. These pharmacotherapies have been approved, based on their effects in increasing abstinence more than placebo. Although these pharmacotherapies, also in combination with psychotherapies, have shown some positive findings, relapse rates are still high in patients with AUD [81]. The first brain stimulation study to test the anticraving efficacy of rTMS was carried out by Mishra and colleagues, who administered high-frequency (10 Hz) rTMS of the right DLPFC in a single-blind, sham-controlled fashion, in 45 patients with AUD [82]. The authors reported that 10 daily sessions of high-frequency rTMS over right DLPFC significantly reduced craving. This study supports the therapeutic potential of rTMS. Hoppner et al. [83] investigated the effect of high-frequency rTMS of the left DLPFC compared to sham stimulation on craving and mood in alcohol-dependent women. Nineteen female detoxified participants were randomized either to a high-frequency rTMS (20 Hz) over the left DLPFC ($N = 10$) or sham stimulations ($N = 9$) for 10 days. There were no significant differences in clinical parameters such as alcohol craving or mood after active rTMS compared to sham stimulation.

Herremans et al. [84] performed a sham-controlled, prospective, single-blind study in order to investigate the effect of single high-frequency rTMS session of the right DLPFC on alcohol craving in the community. Participants ($N = 36$) were alcohol-dependent inpatients. After successful detoxification, participants were allocated to receive one active or one sham rTMS session. The rTMS session (40 trains of 1.9 s at 20 Hz, 110% of MT with a 12-s intertrain interval) was administered the day prior to discharge patients for the weekend. One high-frequency rTMS session delivered to the right DLPFC did not lead to changes in craving (neither immediately after the stimulation session nor in participants' natural environment during the weekend). This study found that application of a single rTMS session had no significant effect on alcohol craving [84]. In another study, repetitive rTMS targeting the dACC using a double cone coil reduced immediate alcohol craving and consumption [85]. In a recent study [50], a small cohort of patients was treated by bilateral dTMS. Clinical and SPECT evaluations were then carried out after 4 weeks of rTMS sessions. Patients that received the real stimulation revealed a reduction in DAT availability at T1, whereas the sham-treated group did not suggest a modulatory effect of deep rTMS on dopaminergic terminals and a potential clinical efficacy in reducing alcohol intake in AUD patients.

Based on these findings, Herremans and Baeken [86] suggested the evaluation of multiple rTMS sessions in larger, randomized, and sham-controlled population samples. Furthermore, randomized controlled studies should be done to evaluate whether patients need stimulation with high or low frequency [86].

Taken together, data regarding the efficacy of rTMS in AUD are still partial and not conclusive. According to the criteria suggested by Brainin et al. [80], there is inadequate evidence to confer a level of recommendation for its effectiveness in the treatment of AUD.

11.3.3 rTMS in Cocaine- and Stimulant-Use Disorder

Cocaine-use disorder (CUD) is a major public health concern, associated with high relapse rates, significant disability, and substantial mortality [87]. Chronic cocaine use is among the most difficult substance-use disorders to treat. Nearly 1 in every 7 people seeking treatment for drug abuse is dependent upon cocaine and short-term cocaine relapse rates can reach up to 75% [88]. Unfortunately, no unequivocally effective pharmacological or psychological therapies have been identified to date. At the moment, there are currently no FDA-approved pharmacotherapies for cocaine- and amphetamine-use disorders.

Advances in understanding the neurobiological underpinnings of cocaine-use disorders have unraveled that chronic cocaine use causes damage and changes in the prefrontal cortex (PFC), [89], including significant brain volume reduction [90, 91], cortical hypoactivity [16, 92, 93], impairment in executive functions, and dysregulation of neurotransmitters systems [94–96]. Thus, targeting the PFC via TMS appears to be a promising intervention. In the first, open-label study testing this hypothesis, high-frequency rTMS of the right (but not left) DLPFC was linked to a reduction of craving in cocaine-addicted subjects [97]. The authors investigated whether a single session of rTMS over DLPFC could reduce cocaine craving among six male participants with CUD, and also assessed effects on mood. Participants received two sessions of high-frequency (10 Hz) rTMS at 90% of MT, to the right and left DLPFC, separated by 1 week. Patients were asked to complete a set of 15 visual analogue scales (VAS) ranging from "not at all" to "more than ever." Each VAS evaluated one of the primary or secondary endpoints on three occasions: 10 min before the intervention and immediately after and 4 h after rTMS session. This research provided the first demonstration that high-frequency rTMS applied over the right DLPFC could reduce craving associated with chronic use of cocaine.

In 2008, Politi and colleagues also performed an open-label study showing that in cocaine users ($n = 36$), 10 sessions of 15-Hz TMS to the left DLPFC (600 pulses, 100% resting MT, rTMT) led to a significant reduction in self-reported craving [98].

Other open-label studies confirmed these preliminary data, suggesting that rTMS of the PFC may determine a reduction in cocaine use and minimize the risk of relapse [97, 99–102, 103]. In a recent open-label study, Pettorruso et al. [104] confirmed the efficacy of high-frequency rTMS of the DLPF in CUD, showing a reduction in psychiatric symptoms that contribute to the overall clinical burden. rTMS appears to elicit its more notable effects on depressive and anxiety symptoms, confirming previous data by the same group, according to which the prohedonic effect of rTMS is crucial and directly related to the reduction of cocaine craving [100]. Future studies that assess cocaine intake after treatment are also required. According to the criteria suggested by Brainin et al. [80], there is still inadequate evidence to confer a level of recommendation for the effectiveness of this treatment.

Methamphetamine (METH) is a psychostimulant of the phenethylamine and amphetamine class of psychoactive drugs and is a widely used illicit drug, also available on the cybermarket [105, 106]. Neurotoxic effects and potentially irreversible loss of neurons and axons have been linked to the repeated exposure to moderate-to-high levels of METH [107]. Moreover, cognitive functioning under methamphetamine administration is linked to cognitive deficits and alteration of fronto-striatal and limbic pathways [107]. At the same time, METH users showed impaired cortical plasticity induced by TMS [108]. Nowadays, available treatments are limited psychosocial interventions and no medications have been approved by the FDA. NIBS have been evaluated as a potential treatment for Methamphetamine-Use Disorder (MUD) in few sham-controlled trials. High-Frequency rTMS on the left DLPFC has been proven to reduce craving [109, 110] and sleep disturbances [111] and to improve cognitive performance [112] in both male [111, 112] and female METH users [109]. At the same time, low-frequency rTMS transiently increased craving when applied on the same site [113]. Interestingly, both high- and low-frequency rTMS applied on both right and left DLPFC showed a significant effect on craving when compared to a control stimulation site (P3, of 10–20 EEG system) [114]. Unfortunately, given the high variability across studies, no recommendation may be highlighted.

11.3.4 rTMS in Opiate-Use Disorder

Recently, increases in opioid addiction, opioid-related morbidity, and opioid-related mortality have been reported in both USA and Europe. While the number of opioid prescriptions doubled in Europe during the last 10 years, nowadays every day 130 patients die from an overdose of prescription opioids in the USA [115]. Treatment for opioid-use disorder typically requires acute detoxification and/or opioid maintenance treatment. The two primary treatments for opioid-use disorder (methadone, buprenorphine) are designed for long-term opioid maintenance therapy. Methadone is a mu-opioid receptor agonist, whereas buprenorphine is a partial mu-opioid receptor agonist (mu agonist-K antagonist). Given that opioid withdrawal increases brain sensitivity to TMS-induced seizures, TMS has not been deeply examined in opioid-dependent patients. However, it is important to note that currently more than 15 different studies evaluating the effects of TMS in OUD have been registered in clinical trial.gov. Moreover, it may be interesting to notice that Nucleus Accumbens (NAcc) stimulation with Deep Brain Stimulation (DBS) was reported to significantly reduce heroin consumption and/or craving in single cases [116–118].

11.3.5 rTMS in Other SUDs

Cannabis is the most recreationally used drug worldwide: recreational users were approximately 3.8% of the world population in 2017. As the number of cannabis users has increased, the potency of cannabis expressed as the amount of THC has increased as well. At the same time, legalization policies led to decreased risk perception. The risk to develop a Cannabis-Use Disorder is around 10% for recreational users and is linked to increased risk of psychiatric and neurological illnesses [119]. As for Stimulants, available treatments for Cannabis-Use Disorders are limited to few effective psychosocial interventions and no medications have been approved. Even if rTMS has been shown to be safe in cannabis-dependent individuals, one single 10-Hz rTMS session on the left DLPFC did not exert any significant changes in craving when compared to sham stimulation [120].

11.3.6   rTMS in Gambling Disorder and Other Behavioral Addictions

Nonsubstance-related addictive disorders are frequently comorbid and share some neurobiological substrates and behavioral manifestations of substance-related addictive disorders. This is particularly true for gambling disorder (GD). It is thus an important question whether neuromodulation could change these neurobiological vulnerabilities, and thereby have clinical value for nonsubstance addictive behaviors as well [121].

GD was recognized as the first behavioral addiction, and as such was reclassified within the category of "Substance-related and Addictive Disorders," in the Diagnostic and Statistical Manual of psychiatric disorders (DSM-5) in 2013. In the ICD-11, gambling disorder was classified within the same supercategory of disorders due to substance use or addictive behaviors. In the DSM-5, gaming disorder was placed in the Appendix as a condition requiring more research. There is abundant evidence on similarities between GD and SUDs regarding genetics, neurobiology, psychological processes, and effectiveness of psychological treatment [122]. In GD, a neurocognitive profile showing diminished executive functioning compared to healthy controls (e.g., diminished response inhibition, cognitive flexibility) was related to differential functioning of the DLPFC and anterior cingulate cortex (ACC), both part of the cognitive control circuitry [123, 124]. Moreover, increased neural cue reactivity and associated self-reported craving are present in the striatum, orbitofrontal cortex, and insular cortex in GD patients compared to healthy controls.

These abnormalities in frontostriatal functioning in GD warrant the question of whether NIBS may be a promising add-on treatment for GD and other nonsubstance-related addictive disorders [125]. Currently, a very limited number of studies have explored TMS correlates in GD. For instance, in a single-session pilot study in nine men pathological gamblers, high-frequency rTMS over MPFC reduced desire to gamble, whereas cTBS over right DLPFC reduced blood pressure, but had no effects on gambling desire [126]. Furthermore, the authors reported that rTMS and cTBS had no effect on impulsive behavior (delay discounting) while both active stimulation protocols improved Stroop interference. Also in a sham-controlled crossover high-frequency rTMS study (left DLPFC), a single session active rTMS diminished craving compared to sham rTMS [127]. Yet in another trial, low-frequency rTMS over the right DLPFC had similar effects as sham stimulation on craving, thus suggesting the occurrence of placebo effect [128]. Recently, a sustained effect (6 months) was described in a GD subject [129], along with a modulation in dopaminergic pathways. In addition, a reduction in gambling-related symptoms has been observed also in GD-CUD comorbid patients [131]. Although preliminary, rTMS shows promise in restoring gambling-related pathophysiological alterations [130], deserving further investigations in well-powered controlled studies. Moreover, rigorously conducted clinical trials are needed to investigate optimal rTMS protocols with the potential to improve cognitive functioning, to diminish craving, and/or to reduce gambling behaviors/relapses in GD. Finally, if we consider GD as a disorder characterized by loss of control with respect to striatal drives such as craving, urgency for gambling, and reward-seeking behaviors, then neuromodulation could be utilized as an intervention aimed at enhancing both cognitive control and the regulation of the reactivity to natural rewards.

11.4 Safety of rTMS in SUDs

The major concern about TMS safety in the treatment of SUDs is related to the risk of inducing seizures [132]. Currently, no evidence supports a TMS-related increased risk of serious or nonserious adverse events in the treatment of addictive disorders. Nonetheless, increased vigilance is always warranted when theoretical concerns exist or in specific patient subgroups with limited prior data. From a safety standpoint, while rTMS has been recently established as a safe therapeutic tool, it is important to take into account that the application of rTMS in addiction is still a nascent field. SUD patients may present with long-lasting adaptations and changes in brain circuits and given that rTMS treatment results in functional changes in brain activity, establishing the safety of rTMS protocols in SUDs patients is a relevant issue and deserves further investigation. Any medical and pharmacological factor independently increasing the risk of a seizure (e.g., stimulant use, alcohol use/withdrawal, benzodiazepine/barbiturate use/withdrawal, opioid use, tramadol use, bupropion in nicotine treatment, other psychopharmacological treatments used for comorbid psychiatric disorders) can in theory synergistically increase brain sensitivity to TMS-induced seizures.

11.5 Current Limitations and Future Perspectives

Based on the rationale we exposed and on the current evidence, rTMS can be classified as probably effective in the treatment of addiction, with a promising effect size for high-frequency rTMS stimulation protocol of the DLPFC mainly in nicotine- and cocaine-use disorders. However, as recently reported by a consensus of experts [125], different points need to be better explored in order to understand which specific protocol could guarantee a better outcome: (1) frequency of stimulation (high vs. low frequency); (2) laterality of stimulation; (3) area of stimulation and the role of neuronavigation; (4) number of stimulations; (5) duration of repetition interval; (6) typology of coil; (7) should TMS be administered in "resting state" or during an "induced state" such as during cue-induced craving inhibition; (8) how should the clinical efficacy of TMS be determined (e.g., drug use behavior, self-reports of craving, cognitive constructs like working memory or executive control, alterations in brain circuits and networks); (9) the role of psychiatric comorbidities other than addiction; (10) should TMS be thought of as a monotherapy or combined with pharmacotherapy and/or behavioral interventions; (11) the relevance of placebo effect and sham stimulations; (12) duration of the positive effect on the long term and the role of long-term sessions (as a relapse prevention strategy); (13) how to phenotypically subtype individuals most likely to benefit from TMS.

Stimulation parameters, such as duration, number of stimulation sessions, stimulation frequency, intensity, target brain region, and interval between treatments, should be investigated to define the dose response of rTMS. Few of these parameters have been systematically investigated for addiction treatment [125]. Among TMS studies, most of them applied 10-Hz or 20-Hz pulses, whereas a minority performed 1 Hz and intermittent and continuous TBS stimulations. Evidence from depression rTMS studies suggest that longer treatment duration and/or higher number of rTMS sessions could contribute to faster clinical improvement and better outcomes [133]. Moreover, the use of multiple rTMS sessions per day may also be a promising therapeutic development, as recently shown in depression samples [134].

Another relevant issue is that of treatment duration. There were only two studies with 1-year follow-up, six studies with 6 months' follow-up, and four studies with 3 months' follow-up. Twelve studies had less than 3 months' follow-up [125]. This is a serious limitation, given that addiction is a chronically relapsing disorder.

There is very little information available from empirical studies to help guide the selection of left- or right-sided targets for neuromodulation approaches in SUDs. Most rTMS studies in SUDs have targeted the left DLPFC (following the pathway that was forged by depression researchers) [125]. In alcohol research, however, there has been a unique emphasis on stimulating the right DLPFC. Thus, the question on laterality in the treatment of addictive disorders should be put in a wider perspective, and be approached from a network perspective, where not only laterality, but also the target location is relevant. However, it has also been assumed that the left DLPFC processes reward-based motivation, whereas the right DLPFC is more involved in withdrawal-related behaviors and self-inhibition [135].

In order to establish protocols for clinically relevant long-lasting effects, an ongoing effort of research has been dedicated to exploring the effects of repeating stimulation, either by applying stimulation daily over several days or weeks, or repeating stimulation within a single daily session, separated by a critical time window [125]. In general, repeating stimulation over multiple days has demonstrated efficacy in various clinical applications, such as treatment of depression using rTMS [136, 137]. With regard to addiction studies, positive evidence also exists for lasting effects of repeated stimulation for smokers [78, 138]. However, even with these promising results, systematic or face-to-face studies comparing different repetition intervals are missing, and are crucially needed in order to determine effective repetition rates and durations. The importance of this issue also underlies the need for determining the optimal repetition intervals between sessions. In studies using TMS, the duration of the repetition interval has been found to be critical in modulating plasticity, while also avoiding homeostatic mechanisms that may limit or counteract plasticity [139–142]. For example, in a study on depression, repeating rTMS twice daily with a 15-min interval between stimulation blocks resulted in superior effects compared to a once daily application with the same number of pulses [143]. In case of addictive disorders, the number of studies investigating the effect of interval timings remains scarce. In summary, although there is promising evidence for persisting and long-lasting effects with repeated stimulation sessions, the relatively large heterogeneity of these studies with regard to stimulation technique, timing, repetition, and montage precludes a clear understanding of how repetition may affect therapeutic outcomes in SUD, warranting a need for systematic research designs [144].

The role of placebo effects and sham stimulations in rTMS is another issue specifically relevant in addiction. Participants and patients typically receive considerable information in advance about TMS and they inevitably speculate about its effects [145]. The occurrence of a placebo effect is therefore at least plausible and should be considered when evaluating rTMS efficacy, especially in light of a recent study reporting that sham rTMS has itself differential effects on neuronal activity on an individual-by-individual basis [146]. Placebo effects have been observed in different psychiatric disorders with a strong neurobiological component, including major depression [147] and obsessive-compulsive disorder (OCD) [148]. SUDs and behavioral addictions are conditions that can be easily complicated by abnormal personality, with histrionic features that can enhance the possibility to observe a placebo effect. Moreover, the external locus of control, a typical cognitive psychological disposition frequently reported in SUDs [149], might emphasize the possibility to see in an external aid (the use of rTMS) the resolution of their disorders. Adequate sham stimulation protocols are therefore a critical factor in clinical trials to ensure that effects can be ascribed specifically to TMS. Sham TMS approaches require further development but may be sufficient in clinical settings in which patients are generally naïve to TMS [145]. There are ongoing efforts by the TMS community to evaluate and revise sham protocols in order to increase rigor across the field [150], "When to stimulate" is another issue that needs to be better defined. As suggested in a recent consensus paper [125], there are four distinct time intervals at which rTMS/tDCS interventions were administered: (1) before the participant sought standard treatment (2), while the subject was treatment seeking but before undergoing standard treatment, (3) within the first month of standard treatment (mainly detoxification and stabilization), and (4) after the initial recovery period (more than 1 month). If the definition of these time intervals appears to be clear, we are still far to know which intervention would benefit the most in terms of efficacy. For safety reason, it is of course advisable to avoid the intoxication phase and the early detoxification, specifically alcohol and opiates withdrawals.

The role of "Outcome Measures" is also of high relevance [125]. Most of the studies used craving as their primary outcome measure. Self-report on a visual analogue scale (VAS) was the most frequently used craving measure, whereas few studies used objective measures such as urine drug tests or breath analyzers. Although a reduction or elimination of the consumption of the drug is the ultimate endpoint for clinical trials research, there are also many other behavioral and biological variables that have been studied extensively and are considered meaningful surrogate endpoints for patients seeking treatment for SUDs (e.g., heightened reactivity to predictive drug cues, perseverative responding, delayed discounting for the drug, response to stress, narrowing of the behavioral repertoire) [151].

Neuromodulatory treatments have also been used for comorbidities with SUDs [152]. One group studying smoking patients with schizophrenia demonstrated that rTMS reduced cigarette cravings compared to sham [153]. Another group using rTMS for comorbid dysthymia and AUD showed decreased alcohol consumption with rTMS [154]. Perhaps a dual benefit of brain stimulation treatments targeting underlying neurobiological factors in SUDs may also extend to deficiencies found in other psychiatric disorders (i.e., nicotinic acetylcholine receptor deficits found in schizophrenia patients, associated with both higher smoking rates and cognitive dysfunction) [155]. Actually, overlapping neurobiological substrates between SUDs and psychiatric disorders [19, 156] have been widely reported.

While neuromodulatory techniques are a promising interventional approach in the treatment of SUDs, most responses are partial and even the well-documented anti-craving effects of rTMS do not necessarily translate into reduced drug use or abstinence [153]. Combining neuromodulation with behavioral and pharmacotherapeutic interventions may ultimately mitigate these shortcomings [157]. Indeed, coupling pharmacological treatments with brain stimulation methods has an advantage of reversing plasticity induced by drugs of abuse by targeting the neurocircuits that maintain addictive behaviors [158]. For instance, nearly 50% of patients become abstinent from cigarettes after treatment with rTMS and concomitant nicotine replacement therapy [159]. Future studies will define optimal augmentation strategies, in order to determine possible rationales to combine neuromodulation and pharmacological interventions. Promising strategies seem to be represented by the simultaneous interaction with glutamate and GABA neurotransmissions [160, 161].

At present, the gap between the knowledge we have about the neurobiology of addiction and the translation in effective treatments remains substantial. Bridging this gap could help increase the efficacy of treatments for those patients who suffer from the serious consequences of these disorders, as well as for their families. The implementation of neuromodulation techniques offers a chance to remodel dysfunctional neural circuits. Moreover, combining these actions with synergistic pharmacological modulation could determine more pronounced and long-lasting effects. Furthermore, also behavioral interventions (i.e., motivational interviewing (MI); cognitive behavioral therapy (CBT); contingency management (CM)) can be used in combination to NIBS. Given that neuromodulation can improve cognitive control/functioning, it may (in part) diminish the risk for relapse by strengthening cognitive control [162, 163], favoring the psychotherapeutic and rehabilitation process in absence of craving perturbations [164].

11.6 Conclusions

Building on data from major depression and OCD (for which TMS is currently FDA approved), we are now beginning to build a foundation of knowledge regarding rTMS utility as a tool to change smoking, drinking, and cocaine use behavior.

At the moment, the best level of effectiveness of rTMS is in the treatment of nicotine and cocaine/stimulant-use disorders. The effects of rTMS sessions on drug craving and consumption provide evidence and support for further TMS studies in the field of addiction research. It is important to note that none of these studies demonstrated complete abstinence from substance use and few studies [73, 83] evaluated craving in real-life scenarios. The outcome observed is still far from being considered fully satisfactory. Variability in cortical excitability may also be linked to genetic characteristics, in the same way that responses to medications can be influenced by genetic variability [165]. A research domain criteria approach able to identify the specific endophenotype that could be better benefit from rTMS is going to be the goal of NIBS in the next years [166, 167].

Future research should identify potential parameters (i.e., duration, number of stimulation treatments, stimulation frequency, intensity, brain region of target, and proximity between treatments) of stimulation in rTMS studies for the most effective and safe treatment of drug addiction. Optimal stimulation parameters are still far from being defined. Rigorous preclinical TMS-dosing studies in various addiction models are needed to comprehensively evaluate the full parameter space of dosing variables.

The data presented in this chapter demonstrate that whereas most of the efforts for rTMS in addiction have been focused on increasing activity in the DLPFC, decreasing activity in the MPFC and ventral striatum may also be a feasible and fruitful target to consider [47]. It seems plausible that either increasing neural firing in the executive control circuit (perhaps via 10-Hz TMS in the DLPFC) or decreasing firing in the limbic circuit in the presence of cues (perhaps via cTBS TMS in the MPFC) may be valuable strategies for decreasing vulnerability to drug-related cues among patients. Convincing evidence also leads to the idea of the insula being a promising brain region to target for addiction with dTMS stimulation [168].

Promising therapeutic development is represented by the use of multiple rTMS sessions per day, as shown in depression studies for accelerated rTMS protocols [134], by the use of appropriate add-on pharmacotherapy [160, 161], and by the concomitant use of other NIBS (tDCS) in the long term, also in terms of cost effectiveness [160, 161].

Future studies should focus on the personalization of the rTMS treatment, as well as on the optimization of stimulation protocols.

Conflict of Interest None.

References

1. Koob GF, Volkow ND. Neurobiology of addiction: a neurocircuitry analysis. Lancet Psychiatry. 2016;3:760–73. https://doi.org/10.1016/S2215-0366(16)00104-8.
2. Koob GF, Volkow ND. Neurocircuitry of addiction. Neuropsychopharmacology. 2010;35:217–38. https://doi.org/10.1038/npp.2009.110.
3. Nestler EJ. Is there a common molecular pathway for addiction? Nat Neurosci. 2005;8:1445–9. https://doi.org/10.1038/nn1578.
4. Robinson TE, Berridge KC. The neural basis of drug craving: an incentive-sensitization theory of addiction. Brain Res Brain Res Rev. 1993;18:247–91.
5. Nestler EJ. Molecular neurobiology of addiction. Am J Addict. 2001;10(3):201–17.
6. Garbusow M, Schad DJ, Sebold M, Friedel E, Bernhardt N, Koch SP, Steinacher B, Kathmann N, Geurts DE, Sommer C, Müller DK, Nebe S, Paul S, Wittchen HU, Zimmermann US, Walter H, Smolka MN, Sterzer P, Rapp MA, Huys QJ, Schlagenhauf F, Heinz A. Pavlovian-to-instrumental transfer effects in the nucleus accumbens relate to relapse in alcohol dependence. Addict Biol. 2016;21(3):719–31. https://doi.org/10.1111/adb.12243
7. Kourrich S, Calu DJ, Bonci A. Intrinsic plasticity: an emerging player in addiction. Nat Rev Neurosci. 2015;16(3):173–84.
8. Di Ciano P, Everitt BJ. Contribution of the ventral tegmental area to cocaine-seeking maintained by a drug-paired conditioned stimulus in rats. Eur J Neurosci. 2004;19(6):1661–7.

9. Kiyatkin EA, Stein EA. Conditioned changes in nucleus accumbens dopamine signal established by intravenous cocaine in rats. Neurosci Lett. 1996;211(2):73–6.
10. Phillips PE, Stuber GD, Heien ML, Wightman RM, Carelli RM. Subsecond dopamine release promotes cocaine seeking. Nature. 2003;422(6932):614-8. Erratum in: Nature. 2003;423(6938):461.
11. Vanderschuren LJ, Di Ciano P, Everitt BJ. Involvement of the dorsal striatum in cue-controlled cocaine seeking. J Neurosci. 2005;25(38):8665–70.
12. Weiss F, Maldonado-Vlaar CS, Parsons LH, Kerr TM, Smith DL, Ben-Shahar O. Control of cocaine-seeking behavior by drug-associated stimuli in rats: effects on recovery of extinguished operant-responding and extracellular dopamine levels in amygdala and nucleus accumbens. Proc Natl Acad Sci U S A. 2000;97(8):4321–6.
13. Everitt BJ, Robbins TW. Neural systems of reinforcement for drug addiction: from actions to habits to compulsion. Nat Neurosci. 2005;8:1481–9.
14. Belin D, Belin-Rauscent A, Murray JE, Everitt BJ. Addiction: failure of control over maladaptive incentive habits. Curr Opin Neurobiol. 2013;23(4):564-72. https://doi.org/10.1016/j.conb.2013.01.025.
15. Volkow ND, Koob G, Baler R. Biomarkers in substance use disorders. ACS Chem Nerosci. 2015;6:522–5. https://doi.org/10.1021/acschemneuro.5b00067.
16. Goldstein RZ, Volkow ND. Dysfunction of the prefrontal cortex in addiction: neuroimaging findings and clinical implications. Nat Rev Neurosci. 2011;12:652.
17. McClure SM, Bickel WK. A dual-systems perspective on addiction: contributions from neuroimaging and cognitive training. Ann N Y Acad Sci. 2014;1327:62–78. https://doi.org/10.1111/nyas.12561.
18. Hayashi T, Ko JH, Strafella AP, Dagher A. Dorsolateral prefrontal and orbitofrontal cortex interactions during self-control of cigarette craving. Proc Natl Acad Sci U S A. 2013;110:4422–7. https://doi.org/10.1073/pnas.1212185110.
19. Dunlop K, Hanlon CA, Downar J. Noninvasive brain stimulation treatments for addiction and major depression. Ann N Y Acad Sci. 2017;1394:31–54. https://doi.org/10.1111/nyas.12985.
20. Eldreth DA, Matochik JA, Cadet JL, Bolla KI. Abnormal brain activity in prefrontal brain regions in abstinent marijuana users. Neuroimage. 2004;23:914–20. https://doi.org/10.1016/j.neuroimage.2004.07.032.
21. Salo R, Ursu S, Buonocore MH, Leamon MH, Carter C. Impaired prefrontal cortical function and disrupted adaptive cognitive control in methamphetamine abusers: a functional magnetic resonance imaging study. Biol Psychiatry. 2009;65:706–9. https://doi.org/10.1016/j.biopsych.2008.11.026.
22. Koob GF, Le Moal M, Se V. Neurobiological mechanisms for opponent motivational processes in addiction. Philos Trans R Soc Lond B Biol Sci. 2008;363(1507):3113–23. https://doi.org/10.1098/rstb.2008.0094.
23. Kwako LE, Momenan R, Litten RZ, Koob GF, Goldman D. Addictions Neuroclinical Assessment: A Neuroscience-Based Framework for Addictive Disorders. Biol Psychiatry. 2016;80(3):179–89. https://doi.org/10.1016/j.biopsych.2015.10.024.
24. Spagnolo PA, Gómez Pérez LJ, Terraneo A, Gallimberti L, Bonci A. Neural correlates of cue- and stress-induced craving in gambling disorders: implications for transcranial magnetic stimulation interventions. Eur J Neurosci. 2019;50(3):2370–2383. https://doi.org/10.1111/ejn.14313.
25. Yücel M, Oldenhof E, Ahmed SH, Belin D, Billieux J, Bowden-Jones H, Carter A, Chamberlain SR, Clark L, Connor J, Daglish M, Dom G, Dannon P, Duka T, Fernandez-Serrano MJ, Field M, Franken I, Goldstein RZ, Gonzalez R, Goudriaan AE, Grant JE, Gullo MJ, Hester R, Hodgins DC, Le Foll B, Lee RSC, Lingford- Hughes A, Lorenzetti V, Moeller SJ, Munafò MR, Odlaug B, Potenza MN, Segrave R, Sjoerds Z, Solowij N, van den Brink W, van Holst RJ, Voon V, Wiers R, Fontenelle LF, Verdejo-Garcia A. A transdiagnostic dimensional approach towards a neuropsychological assessment for addiction: an international Delphi consensus study. Addiction. 2019;114(6):1095–1109. https://doi.org/10.1111/add.14424.
26. Achab S, Khazaal Y. Psychopharmacological treatment in pathological gambling: a critical review. Curr Pharm Des. 2011;17:1389–95. https://doi.org/10.2174/138161211796150774.

27. Bolt DM, Piper ME, Theobald WE, Baker TB. Why two smoking cessation agents work better than one: role of craving suppression. J Consult Clin Psychol. 2012;80:54–65. https://doi.org/10.1037/a0026366.
28. Mariani JJ, Levin FR. Psychostimulant treatment of cocaine dependence. Psychiatr Clin North Am. 2012;35:425–39. https://doi.org/10.1016/j.psc.2012.03.012.
29. Muller CA, Schafer M, Banas R, Heimann HM, Volkmar K, Forg A, Heinz A, Hein J. A combination of levetiracetam and tiapride for outpatient alcohol detoxification: a case series. J Addict Med. 2011;5:153–6. https://doi.org/10.1097/ADM.0b013e3181ec5f81.
30. McHugh RK, Hearon BA, Otto MW. Cognitive-behavioral therapy for substance use disorders. Psychiatr Clin North Am. 2010;33:511–25.
31. Chen AC, Oathes DJ, Chang C, Bradley T, Zhou ZW, Williams LM, Glover GH, Deisseroth K, Etkin A. Causal interactions between fronto-parietal central executive and default-mode networks in humans. Proc Natl Acad Sci U S A. 2013;110(49):19944–9. https://doi.org/10.1073/pnas.1311772110.
32. Jasinska AJ, Chen BT, Bonci A, Stein EA. Dorsal medial prefrontal cortex (MPFC) circuitry in rodent models of cocaine use: implications for drug addiction therapies. Addict Biol. 2015;20:215–26. https://doi.org/10.1111/adb.12132.
33. Balleine BW, Dickinson A. Goal-directed instrumental action: contingency and incentive learning and their cortical substrates. Neuropharmacology. 1998;37:407–19. https://doi.org/10.1016/s0028-3908(98)00033-1.
34. Gass JT, Chandler LJ. The plasticity of extinction: contribution of the prefrontal cortex in treating addiction through inhibitory learning. Front Psych. 2013;4:46. https://doi.org/10.3389/fpsyt.2013.00046.
35. Papaleo F, Erickson L, Liu G, Chen J, Weinberger DR. Effects of sex and COMT genotype on environmentally modulated cognitive control in mice. Proc Natl Acad Sci U S A. 2012;109:20160–5. https://doi.org/10.1073/pnas.1214397109.
36. Rorie AE, Newsome WT. A general mechanism for decision-making in the human brain? Trends Cogn Sci. 2005;9:41–3. https://doi.org/10.1016/j.tics.2004.12.007.
37. Knoch D, Gianotti LRR, Pascual-Leone A, Treyer V, Regard M, Hohmann M, Brugger P. Disruption of right prefrontal cortex by low-frequency repetitive transcranial magnetic stimulation induces risk-taking behavior. J Neurosci. 2006;26:6469–72. https://doi.org/10.1523/JNEUROSCI.0804-06.2006.
38. Haber SN, Knutson B. The reward circuit: linking primate anatomy and human imaging. Neuropsychopharmacology. 2010;35:4–26. https://doi.org/10.1038/npp.2009.129.
39. Seeley WW, Menon V, Schatzberg AF, Keller J, Glover GH, Kenna H, et al. Dissociable intrinsic connectivity networks for salience processing and executive control. J Neurosci. 2007;27:2349–56.
40. Raichle ME. The brain's default mode network. Annu Rev Neurosci. 2015;38:433–47. https://doi.org/10.1146/annurev-neuro-071013-014030.
41. Spronk DB, van Wel JHP, Ramaekers JG, Verkes RJ. Characterizing the cognitive effects of cocaine: a comprehensive review. Neurosci Biobehav Rev. 2013;37:1838–59. https://doi.org/10.1016/j.neubiorev.2013.07.003.
42. Bechara A, Damasio H, Tranel D, Damasio AR. The Iowa gambling task and the somatic marker hypothesis: some questions and answers. Trends Cogn Sci. 2005;9:154–9. https://doi.org/10.1016/j.tics.2005.02.002.
43. Bickel WK, Miller ML, Yi R, Kowal BP, Lindquist DM, Pitcock JA. Behavioral and neuroeconomics of drug addiction: competing neural systems and temporal discounting processes. Drug Alcohol Depend. 2007;90(Suppl 1):S85–91. https://doi.org/10.1016/j.drugalcdep.2006.09.016.
44. Childress AR, Mozley PD, McElgin W, Fitzgerald J, Reivich M, O'Brien CP. Limbic activation during cue-induced cocaine craving. Am J Psychiatry. 1999;156:11–8. https://doi.org/10.1176/ajp.156.1.11.
45. Hu Y, Salmeron BJ, Gu H, Stein EA, Yang Y. Impaired functional connectivity within and between frontostriatal circuits and its association with compulsive drug use and trait impulsivity in cocaine addiction. JAMA Psychiat. 2015;72:584–92. https://doi.org/10.1001/jamapsychiatry.2015.1.

46. Volkow ND, Koob GF, McLellan AT. Neurobiologic advances from the brain disease model of addiction. N Engl J Med. 2016;374:363–71. https://doi.org/10.1056/NEJMra1511480.
47. Hanlon CA, Dowdle LT, Henderson JS. Modulating neural circuits with transcranial magnetic stimulation: implications for addiction treatment development. Pharmacol Rev. 2018;70:661–83. https://doi.org/10.1124/pr.116.013649.
48. Strafella AP, Paus T, Barrett J, Dagher A. Repetitive transcranial magnetic stimulation of the human prefrontal cortex induces dopamine release in the caudate nucleus. J Neurosci. 2001;21:RC157.
49. Cho SS, Strafella AP. rTMS of the left dorsolateral prefrontal cortex modulates dopamine release in the ipsilateral anterior cingulate cortex and orbitofrontal cortex. PLoS One. 2009;4:e6725. https://doi.org/10.1371/journal.pone.0006725.
50. Addolorato G, Antonelli M, Cocciolillo F, Vassallo GA, Tarli C, Sestito L, Mirijello A, Ferrulli A, Pizzuto DA, Camardese G, Miceli A, Diana M, Giordano A, Gasbarrini A, Di Giuda D. Deep transcranial magnetic stimulation of the dorsolateral prefrontal cortex in alcohol use disorder patients: effects on dopamine transporter availability and alcohol intake. Eur Neuropsychopharmacol. 2017;27:450–61. https://doi.org/10.1016/j.euroneuro. 2017.03.008.
51. Vanderschuren LJ, Kalivas PW. Alterations in dopaminergic and glutamatergic transmission in the induction and expression of behavioral sensitization: a critical review of preclinical studies. Psychopharmacology (Berl). 2000;151:99–120. https://doi.org/10.1007/s002130000493.
52. Kalivas PW, O'Brien C. Drug addiction as a pathology of staged neuroplasticity. Neuropsychopharmacology. 2008;33:166–80. https://doi.org/10.1038/sj.npp.1301564.
53. Diana M. The dopamine hypothesis of drug addiction and its potential therapeutic value. Front Psych. 2011;2:64. https://doi.org/10.3389/fpsyt.2011.00064.
54. Gersner R, Kravetz E, Feil J, Pell G, Zangen A. Long-term effects of repetitive transcranial magnetic stimulation on markers for neuroplasticity: differential outcomes in anesthetized and awake animals. J Neurosci. 2011;31:7521–6. https://doi.org/10.1523/JNEUROSCI.6751-10.2011.
55. Cirillo G, Di Pino G, Capone F, Ranieri F, Florio L, Todisco V, Tedeschi G, Funke K, Di Lazzaro V. Neurobiological after-effects of non-invasive brain stimulation. Brain Stimul. 2017;10:1–18. https://doi.org/10.1016/j.brs.2016.11.009.
56. Diana M, Raij T, Melis M, Nummenmaa A, Leggio L, Bonci A. Rehabilitating the addicted brain with transcranial magnetic stimulation. Nat Rev Neurosci. 2017;18:685 93. https://doi.org/10.1038/nrn.2017.113.
57. Argilli E, Sibley DR, Malenka RC, England PM, Bonci A. Mechanism and time course of cocaine-induced long term potentiation in the ventral tegmental area. J Neurosci. 2008;28:9092–100. https://doi.org/10.1523/JNEUROSCI.1001-08.2008.
58. McDonnell MN, Orekhov Y, Ziemann U. The role of GABA(B) receptors in intracortical inhibition in the human motor cortex. Exp Brain Res. 2006;173(1):86–93.
59. Daskalakis ZJ, Moller B, Christensen BK, Fitzgerald PB, Gunraj C, Chen R. The effects of repetitive transcranial magnetic stimulation on cortical inhibition in healthy human subjects. Exp Brain Res. 2006;174:403–12. https://doi.org/10.1007/s00221-006-0472-0.
60. Di Nicola M, Martinotti G, Tedeschi D, Frustaci A, Mazza M, Sarchiapone M, Pozzi G, Bria P, Janiri L. Pregabalin in outpatient detoxification of subjects with mild-to-moderate alcohol withdrawal syndrome. Hum Psychopharmacol. 2010;25:268–75. https://doi.org/10.1002/hup.1098.
61. Martinotti G, Di Nicola M, Romanelli R, Andreoli S, Pozzi G, Moroni N, Janiri L. High and low dosage oxcarbazepine versus naltrexone for the prevention of relapse in alcohol-dependent patients. Hum Psychopharmacol. 2007;22:149–56. https://doi.org/10.1002/hup.833.
62. Martinotti G, Di Nicola M, Tedeschi D, Mazza M, Janiri L, Bria P. Efficacy and safety of pregabalin in alcohol dependence. Adv Ther. 2008;25(6):608–18.
63. Spagnolo PA, Goldman D. Neuromodulation interventions for addictive disorders: challenges, promise, and roadmap for future research. Brain. 2017;140:1183–203. https://doi.org/10.1093/brain/aww284.

64. Zhang X, Mei Y, Liu C, Yu S. Effect of transcranial magnetic stimulation on the expression of c-Fos and brain-derived neurotrophic factor of the cerebral cortex in rats with cerebral infarct. J Huazhong Univ Sci Technolog Med Sci. 2007;27:415–8. https://doi.org/10.1007/s11596-007-0416-3.

65. Ghitza UE, Zhai H, Wu P, Airavaara M, Shaham Y, Lu L. Role of BDNF and GDNF in drug reward and relapse: a review. Neurosci Biobehav Rev. 2010;35:157–71. https://doi.org/10.1016/j.neubiorev.2009.11.009.

66. Ricci V, Martinotti G, Gelfo F, Tonioni F, Caltagirone C, Bria P, Angelucci F. Chronic ketamine use increases serum levels of brain-derived neurotrophic factor. Psychopharmacology (Berl). 2011;215(1):143–8.

67. Zhang JJQ, Fong KNK, Ouyang R-G, Siu AMH, Kranz GS. Effects of repetitive transcranial magnetic stimulation (rTMS) on craving and substance consumption in patients with substance dependence: a systematic review and meta-analysis. Addiction. 2019;114(12):2137–49. https://doi.org/10.1111/add.14753.

68. Bellamoli E, Manganotti P, Schwartz RP, Rimondo C, Gomma M, Serpelloni G. rTMS in the treatment of drug addiction: an update about human studies. Behav Neurol. 2014;2014:815215. https://doi.org/10.1155/2014/815215.

69. Roth Y, Zangen A, Hallett M. A coil design for transcranial magnetic stimulation of deep brain regions. J Clin Neurophysiol. 2002;19:361–70.

70. Hanlon CA, Dowdle LT, Austelle CW, DeVries W, Mithoefer O, Badran BW, George MS. What goes up, can come down: novel brain stimulation paradigms may attenuate craving and craving-related neural circuitry in substance dependent individuals. Brain Res. 2015;1628:199–209. https://doi.org/10.1016/j.brainres.2015.02.053.

71. Hanlon CA, Dowdle LT, Correia B, Mithoefer O, Kearney-Ramos T, Lench D, Griffin M, Anton RF, George MS. Left frontal pole theta burst stimulation decreases orbitofrontal and insula activity in cocaine users and alcohol users. Drug Alcohol Depend. 2017;178:310–7. https://doi.org/10.1016/j.drugalcdep.2017.03.039.

72. Johann M, Wiegand R, Kharraz A, Bobbe G, Sommer G, Hajak G, Wodarz N, Eichhammer P. Repetitiv transcranial magnetic stimulation in nicotine dependence. Psychiatr Prax. 2003;30:129–31. https://doi.org/10.1055/s-2003-39733.

73. Eichhammer P, Johann M, Kharraz A, Binder H, Pittrow D, Wodarz N, Hajak G. High-frequency repetitive transcranial magnetic stimulation decreases cigarette smoking. J Clin Psychiatry. 2003;64:951–3. https://doi.org/10.4088/jcp.v64n0815.

74. Barr MS, Fitzgerald PB, Farzan F, George TO, Daskalakis J. Transcranial magnetic stimulation to understand the pathophysiology and treatment of substance use disorders. Curr Drug Abuse Rev. 2008;1(3):328–39.

75. Amiaz R, Levy D, Vainiger D, Grunhaus L, Zangen A. Repeated high-frequency transcranial magnetic stimulation over the dorsolateral prefrontal cortex reduces cigarette craving and consumption. Addiction. 2009;104:653–60. https://doi.org/10.1111/j.1360-0443.2008.02448.x.

76. Wing VC, Bacher I, Wu BS, Daskalakis ZJ, George TP. High frequency repetitive transcranial magnetic stimulation reduces tobacco craving in schizophrenia. Schizophr Res. 2012;139(1-3):264–6. https://doi.org/10.1016/j.schres.2012.03.006.

77. Rose JE, McClernon FJ, Froeliger B, Behm FM, Preud'homme X, Krystal AD. Repetitive transcranial magnetic stimulation of the superior frontal gyrus modulates craving for cigarettes. Biol Psychiatry. 2011;70:794–9. https://doi.org/10.1016/j.biopsych.2011.05.031.

78. Dinur-Klein L, Dannon P, Hadar A, Rosenberg O, Roth Y, Kotler M, Zangen A. Smoking cessation induced by deep repetitive transcranial magnetic stimulation of the prefrontal and insular cortices: a prospective, randomized controlled trial. Biol Psychiatry. 2014;76:742–9. https://doi.org/10.1016/j.biopsych.2014.05.020.

79. Naqvi NH, Gaznick N, Tranel D, Bechara A. The insula: a critical neural substrate for craving and drug seeking under conflict and risk. Ann N Y Acad Sci. 2014;1316:53-70. https://doi.org/10.1111/nyas.12415.

80. Brainin M, Barnes M, Baron J-C, Gilhus NE, Hughes R, Selmaj K, Waldemar G. Guidance for the preparation of neurological management guidelines by EFNS scientific task

forces—revised recommendations 2004. Eur J Neurol. 2004;11:577–81. https://doi.org/10.1111/j.1468-1331.2004.00867.x.

81. Soyka M, Müller CA. Pharmacotherapy of alcoholism—an update on approved and off-label medications. Expert Opin Pharmacother. 2017;18(12):1187–99.

82. Mishra BR, Nizamie SH, Das B, Praharaj SK. Efficacy of repetitive transcranial magnetic stimulation in alcohol dependence: a sham-controlled study. Addiction. 2010;105:49–55. https://doi.org/10.1111/j.1360-0443.2009.02777.x.

83. Hoppner J, Broese T, Wendler L, Berger C, Thome J. Repetitive transcranial magnetic stimulation (rTMS) for treatment of alcohol dependence. World J Biol Psychiatry. 2011;12(Suppl 1):57–62. https://doi.org/10.3109/15622975.2011.598383.

84. Herremans SC, Baeken C, Vanderbruggen N, Vanderhasselt MA, Zeeuws D, Santermans L, De Raedt R. No influence of one right-sided prefrontal HF-rTMS session on alcohol craving in recently detoxified alcohol-dependent patients: results of a naturalistic study. Drug Alcohol Depend. 2012;120:209–13. https://doi.org/10.1016/j.drugalcdep.2011.07.021.

85. De Ridder D, Vanneste S, Kovacs S, Sunaert S, Dom G. Transient alcohol craving suppression by rTMS of dorsal anterior cingulate: an fMRI and LORETA EEG study. Neurosci Lett. 2011;496:5–10. https://doi.org/10.1016/j.neulet.2011.03.074.

86. Herremans SC, Baeken C. The current perspective of neuromodulation techniques in the treatment of alcohol addiction: a systematic review. Psychiatr Danub. 2012;24(Suppl 1):S14–20.

87. Reitox National Drug Information Centre-Italy—EMCDDA. National Report to EMCDDA 2013—Italy. 2014.

88. Sinha R. New findings on biological factors predicting addiction relapse vulnerability. Curr Psychiatry Rep. 2011;13(5):398–405. https://doi.org/10.1007/s11920-011-0224-0.

89. Volkow ND, Fowler JS, Wang G-J, Swanson JM. Dopamine in drug abuse and addiction: results from imaging studies and treatment implications. Mol Psychiatry. 2004;9:557–69. https://doi.org/10.1038/sj.mp.4001507.

90. Matochik JA, London ED, Eldreth DA, Cadet J-L, Bolla KI. Frontal cortical tissue composition in abstinent cocaine abusers: a magnetic resonance imaging study. Neuroimage. 2003;19:1095–102.

91. Moreno-López L, Stamatakis EA, Fernández-Serrano MJ, Gómez-Río M, Rodríguez-Fernández A, Pérez-García M, Verdejo-García A. Neural correlates of the severity of cocaine, heroin, alcohol, MDMA and cannabis use in polysubstance abusers: a resting-PET brain metabolism study. PLoS One. 2012;7:e39830. https://doi.org/10.1371/journal.pone.0039830.

92. Goldstein RZ, Volkow ND. Drug addiction and its underlying neurobiological basis: neuroimaging evidence for the involvement of the frontal cortex. Am J Psychiatry. 2002;159:1642–52. https://doi.org/10.1176/appi.ajp.159.10.1642.

93. Kaufman JN, Ross TJ, Stein EA, Garavan H. Cingulate hypoactivity in cocaine users during a GO-NOGO task as revealed by event-related functional magnetic resonance imaging. J Neurosci. 2003;23:7839–43.

94. Ke Y, Streeter CC, Nassar LE, Sarid-Segal O, Hennen J, Yurgelun-Todd DA, Awad LA, Rendall MJ, Gruber SA, Nason A, Mudrick MJ, Blank SR, Meyer AA, Knapp C, Ciraulo DA, Renshaw PF. Frontal lobe GABA levels in cocaine dependence: a two-dimensional, J-resolved magnetic resonance spectroscopy study. Psychiatry Res. 2004;130:283–93. https://doi.org/10.1016/j.pscychresns.2003.12.001.

95. Licata SC, Renshaw PF. Neurochemistry of drug action: insights from proton magnetic resonance spectroscopic imaging and their relevance to addiction. Ann N Y Acad Sci. 2010;1187:148–71. https://doi.org/10.1111/j.1749-6632.2009.05143.x.

96. Volkow ND, Fowler JS, Wang G-J. The addicted human brain: insights from imaging studies. J Clin Invest. 2003;111:1444–51. https://doi.org/10.1172/JCI18533.

97. Camprodon JA, Martínez-Raga J, Alonso-Alonso M, Shih M-C, Pascual-Leone A. One session of high frequency repetitive transcranial magnetic stimulation (rTMS) to the right prefrontal cortex transiently reduces cocaine craving. Drug Alcohol Depend. 2007;86:91–4. https://doi.org/10.1016/j.drugalcdep.2006.06.002.

98. Politi E, Fauci E, Santoro A, Smeraldi E. Daily sessions of transcranial magnetic stimulation to the left prefrontal cortex gradually reduce cocaine craving. Am J Addict. 2008;17(4):345–6. https://doi.org/10.1080/10550490802139283.

99. Martinez D, Urban N, Grassetti A, Chang D, Hu MC, Zangen A, Levin FR, Foltin R, Nunes EV. Transcranial magnetic stimulation of medial prefrontal and cingulate cortices reduces cocaine self-administration: a pilot study. Front Psych. 2018;9:10–5. https://doi.org/10.3389/fpsyt.2018.00080.

100. Pettorruso M, Spagnolo PA, Leggio L, Janiri L, Di Giannantonio M, Gallimberti L, Bonci A, Martinotti G. Repetitive transcranial magnetic stimulation of the left dorsolateral prefrontal cortex may improve symptoms of anhedonia in individuals with cocaine use disorder: a pilot study. Brain Stimul. 2018;11:1195–7. https://doi.org/10.1016/j.brs.2018.06.001.

101. Rapinesi C, Del Casale A, Di Pietro S, Ferri VR, Piacentino D, Sani G, Raccah RN, Zangen A, Ferracuti S, Vento AE, Angeletti G, Brugnoli R, Kotzalidis GD, Girardi P. Add-on high frequency deep transcranial magnetic stimulation (dTMS) to bilateral prefrontal cortex reduces cocaine craving in patients with cocaine use disorder. Neurosci Lett. 2016;629:43–7. https://doi.org/10.1016/j.neulet.2016.06.049.

102. Terraneo A, Leggio L, Saladini M, Ermani M, Bonci A, Gallimberti L. Transcranial magnetic stimulation of dorsolateral prefrontal cortex reduces cocaine use: a pilot study. Eur Neuropsychopharmacol. 2016;26(1):37–44.

103. Sanna A, Fattore L, Badas P, Corona G, Cocco V, Diana M. Intermittent Theta burst stimulation of the prefrontal cortex in cocaine use disorder: a pilot study. Front Neurosci. 2019;13:765.

104. Pettorruso M, Martinotti G, Santacroce R, Montemitro C, Fanella F, Di Giannantonio M. rTMS reduces psychopathological burden and cocaine consumption in treatment-seeking subjects with cocaine use disorder: an open label, feasibility study. Front Psych. 2019b;10:1–9. https://doi.org/10.3389/fpsyt.2019.00621.

105. Corkery JM, Schifano F, Martinotti G. Pharmacology influencing practice, policy and the law. Br J Clin Pharmacol. 2019; https://doi.org/10.1111/bcp.14183.

106. Schifano F, Leoni M, Martinotti G, Rawaf S, Rovetto F. Importance of cyberspace for the assessment of the drug abuse market: preliminary results from the Psychonaut 2002 project. Cyberpsychol Behav. 2003;6(4):405–10.

107. Courtney KE, Ray LA. Methamphetamine: an update on epidemiology, pharmacology, clinical phenomenology, and treatment literature. Drug Alcohol Depend. 2014;143:11–21. https://doi.org/10.1016/j.drugalcdep.2014.08.003.

108. Du X, Yu C, Hu Z-Y, Zhou D-S. Commentary: methamphetamine abuse impairs motor cortical plasticity and function. Front Hum Neurosci. 2017;11:562. https://doi.org/10.3389/fnhum.2017.00562.

109. Liu T, Li Y, Shen Y, Liu X, Yuan T. Progress in Neuropsychopharmacology & Biological Psychiatry Gender does not matter: add-on repetitive transcranial magnetic stimulation treatment for female methamphetamine dependents. Prog Neuropsychopharmacol Biol Psychiatry. 2019;92:70–5. https://doi.org/10.1016/j.pnpbp.2018.12.018.

110. Su H, Zhong N, Gan H, Wang J, Han H, Chen T, Li X, Ruan X, Zhu Y, Jiang H, Zhao M. High frequency repetitive transcranial magnetic stimulation of the left dorsolateral prefrontal cortex for methamphetamine use disorders: a randomised clinical trial. Drug Alcohol Depend. 2017;175:84–91. https://doi.org/10.1016/j.drugalcdep.2017.01.037.

111. Lin J, Liu X, Li H, Yu L, Shen M, Lou Y, Xie S, Chen J, Zhang R, Yuan T-F. Chronic repetitive transcranial magnetic stimulation (rTMS) on sleeping quality and mood status in drug dependent male inpatients during abstinence. Sleep Med. 2019;58:7–12. https://doi.org/10.1016/j.sleep.2019.01.052.

112. Liang Q, Lin J, Yang J, Li X, Chen Y, Meng X, Yuan J. Intervention effect of repetitive TMS on behavioral adjustment after error commission in long-term methamphetamine addicts: evidence from a two-choice oddball task. Neurosci Bull. 2018;34:449–56. https://doi.org/10.1007/s12264-018-0205-y.

113. Li X, Malcolm RJ, Huebner K. Low frequency repetitive transcranial magnetic stimulation of the left dorsolateral prefrontal cortex transiently increases cue-induced craving for methamphetamine: a preliminary study. Drug Alcohol Depend. 2013;133:641–6.
114. Liu Q, Shen Y, Cao X, Li Y. Brief report: either at left or right, both high and low frequency rTMS of dorsolateral prefrontal cortex decreases Cue induced craving for methamphetamine. Am J Addict. 2017;26(8):776–9. https://doi.org/10.1111/ajad.12638.
115. Verhamme KMC, Bohnen AM. Are we facing an opioid crisis in Europe? Lancet Public Health. 2019;4(10):e483–4. https://doi.org/10.1016/S2468-2667(19)30156-2.
116. Kuhn J, Moller M, Treppmann JF, Bartsch C, Lenartz D, Gruendler TOJ, Maarouf M, Brosig A, Barnikol UB, Klosterkotter J, Sturm V. Deep brain stimulation of the nucleus accumbens and its usefulness in severe opioid addiction. Mol Psychiatry. 2014;19(2):145–6. https://doi.org/10.1038/mp.2012.196.
117. Valencia-Alfonso C-E, Luigjes J, Smolders R, Cohen MX, Levar N, Mazaheri A, van den Munckhof P, Schuurman PR, van den Brink W, Denys D. Effective deep brain stimulation in heroin addiction: a case report with complementary intracranial electroencephalogram. Biol Psychiatry. 2012; https://doi.org/10.1016/j.biopsych.2011.12.013.
118. Zhou H, Xu J, Jiang J. Deep brain stimulation of nucleus accumbens on heroin-seeking behaviors: a case report. Biol Psychiatry. 2011;69(11):e41–2. https://doi.org/10.1016/j.biopsych.2011.02.012.
119. Kroon E, Kuhns L, Hoch E, Cousijn J. Heavy cannabis use, dependence and the brain: a clinical perspective. Addiction. 2019;115:559–72. https://doi.org/10.1111/add.14776.
120. Sahlem GL, Baker NL, George MS, Malcolm RJ, McRae-Clark AL. Repetitive transcranial magnetic stimulation (rTMS) administration to heavy cannabis users. Am J Drug Alcohol Abuse. 2018;44:47–55. https://doi.org/10.1080/00952990.2017.1355920.
121. Spagnolo PA, Gómez Pérez LJ, Terraneo A, Gallimberti L, Bonci A. Neural correlates of cue- and stress-induced craving in gambling disorders: implications for transcranial magnetic stimulation interventions. Eur J Neurosci. 2019;50(3):2370–83.
122. Goudriaan AE, Yucel M, van Holst RJ. Getting a grip on problem gambling: what can neuroscience tell us? Front Behav Neurosci. 2014;8:141. https://doi.org/10.3389/fnbeh.2014.00141.
123. Moccia L, Pettorruso M, De Crescenzo F, De Risio L, di Nuzzo L, Martinotti G, Bifone A, Janiri L, Di Nicola M. Neural correlates of cognitive control in gambling disorder: a systematic review of fMRI studies. Neurosci Biobehav Rev. 2017;78:104–16. https://doi.org/10.1016/j.neubiorev.2017.04.025.
124. van Holst RJ, van den Brink W, Veltman DJ, Goudriaan AE. Why gamblers fail to win: a review of cognitive and neuroimaging findings in pathological gambling. Neurosci Biobehav Rev. 2010;34:87–107. https://doi.org/10.1016/j.neubiorev.2009.07.007.
125. Ekhtiari H, Tavakoli H, Addolorato G, Baeken C, Bonci A, Campanella S, Castelo-Branco L, Challet-Bouju G, Clark VP, Claus E, Dannon PN, Del Felice A, den Uyl T, Diana M, di Giannantonio M, Fedota JR, Fitzgerald P, Gallimberti L, Grall-Bronnec M, Herremans SC, Herrmann MJ, Jamil A, Khedr E, Kouimtsidis C, Kozak K, Krupitsky E, Lamm C, Lechner WV, Madeo G, Malmir N, Martinotti G, McDonald WM, Montemitro C, Nakamura-Palacios EM, Nasehi M, Noël X, Nosratabadi M, Paulus M, Pettorruso M, Pradhan B, Praharaj SK, Rafferty H, Sahlem G, Salmeron BJ, Sauvaget A, Schluter RS, Sergiou C, Shahbabaie A, Sheffer C, Spagnolo PA, Steele VR, Yuan T, van Dongen JDM, Van Waes V, Venkatasubramanian G, Verdejo-García A, Verveer I, Welsh JW, Wesley MJ, Witkiewitz K, Yavari F, Zarrindast M-R, Zawertailo L, Zhang X, Cha Y-H, George TP, Frohlich F, Goudriaan AE, Fecteau S, Daughters SB, Stein EA, Fregni F, Nitsche MA, Zangen A, Bikson M, Hanlon CA. Transcranial electrical and magnetic stimulation (tES and TMS) for addiction medicine: a consensus paper on the present state of the science and the road ahead. Neurosci Biobehav Rev. 2019;104:118–40. https://doi.org/10.1016/j.neubiorev.2019.06.007.
126. Zack M, Cho SS, Parlee J, Jacobs M, Li C, Boileau I, Strafella A. Effects of high frequency repeated transcranial magnetic stimulation and continuous theta burst stimulation on gam-

bling reinforcement, delay discounting, and Stroop interference in men with pathological gambling. Brain Stimul. 2016;9:867–75. https://doi.org/10.1016/j.brs.2016.06.003.

127. Gay A, Boutet C, Sigaud T, Kamgoue A, Sevos J, Brunelin J, Massoubre C. A single session of repetitive transcranial magnetic stimulation of the prefrontal cortex reduces cue-induced craving in patients with gambling disorder. Eur Psychiatry. 2017;41:68–74. https://doi.org/10.1016/j.eurpsy.2016.11.001.

128. Sauvaget A, Bulteau S, Guilleux A, Leboucher J, Pichot A, Valriviere P, Vanelle J-M, Sebille-Rivain V, Grall-Bronnec M. Both active and sham low-frequency rTMS single sessions over the right DLPFC decrease cue-induced cravings among pathological gamblers seeking treatment: a randomized, double-blind, sham-controlled crossover trial. J Behav Addict. 2018;7:126–36. https://doi.org/10.1556/2006.7.2018.14.

129. Pettorruso M, Di Giuda D, Martinotti G, Cocciolillo F, De Risio L, Montemitro C, Camardese G, Di Nicola M, Janiri L, di Giannantonio M. Dopaminergic and clinical correlates of high-frequency repetitive transcranial magnetic stimulation in gambling addiction: a SPECT case study. Addict Behav. 2019a;93:246–9. https://doi.org/10.1016/j.addbeh.2019.02.013.

130. Pettorruso M, Martinotti G, Montemitro C, De Risio L, Spagnolo PA, Gallimberti L, Fanella F, Bonci A, Di Giannantonio M; Brainswitch Study Group. Multiple Sessions of High-Frequency Repetitive Transcranial Magnetic Stimulation as a Potential Treatment for Gambling Addiction: A 3-Month, Feasibility Study. Eur Addict Res. 2020;26(1):52-56. https://doi.org/10.1159/000504169.

131. Cardullo S, Gomez Perez LJ, Marconi L, Terraneo A, Gallimberti L, Bonci A, Madeo G. Clinical improvements in comorbid gambling/cocaine use disorder (GD/CUD) patients undergoing repetitive transcranial magnetic stimulation (rTMS). J Clin Med. 2019;8:768. https://doi.org/10.3390/jcm8060768.

132. Rossi S, De Capua A, Tavanti M, Calossi S, Polizzotto NR, Mantovani A, Falzarano V, Bossini L, Passero S, Bartalini S, Ulivelli M. Dysfunctions of cortical excitability in drug-naive post-traumatic stress disorder patients. Biol Psychiatry. 2009;66:54–61. https://doi.org/10.1016/j.biopsych.2009.03.008.

133. Schulze L, Feffer K, Lozano C, Giacobbe P, Daskalakis ZJ, Blumberger DM, Downar J. Number of pulses or number of sessions? An open-label study of trajectories of improvement for once-vs twice-daily dorsomedial prefrontal rTMS in major depression. Brain Stimul. 2018;11:327–36. https://doi.org/10.1016/j.brs.2017.11.002.

134. Baeken C, Vanderhasselt M-A, Remue J, Herremans S, Vanderbruggen N, Zeeuws D, Santermans L, De Raedt R. Intensive HF-rTMS treatment in refractory medication-resistant unipolar depressed patients. J Affect Disord. 2013;151:625–31. https://doi.org/10.1016/j.jad.2013.07.008.

135. Balconi M, Finocchiaro R, Canavesio Y. Reward-system effect (BAS rating), left hemispheric "unbalance" (alpha band oscillations) and decisional impairments in drug addiction. Addict Behav. 2014;39:1026–32. https://doi.org/10.1016/j.addbeh.2014.02.007.

136. Rapinesi C, Bersani FS, Kotzalidis GD, Imperatori C, Del Casale A, Di Pietro S, Ferri VR, Serata D, Raccah RN, Zangen A, Angeletti G, Girardi P. Maintenance deep transcranial magnetic stimulation sessions are associated with reduced depressive relapses in patients with unipolar or bipolar depression. Front Neurol. 2015;6:16. https://doi.org/10.3389/fneur.2015.00016.

137. Senova S, Cotovio G, Pascual-Leone A, Oliveira-Maia AJ. Durability of antidepressant response to repetitive transcranial magnetic stimulation: systematic review and meta-analysis. Brain Stimul. 2019;12:119–28. https://doi.org/10.1016/j.brs.2018.10.001.

138. Dieler AC, Dresler T, Joachim K, Deckert J, Herrmann MJ, Fallgatter AJ. Can intermittent theta burst stimulation as add-on to psychotherapy improve nicotine abstinence? Results from a pilot study. Eur Addict Res. 2014;20:248–53. https://doi.org/10.1159/000357941.

139. Goldsworthy MR, Pitcher JB, Ridding MC. Neuroplastic modulation of inhibitory motor cortical networks by spaced theta burst stimulation protocols. Brain Stimul. 2013;6:340–5. https://doi.org/10.1016/j.brs.2012.06.005.

140. Monte-Silva K, Kuo M-F, Hessenthaler S, Fresnoza S, Liebetanz D, Paulus W, Nitsche MA. Induction of late LTP-like plasticity in the human motor cortex by repeated non-invasive brain stimulation. Brain Stimul. 2013;6:424–32. https://doi.org/10.1016/j.brs.2012.04.011.
141. Thickbroom GW. Transcranial magnetic stimulation and synaptic plasticity: experimental framework and human models. Exp Brain Res. 2007;180:583–93. https://doi.org/10.1007/s00221-007-0991-3.
142. Tse NY, Goldsworthy MR, Ridding MC, Coxon JP, Fitzgerald PB, Fornito A, Rogasch NC. The effect of stimulation interval on plasticity following repeated blocks of intermittent theta burst stimulation. Sci Rep. 2018;8:8526. https://doi.org/10.1038/s41598-018-26791-w.
143. Modirrousta M, Meek BP, Wikstrom SL. Efficacy of twice-daily vs once-daily sessions of repetitive transcranial magnetic stimulation in the treatment of major depressive disorder: a retrospective study. Neuropsychiatr Dis Treat. 2018;14:309–16. https://doi.org/10.2147/NDT.S151841.
144. Trojak B, Sauvaget A, Fecteau S, Lalanne L, Chauvet-Gelinier J-C, Koch S, Bulteau S, Zullino D, Achab S. Outcome of non-invasive brain stimulation in substance use disorders: a review of randomized sham-controlled clinical trials. J Neuropsychiatry Clin Neurosci. 2017;29:105–18. https://doi.org/10.1176/appi.neuropsych.16080147.
145. Duecker F, Sack AT. Rethinking the role of sham TMS. Front Psychol. 2015;6:210. https://doi.org/10.3389/fpsyg.2015.00210.
146. Cunningham AD, Jacqueline Cavendish J, Sankarasubramanian V, Potter-Baker KA, Machado AJ, Plow EB. The influence of sham repetitive transcranial magnetic stimulation on commonly collected TMS metrics in patients with chronic stroke. Brain Stimul. 2017;10(4):e24–5.
147. Brunoni AR, Sampaio-Junior B, Moffa AH, Aparicio LV, Gordon P, Klein I, Rios RM, Razza LB, Loo C, Padberg F, Valiengo L. Noninvasive brain stimulation in psychiatric disorders: a primer. Rev Bras Psiquiatr. 2019;41:70–81. https://doi.org/10.1590/1516-4446-2017-0018.
148. Mansur CG, Myczkowki ML, de Barros Cabral S, Sartorelli MC, Bellini BB, Dias AM, Bernik MA, Marcolin MA. Placebo effect after prefrontal magnetic stimulation in the treatment of resistant obsessive-compulsive disorder: a randomized controlled trial. Int J Neuropsychopharmacol. 2011;14(10):1389–97 . Epub 2011 Apr 18. https://doi.org/10.1017/S1461145711000575.
149. Ersche KD, Turton AJ, Croudace T, Stochl J. Who do you think is in control in addiction? A pilot study on drug related locus of control beliefs. Addict Disord Their Treat 2012;11:173–223. https://doi.org/10.1097/ADT.0b013e31823da151.
150. Opitz A, Legon W, Mueller J, Barbour A, Paulus W, Tyler WJ. Is sham cTBS real cTBS? The effect on EEG dynamics. Front Hum Neurosci. 2015;8:1043. https://doi.org/10.3389/fnhum.2014.01043.
151. Beveridge TJR, Smith HR, Nader MA, Porrino LJ. Abstinence from chronic cocaine self-administration alters striatal dopamine systems in rhesus monkeys. Neuropsychopharmacology. 2009;34:1162–71. https://doi.org/10.1038/npp.2008.135.
152. Coles AS, Kozak K, George TP. A review of brain stimulation methods to treat substance use disorders. Am J Addict. 2018;27(2):71-91. https://doi.org/10.1111/ajad.12674.
153. Wing VC, Barr MS, Wass CE, Lipsman N, Lozano AM, Daskalakis ZJ, George TP. Brain stimulation methods to treat tobacco addiction. Brain Stimul. 2013;6:221–30. https://doi.org/10.1016/j.brs.2012.06.008.
154. Ceccanti M, Inghilleri M, Attilia ML, Raccah R, Fiore M, Zangen A, Ceccanti M. Deep TMS on alcoholics: effects on cortisolemia and dopamine pathway modulation. A pilot study. Can J Physiol Pharmacol. 2015;93:283–90. https://doi.org/10.1139/cjpp-2014-0188.
155. Lucatch AM, Lowe DJE, Clark RC, Kozak K, George TP. Neurobiological determinants of tobacco smoking in schizophrenia. Front Psych. 2018;9:672. https://doi.org/10.3389/fpsyt.2018.00672.
156. Martinotti G, Santacroce R, Pettorruso M, Montemitro C, Spano MC, Lorusso M, di Giannantonio M, Lerner AG. Hallucinogen Persisting Perception Disorder: Etiology, Clinical

Features, and Therapeutic Perspectives. Brain Sci. 2018 Mar 16;8(3). pii: E47. https://doi. org/10.3390/brainsci8030047.

157. Spagnolo PA, Montemitro C, Pettorruso M, Martinotti G, Di Giannantonio M. Better Together? Coupling Pharmacotherapies and Cognitive Interventions With Non-invasive Brain Stimulation for the Treatment of Addictive Disorders. Front Neurosci. 2020 Jan 10;13:1385. https://doi.org/10.3389/fnins.2019.01385.

158. Salling MC, Martinez D. Brain stimulation in addiction. Neuropsychopharmacology. 2016;41:2798–809. https://doi.org/10.1038/npp.2016.80.

159. Trojak B, Meille V, Achab S, Lalanne L, Poquet H, Ponavoy E, Blaise E, Bonin B, Chauvet-Gelinier J-C. Transcranial magnetic stimulation combined with nicotine replacement therapy for smoking cessation: a randomized controlled trial. Brain Stimul. 2015;8:1168–74. https:// doi.org/10.1016/j.brs.2015.06.004.

160. Martinotti G, Lupi M, Montemitro C, Miuli A, Di Natale C, Spano MC, Mancini V, Lorusso M, Stigliano G, Tambelli A, Di Carlo F, Di Caprio L, Fraticelli S, Chillemi E, Pettorruso M, Sepede G, di Giannantonio M. Transcranial direct current stimulation reduces craving in substance use disorders: a double-blind, placebo-controlled study. J ECT. 2019a;35(3):207–11. https://doi.org/10.1097/YCT.0000000000000580.

161. Martinotti G, Montemitro C, Pettorruso M, Viceconte D, Alessi MC, Di Carlo F, Lucidi L, Picutti E, Santacroce R, Di Giannantonio M. Augmenting pharmacotherapy with neuromodulation techniques for the treatment of bipolar disorder: a focus on the effects of mood stabilizers on cortical excitability. Expert Opin Pharmacother. 2019b:1–14. https://doi.org/1 0.1080/14656566.2019.1622092.

162. Jansen JM, Daams JG, Koeter MWJ, Veltman DJ, van den Brink W, Goudriaan AE. Effects of non-invasive neurostimulation on craving: a meta-analysis. Neurosci Biobehav Rev. 2013;37:2472–80. https://doi.org/10.1016/j.neubiorev.2013.07.009.

163. Schluter RS, Daams JG, van Holst RJ, Goudriaan AE. Effects of non-invasive neuromodulation on executive and other cognitive functions in addictive disorders: a systematic review. Front Neurosci. 2018;12:642. https://doi.org/10.3389/fnins.2018.00642.

164. Pettorruso M, di Giannantonio M, De Risio L, Martinotti G, Koob GF. A light in the darkness: repetitive transcranial magnetic stimulation (rTMS) to treat the hedonic dysregulation of addiction. J Addict Med. 2019; https://doi.org/10.1097/ADM.0000000000000575.

165. Sturgess JE, George TP, Kennedy JL, Heinz A, Muller DJ. Pharmacogenetics of alcohol, nicotine and drug addiction treatments. Addict Biol. 2011;16:357–76. https://doi. org/10.1111/j.1369-1600.2010.00287.x.

166. Spano MC, Lorusso M, Pettorruso M, Zoratto F, Di Giuda D, Martinotti G, di Giannantonio M. Anhedonia across borders: Transdiagnostic relevance of reward dysfunction for noninvasive brain stimulation endophenotypes. CNS Neurosci Ther. 2019 Nov;25(11):1229–36. https://doi.org/10.1111/cns.13230.

167. Pettorruso M, Martinotti G, Montemitro C, Miuli A, Spano MC, Lorusso M, Vellante F, di Giannantonio M. Craving and Other Transdiagnostic Dimensions in Addiction: Toward Personalized Neuromodulation Treatments. J ECT. 2020;6. https://doi.org/10.1097/YCT.0000000000000643.

168. Ibrahim C, Rubin-Kahana DS, Pushparaj A, Musiol M, Blumberger DM, Daskalakis ZJ, Zangen A, Le Foll B. The insula: a brain stimulation target for the treatment of addiction. Front Pharmacol. 2019;10:720. https://doi.org/10.3389/fphar.2019.00720.

Transcranial Magnetic Stimulation in Dementia: From Pathophysiology to Treatment

12

Giacomo Koch

12.1 Introduction

Alzheimer's disease (AD) is one of the most devastating forms of dementia, being considered a remarkable problem due to the ageing of the population. It is nowadays considered as one of the most serious medical, economic, and social emergencies faced by our society, and it is predicted to become even more problematic over the next decades. Unfortunately, there are no effective treatments, and patients diagnosed with AD face an uncertain future, caused by the current inability to predict the course of the disease. The only approved treatment for AD is indeed based on standard cholinergic and glutamatergic drugs, whose clinical efficacy is overall negligible and debated. Since the 1990s, symptomatic therapies have been available, which moderately improve cognition and function. The most frequently prescribed treatments for AD are Acetylcholinesterase Inhibitors (AchEIs) and memantine. These therapies may provide transient relief from some symptoms (6–12 months in most cases), but are unable to reduce the progressive decline of everyday activities, communication, and social behavior [1]. In addition, the current treatments are not effective for everyone: it is estimated that only approximately 40–70% of the patients benefit from current treatments. Based on this, and on the significant limitations of the current treatment options, more effective symptomatic therapies, particularly in the earlier stages of AD, are needed. Nonetheless, recent clinical trials based on new "putative" disease-modifying drugs have failed in reaching their principal clinical outcome.

G. Koch (✉)

Non-invasive Brain Stimulation Unit, Department of Clinical and Behavioral Neurology, IRCCS Santa Lucia Foundation, Rome, Italy

Department of Psychology, eCampus University, Novedrate, Italy
e-mail: g.koch@hsantalucia.it

So far, relatively well-defined criteria have been identified for the diagnosis of early AD, based on patients' clinical presentation and biomarkers' profile. In particular, recent consensus was found on the necessity to determine the presence of beta-amyloid- and tau-related pathology. Evidence of these abnormalities may be identified either by cerebrospinal fluid (CSF) sampling or Positron Emission Tomography (PET) imaging, using specific ligands [2]. Nonetheless, the clinical course of AD remains largely variable at single subject level. This is mainly due to the modest understanding we presently have of AD pathophysiology. Critically, the mechanisms determining the severity of AD progression, and those counteracting it, are largely unknown, thus preventing any consistent prognostic estimate at the individual patient level. Thus, there is a critical demand to explore other paths that may expand our knowledge on the pathophysiological changes occurring in AD, especially in the early phases of the disease, when the first minimal signs appear or even before.

In this perspective, I review the emerging contribution of transcranial magnetic stimulation (TMS), a noninvasive brain stimulation method that may allow to determine new key pathophysiological features characterizing the different forms of dementia. Moreover, I will consider the application of repetitive sessions of noninvasive brain stimulation such as repetitive TMS (rTMS) as a new promising therapeutic strategy to slow down the progression of cognitive decline.

12.2   Synaptic Dysfunction in AD

The aggregation and deposition of amyloid-β (Aβ) and tau proteins are two fundamental factors recognized in AD pathogenesis. These pathological processes are thought to start many years before the onset of cognitive impairment. However, the first signs of cognitive damage appear only when a substantial synaptic loss has occurred in vulnerable brain regions [3].

CSF concentrations of beta-amyloid 1–42, total tau (t-tau), and phosphorylated tau (p-tau) proteins have been recently put forward as a useful tool for AD diagnosis and phenotyping. Notably, AD patients with higher levels of CSF t-tau and p-tau have been reported to exhibit a more malignant disease course [4]. Recently, growing evidence has shown that the accumulation of tau pathology is highly associated with functional and structural weakening of AD brains [5]. Moreover, it has been established that the gathering of "tangles" correlates with patients' level of cognitive deterioration, while beta-amyloid requires the presence of tau proteins to develop its toxicity. Thus, the progressive neuronal and synaptic loss mirrors the cumulative result of different pathologic substrates in AD and, therefore, may provide the best marker to follow disease progression. However, it has to be taken into account that synaptic dysfunction is an initial and noticeable pathological feature of AD preceding neuronal loss in numerous brain areas. In basic science studies, earlier investigations have mainly focused on the direct toxic effects of beta-amyloid into AD-related synaptic damages. Only recently, an emergent role of tau was established [6]. It was shown that tau overexpression is able to induce synaptic degeneration even in the absence of neurofibrillary tangles. This synaptic dysfunction has been directly associated with the onset of early memory impairments observed in patients with AD [7].

Actually, although several AD biomarkers are widely applied and considered useful for diagnosis, sufficient accuracy is still lacking in evaluating disease severity and predicting disease progression and response to therapy both considering CSF and neuroimaging parameters, such as hippocampal atrophy/whole brain volume [7]. In particular, the use of a single biomarker provides too limited information to define the complex underlying severity of disease across its entire range, from pre-clinical to clinical phases of AD. Moreover, AD biomarkers assessment is routinely performed by means of invasive and/or high-cost procedures, limiting their use in clinical practice. Indeed, the evidence provided by brain imaging methods is merely correlative. Thus, several efforts are underway to combine multiple biomarkers to predict the severity of AD, with the major difficulty in tracking the temporally different evolution of each biomarker throughout the disease course [7].

In recent years, growing evidence has highlighted the notion that loss of synaptic density could be an early event antecedent to neuronal degeneration, suggesting that the impairment of synaptic plasticity mechanisms should play a key role in the pathogenesis of AD [3]. Notably, in various efforts to find semiquantitative correlations between the progressive cognitive impairment and brain pathological alterations, the strongest relationship has been found between the loss of synaptic density and the degree of cognitive impairment in AD. Thus, the impairment of synaptic transmission due to toxic oligomeric species [8] could predict disease severity more precisely than neuronal loss, which is considered a more tardive event. This evidence finds support on experimental studies showing that Aβ peptides and tau proteins can interfere with physiological mechanisms of neuronal synaptic plasticity in AD animal models. In particular, it has been demonstrated that these molecules influence hippocampal long-term potentiation (LTP) [9], which is related to memory impairment occurring in AD.

These altered mechanisms have been linked to different alterations occurring at different levels of observation, including spine shrinkage, neuronal network disarrangement, and cell death [10]. Taken together, this evidence suggests that synaptic dysfunction, occurring at different levels of brain activity, could represent a key driver of AD-related cognitive decline.

Despite this promising evidence, so far it has not been possible to quantify synaptic functioning (or dysfunction) directly in vivo in AD patients. Different in vivo techniques, such as 18F-fluorodeoxyglucose positron emission tomography (FDG-PET) [11], functional magnetic resonance imaging (fMRI) [12] and electroencephalography (EEG), have been used in order to provide useful biomarkers for synaptic dysfunction and network connectivity in AD progression [13]. However, FDG-PET and fMRI techniques provide only an indirect estimate of synaptic dysfunction, being limited by a low temporal resolution that does not allow to track synaptic activity at the physiological time scale in which neuronal interactions occur (i.e., in the range of milliseconds). Indeed, imaging methods infer alterations of synaptic activity as a consequence of slow and subtle changes in metabolic parameters, such as blood-oxygen-level-dependent contrast imaging (BOLD) used in fMRI. These signals are indeed relative, and not individually quantitative, and observe changes in blood oxygenations occurring across several seconds, being very far from real-time synaptic activity. Moreover, despite all the advances in imaging of AD in the research setting, there is a lack of translation of these methodologies into the clinical practice. Most imaging biomarkers have not been validated in unselected patient cohorts and participants in large AD studies are not representative of the general population. These techniques require special facilities and expertise to perform and interpret. The paucity of standard acquisition and analysis methods between different centers makes the widespread adoption of them even more challenging. In addition, some of the new imaging modalities are still too expensive to be considered cost effective in a community setting or in nonspecialized centers.

12.3   TMS to Measure Synaptic Dysfunction in AD

On the other hand, TMS-based methods provide the possibility to evaluate in real time the brain electrical activity in the healthy and pathological conditions. It is based on the principle that brain stimulation can be induced by generating a brief, high-intensity magnetic field by passing a brief electric current through a magnetic coil. When a substantial electrical current is induced in a stimulating coil, this is able to produce a transient time-variable magnetic field. When a magnetic field of this sort and sufficient strength is applied to the brain, it can induce an electrical current in the brain producing firing of groups of nerve cells. When stimulation of this sort is applied repeatedly, it will progressively change brain activity. The discovery and practical application of these basic techniques has led to the widespread use of TMS in neuroscientific and clinical applications [14]. Within this background, TMS-based approach may represent a valid tool to overcome the problems limiting other imaging techniques to track dysfunction of synaptic activity in incipient dementia [15–17].

Depending on the adopted protocol, it is possible to test key physiological aspects of synaptic activity at different levels of local and global complexity. TMS allows (1) to investigate in detail the properties of local interneural networks that are mediated by specific neurotransmitters [18], (2) to determine the capability of specific areas of the brain to form cortical plasticity [19], (3) to assess the ongoing oscillatory activity of a specific area or across broader and more distributed brain networks [20] and (4) to establish causal relationships between stimulation and subsequent changes in cerebral function and behavioral outcome, by combining measurements of network-based neural activity [21].

For instance, paired pulse TMS protocols applied over specific areas of the brain (e.g., the primary motor cortex) allow to evaluate in vivo the activity of different intracortical circuits such as short intracortical inhibition (SICI), reflecting GABAergic neurotransmission, and short afferent inhibition (SAI) probing cholinergic neurotransmission in AD patients [22, 23]. SICI is measured by paired-pulse TMS: a subthreshold conditioning stimulus and a suprathreshold test stimulus are applied at short interstimulus intervals of 1–5 ms through the same stimulating coil [24]. It has been hypothesized that SICI represents short-lasting inhibitory postsynaptic potentials (IPSPs) in corticospinal neurons through activation of a low-threshold cortical inhibitory circuit [24]. SAI refers to a MEP inhibition in a hand muscle produced by a conditioning afferent electrical stimulus applied to the median or ulnar nerve at the wrist approximately 20 ms prior to focal TMS of the hand area of the contralateral motor cortex. AchEIs increasing the availability of acetylcholine in the synaptic cleft were observed to normalize the abnormally reduced SAI in patients with Alzheimer's disease [25], while nicotine was found to increase SAI in healthy nonsmoking subjects [26]. These data are consistent with the view that SAI represents central cholinergic activity controlled by inhibitory circuits separate from those underlying SICI.

Depending on their specific frequency and/or patterning, different rTMS protocols result in excitatory or inhibitory after-effects lasting several minutes, which have been linked to LTP or to long-term depression (LTD). Repetitive TMS over the primary motor area can be used to measure in vivo cortical plasticity mechanisms such as LTP, which is considered the main neurophysiological correlate for learning and memory [19, 27]. Theta burst stimulation (TBS) is a novel form of rTMS that was developed recently to match theta burst patterns of stimulation commonly used to induce plasticity in animal brain slices. Intermittent TBS (iTBS) enhances cortical excitability for up to 1 h inducing LTP. These after-effects are thought to reflect rTMS influences on the strength of glutamatergic synapses via NMDA receptor, AMPA receptor, and calcium channel effects [28]. Long-lasting influences on the brain depend on changing synaptic strength or causing anatomical changes such as alterations in dendritic spines or sprouting. Since the anatomical changes may well be a secondary consequence of prolonged changes of synaptic strength, the basic logic of TMS stimulation is to change synaptic strength [29].

The combination of TMS with EEG (TMS-EEG) has provided an emergent method to directly probe local and widespread cortical dynamics, through the recording of TMS-evoked potentials (TEPs) [30]. TEPs have the great advantage to be highly reproducible, demonstrating consistency over time, but also to be extremely sensitive to changes in brain state. Moreover, TMS-EEG allows to investigate brain oscillatory activity within a specific area and between anatomically distinct brain regions, which is relevant when considering AD as a disconnection syndrome. TMS-EEG can indeed verify challenging aspect of the clinical assessment of brain disorders independently from patients' ability to interact with the external environment. Theoretical considerations suggest that efficient brain activity involves complex patterns that are, at once, distributed among interacting cortical areas (integrated) and differentiated in space and time (information-rich).

rTMS can also be applied to establish causal relationships between stimulation and subsequent changes in cerebral function and behavioral outcome, for instance by combining fMRI measurements of network-based neural activity. In this scenario, trains of rTMS can be applied over a certain brain area, presumably a key node of a certain network and the induced changes in connectivity may be analyzed by means of resting-state fMRI. These two complementary tools can be combined to optimally study brain connectivity and manipulate distributed brain networks. Important clinical applications include using resting-state fMRI to guide target selection for TMS and using TMS to modulate pathological network interactions identified with resting-state fMRI. The combination of TMS and resting-state fMRI has the potential to accelerate the translation of both techniques into the clinical realm and promises a new approach to the diagnosis and treatment of neurological and psychiatric diseases that demonstrate network pathology [21].

12.4   TMS-Based Biomarkers in AD

On the basis of this background, we and others recently introduced the notion that TMS can be considered a novel tool to shape early features of synaptic dysfunction at different levels of complexity in patients with dementia. We recently showed that a systematic TMS-based assessment of GABAergic and cholinergic neurotransmission reliably distinguishes AD patients from those with frontotemporal dementia (FTD) and age-matched healthy controls (HC) and, therefore, TMS could represent a sensible diagnostic tool for clinical practice. Short-latency afferent inhibition (SAI), assessing the function of cholinergic circuits indirectly, has been found to be impaired in patients with AD; conversely, short-interval intracortical inhibition (SICI) and intracortical facilitation (ICF), markers of γ-aminobutyric acid type A (GABAA)ergic and glutamatergic neurotransmission, respectively, have been found to be impaired in patients with FTD [23]. These findings stemmed from the evidence that AD is defined by both amyloid deposits and a well-established cholinergic deficit, whereas in FTD, abnormalities in glutamatergic and GABAergic neurotransmission have been reported. Thus, the assessment of TMS intracortical connectivity holds promise to be a useful tool in the differential diagnosis of neurodegenerative diseases, being free from strict exclusion criteria, not time consuming, and inexpensive. However, its clinical value needs to be further demonstrated, also taking into consideration that both conditions may show several overlapping features, such as amyloid positivity in FTD, cholinergic deficits in FTD, or glutamatergic overexpression in AD [31].

On the other hand, we were among the first to demonstrate that LTP-like cortical plasticity is consistently impaired in AD patients, as assessed with iTBS protocol applied over the primary motor cortex [27]. The motor cortex is considered a reliable model to investigate early changes in cortical plasticity and central cholinergic transmission occurring in AD patients who are affected only at later stages of the disease, when AD becomes clinically manifest. Cortical plasticity is regarded as the principal biological mechanism for learning and memory. In humans, it can be assessed by noninvasive rTMS [19], in strict analogy with the hippocampal plasticity assessable in animal models. In the case of AD, synaptic loss is the strongest pathophysiological correlate of cognitive decline, indicating that synaptic degeneration has a central role in the development of dementia [32]. Experimental animal models showed that accumulation of soluble Aβ oligomers specifically blocks mechanisms of cortical plasticity such as hippocampal LTP, which is regarded as an electrophysiological correlate of learning and memory [33]. In contrast, these oligomers have been shown to electrically facilitate evoked LTD [34]. These events can, in turn, induce changes in the conformation of tau proteins, leading to further detrimental effects on synaptic plasticity and cognition.

Similar mechanisms of cortical plasticity can be investigated in vivo and noninvasively in humans, although the plasticity-induction procedures adopted are not completely identical in humans and animals. As discussed earlier, repetitive TMS over the primary motor area can be used to measure in vivo cortical plasticity mechanisms such as LTP.

In the context of AD, TMS applied over the motor cortex is considered a reliable model to investigate early changes in cortical plasticity and central cholinergic transmission occurring early in the disease [35].

In general AD patients, as opposed to HCs, are characterized by a weakened LTP-like cortical plasticity together with an impairment of SAI, putative biomarker of central cholinergic transmission [27]. In a large cohort of newly diagnosed sporadic AD patients, it was found that overall AD patients show after iTBS an impairment of LTP-like cortical plasticity, forming a paradoxical LTD in comparison to HCs. Moreover, SAI was impaired in AD showing a strong association with the individual age of subjects rather than with disease age of onset, while there was no association between age of onset and impairment of cortical plasticity. Thus, it was argued that cortical LTP disruption is a central mechanism of AD that is independent of age of onset [17]. Moreover, LTP-like cortical plasticity impairment is selectively associated with a less efficient verbal memory, but not to other cognitive functions, independent from biomarkers and other demographic and clinical factors [36]. Remarkably, LTP-like cortical plasticity is the most powerful TMS measurement in identifying AD patients among different neurophysiological parameters [37]. Motta et al. used TMS-based parameters to evaluate LTP-like cortical plasticity and cholinergic activity as measured by short afferent inhibition (SAI) in 60 newly diagnosed patients with AD and 30 HCs. Receiver-operating characteristic (ROC) curves were used to assess TMS ability in discriminating patients with AD from HCs. It was found that the area under the ROC curve was 0.90 for LTP-like cortical plasticity, indicating an excellent accuracy of this parameter in detecting AD pathology.

Apart from determining the diagnostic accuracy of TMS, we also showed that LTP-like cortical plasticity is able to predict cognitive decline in AD patients. The probability of a faster cognitive decline increased with every point decrease of LTP-like cortical plasticity, suggesting that the level of cortical plasticity evaluated at early stages of the disease is strictly linked to the subsequent clinical worsening in these patients. This finding is supported by experimental works showing that synaptic loss is the strongest pathophysiological correlate of cognitive decline, pointing to synaptic degeneration as a central mechanism in the dementia [37]. Furthermore, more impaired LTP-like cortical plasticity was associated with higher t-tau, but not 1–42 Aβ CSF levels. Aβ peptides exist in several soluble forms (oligomers) that can be released in the extracellular space where they may induce direct detrimental effects on neuronal transmission. However, consistent with previous findings, Aβ

1–42 fragments detected in the CSF of AD patients did not correlate with measures of cortical plasticity. In particular, we found that high tau CSF levels were associated with a paradoxical response toward LTD-like cortical plasticity instead of the expected LTP-like cortical. The same patients underwent a faster clinical progression [16]. These results suggest that more aggressive tau pathology is associated with prominent LTD-like mechanisms of cortical plasticity and faster cognitive decline. In this complex picture, synaptic dysfunction is likely to be influenced also by genetic factors. For instance, there is a strong relationship between Apolipoprotein E (APOE) polymorphisms and cortical plasticity, since APOE is known to regulate both beta-amyloid clearance/aggregation and tau-related microtubule stabilization, being strictly linked with altered mechanisms of synaptic plasticity. In a recent work from our group, it was found that the presence of APOE polymorphisms implies different mechanisms of CSF tau-related dysfunction in AD patients [38]. Indeed, high CSF tau levels are associated with impaired cortical plasticity and more aggressive disease progression only in AD patients carrying APOE4, but not APOE3 genotype. In parallel, CSF tau levels influence apoptosis in normal human astrocytes when incubated with CSF collected from AD patients with APOE4, but not APOE3 genotype. Taken together, these findings reveal that CSF tau levels are linked to cortical plasticity, cognitive decline, and astrocyte survival only when associated with APOE4 genotype [38].

In the field of dementia, TMS-EEG has been scarcely used. So far, in AD patients, only a few TMS-EEG studies investigated cortical correlates of cognitive impairment. Although the findings of these studies highlighted an association of cortical activity changes with cognitive decline and showed good specificity and sensitivity in identifying healthy subjects from those with cognitive impairment, the potential of TMS-EEG in tracking longitudinally disease progression was not investigated [39]. In the context of AD, we recently showed that innovative combined TMS-EEG protocols provide the possibility to directly measure cortical functional activity in cognitive-related areas, such as the dorsolateral prefrontal cortex (DLPFC) or the posterior parietal cortex (PPC), extending the potential role of TMS-based biomarkers in assessing the effects of therapies on cortical activity outside the primary motor cortex [40].

The detection of novel TMS-EEG markers of synaptic dysfunction (in terms of cortical excitability, connectivity, and oscillation) might contribute to provide additional predictive biomarkers of response to therapies in AD.

12.5 TMS-Based Therapeutics in AD

To date, the mainstream treatment for AD patients is represented only by cholinergic and glutamatergic drugs. However, pharmacological treatments have limited efficacy and are accompanied by adverse side effects. For this, it is of great importance to develop alternative therapeutic approaches. Recently, different forms of noninvasive brain stimulation techniques (e.g., TMS) have been applied to patients with AD in order to improve cognitive decline and behavioral disorders. In recent years, treatments based on multiple sessions of rTMS have represented a promising tool for influencing cognition in people with neurodegenerative diseases. This procedure is noninvasive and painless, and it does not require the use of anesthesia or pharmacological substances. The key principle of rTMS is based not only on regularly "repeated" stimulation of a focal cortical area but also on "accelerated" stimulation with multiple sessions and stimuli, leading to long-lasting modulation of the brain plasticity. From a neurobiological perspective, rTMS could induce relevant clinical improvement by promoting changes in synaptic plasticity. Synaptic plasticity is the most important biological mechanism accounting for learning and memory; in particular, LTP is considered as a main neurophysiological correlate of these cognitive functions [36]. We recently demonstrated that AD patients showed a disruption in LTP-like cortical plasticity since the early stages of the disease [37]. In this context, high-frequency rTMS could enhance LTP-like cortical plasticity, thus resulting in changes both at local and network levels as revealed by TMS-EGG and fMRI studies.

Until now, several studies have exclusively explored the effects of intensive treatments, lasting 2 weeks. Recently, safety and efficacy of maintenance with rTMS treatment in early AD patients showed a long-term trend with less cognitive decline than would be expected [41]. Noninvasive brain stimulation methods have been recently proposed as a novel approach to improve cognitive functions in patients with dementia, targeting the prefrontal cortex as a key area to be stimulated [42–45]. Moreover, novel interesting approaches are considering the possibility to stimulate in the same patients more areas such as the right and left DLPFC, Broca and Wernicke areas, and the right and left parietal somatosensory association cortex in conjunction with active cognitive training targeting these same brain regions [46].

However, since the early stages of AD, prominent neuropathological abnormalities (i.e., β-amyloid plaques and neurofibrillary tangles) involve posterior cortical regions of the brain, including the precuneus (PC), the posterior cingulate, the retrosplenial, and lateral PPC. Moreover, there is an initial disruption of medial frontoparietal functional connectivity. Specifically, AD patients show alterations of the so-called default mode network (DMN), for which the PC is a key node [47]. Interestingly, at early clinical stages of AD, disconnection of the PC precedes (and probably contributes to) the occurrence of regional brain atrophy, which becomes prominent at later disease stages [48]. This means that the PC is a vulnerable region for the transitional stage toward dementia, which may be targeted by tailored interventions. Indeed, AD patients often show a reduction of PC cortical thickness accompanied by an abnormal activation during memory tasks and decreased functional connectivity. This is especially relevant since the activity of the PC is considered necessary for episodic memory retrieval [49], whose impairment represents the clinical onset of typical AD. Thus, the PC represents an ideal target for interventions aimed at slowing down and potentially counteracting memory decline in AD patients.

This hypothesis finds support in a recent experimental work performed in healthy subjects showing that TMS [50] was effective in modulating short- and long-term memory functions when applied over the PPC and PC. Following this line of evidence, we recently showed that 20-Hz rTMS was able to increase long-term memory performance and to potentiate the cortical activity of the PC. This provides novel evidence that noninvasive treatment of network dysfunction, through stimulation of the PC, represents a potentially efficacious strategy to improve cognitive dysfunction in AD. We showed that high-frequency excitatory rTMS improved long-term memory in patients with AD, by modulating both local neural activity and the connections with parietal, frontal and temporal areas.

However, the effects were only evaluated in a short-term course temporal window of 2 weeks. Sham-controlled rTMS trials are needed to explore whether rTMS may have a clinical impact in modifying the course of AD when applied over clinically relevant periods of 6–12 months.

12.6   Conclusions

TMS is contributing to shape the characteristics of synaptic dysfunction in AD patients, helping to increase diagnostic accuracy, and providing relevant clinical information in terms of disease progression and response to therapy.

On the other hand, there is a great interest in developing novel rTMS protocols that may have the potential to improve cognitive functions in patients with mild dementia and eventually slow down cognitive decline, if applied during a long-term period of several months.

References

1. Howard R, McShane R, Lindesay J, Ritchie C, Baldwin A, Barber R, Burns A, Dening T, Findlay D, Holmes C, Hughes A. Donepezil and memantine for moderate-to-severe Alzheimer's disease. N Engl J Med. 2012;366(10):893–903.
2. Dubois B, Hampel H, Feldman HH, Scheltens P, Aisen P, Andrieu S, Bakardjian H, Benali H, Bertram L, Blennow K, Broich K. Preclinical Alzheimer's disease: definition, natural history, and diagnostic criteria. Alzheimers Dement. 2016;12(3):292–323.
3. Jack CR Jr, Knopman DS, Jagust WJ, Petersen RC, Weiner MW, Aisen PS, Shaw LM, Vemuri P, Wiste HJ, Weigand SD, Lesnick TG. Tracking pathophysiological processes in Alzheimer's disease: an updated hypothetical model of dynamic biomarkers. Lancet Neurol. 2013;12(2):207–16.
4. Wallin ÅK, Blennow K, Zetterberg H, Londos E, Minthon L, Hansson O. CSF biomarkers predict a more malignant outcome in Alzheimer disease. Neurology. 2010;74(19):1531–7.
5. Cho H, Choi JY, Hwang MS, Kim YJ, Lee HM, Lee HS, Lee JH, Ryu YH, Lee MS, Lyoo CH. In vivo cortical spreading pattern of tau and amyloid in the Alzheimer disease spectrum. Ann Neurol. 2016;80(2):247–58.
6. Yin Y, Gao D, Wang Y, Wang ZH, Wang X, Ye J, Wu D, Fang L, Pi G, Yang Y, Wang XC. Tau accumulation induces synaptic impairment and memory deficit by calcineurin-mediated inactivation of nuclear CaMKIV/CREB signaling. Proc Natl Acad Sci. 2016;113(26):E3773–81.
7. Scheff SW, Price DA, Schmitt FA, DeKosky ST, Mufson EJ. Synaptic alterations in CA1 in mild Alzheimer disease and mild cognitive impairment. Neurology. 2007;68(18):1501–8.
8. Selkoe DJ. The therapeutics of Alzheimer's disease: where we stand and where we are heading. Ann Neurol. 2013;74(3):328–36.

9. Selkoe DJ. Alzheimer's disease is a synaptic failure. Science. 2002;298(5594):789–91.
10. Lasagna-Reeves CA, de Haro M, Hao S, Park J, Rousseaux MW, Al-Ramahi I, Jafar-Nejad P, Vilanova-Velez L, See L, De Maio A, Nitschke L. Reduction of Nuak1 decreases tau and reverses phenotypes in a tauopathy mouse model. Neuron. 2016;92(2):407–18.
11. Mosconi L, Pupi A, De Leon MJ. Brain glucose hypometabolism and oxidative stress in preclinical Alzheimer's disease. Ann N Y Acad Sci. 2008;1147:180.
12. Brickman AM, Small SA, Fleisher A. Pinpointing synaptic loss caused by Alzheimer's disease with fMRI. Behav Neurol. 2009;21(1–2):93–100.
13. Cook IA, Leuchter AF. Synaptic dysfunction in Alzheimer's disease: clinical assessment using quantitative EEG. Behav Brain Res. 1996;78(1):15–23.
14. Fitzgerald PB, Daskalakis ZJ. Repetitive transcranial magnetic stimulation treatment for depressive disorders: a practical guide. Berlin: Springer Science & Business Media; 2013.
15. Cantone M, Di Pino G, Capone F, Piombo M, Chiarello D, Cheeran B, Pennisi G, Di Lazzaro V. The contribution of transcranial magnetic stimulation in the diagnosis and in the management of dementia. Clin Neurophysiol. 2014;125(8):1509–32.
16. Koch G, Di Lorenzo F, Del Olmo MF, Bonnì S, Ponzo V, Caltagirone C, Bozzali M, Martorana A. Reversal of LTP-like cortical plasticity in Alzheimer's disease patients with tau-related faster clinical progression. J Alzheimers Dis. 2016;50(2):605–16.
17. Di Lorenzo F, Ponzo V, Bonnì S, Motta C, Negrão Serra PC, Bozzali M, Caltagirone C, Martorana A, Koch G. Long-term potentiation–like cortical plasticity is disrupted in Alzheimer's disease patients independently from age of onset. Ann Neurol. 2016;80(2):202–10.
18. Ziemann U. 1. Neuromodulation of motor learning in health and after stroke. Clin Neurophysiol. 2012;3(123):e9.
19. Huang YZ, Edwards MJ, Rounis E, Bhatia KP, Rothwell JC. Theta burst stimulation of the human motor cortex. Neuron. 2005;45(2):201–6.
20. Rosanova M, Casali A, Bellina V, Resta F, Mariotti M, Massimini M. Natural frequencies of human corticothalamic circuits. J Neurosci. 2009;29(24):7679–85.
21. Fox MD, Halko MA, Eldaief MC, Pascual-Leone A. Measuring and manipulating brain connectivity with resting state functional connectivity magnetic resonance imaging (fcMRI) and transcranial magnetic stimulation (TMS). NeuroImage. 2012;62(4):2232–43.
22. Di Lazzaro V, Rothwell JC. Corticospinal activity evoked and modulated by non-invasive stimulation of the intact human motor cortex. J Physiol. 2014;592(19):4115–28.
23. Benussi A, Di Lorenzo F, Dell'Era V, Cosseddu M, Alberici A, Caratozzolo S, Cotelli MS, Micheli A, Rozzini L, Depari A, Flammini A, Ponzo V, Martorana A, Caltagirone C, Padovani A, Koch G, Borroni B. Transcranial magnetic stimulation distinguishes Alzheimer disease from frontotemporal dementia. Neurology. 2017;89(7):665–72.
24. Kujirai T, Caramia MD, Rothwell JC, Day BL, Thompson PD, Ferbert A, Wroe S, Asselman P, Marsden CD. Corticocortical inhibition in human motor cortex. J Physiol. 1993;471(1):501–19.
25. Di Lazzaro V, Oliviero A, Pilato F, Saturno E, Dileone M, Marra C, Daniele A, Ghirlanda S, Gainotti G, Tonali PA. Motor cortex hyperexcitability to transcranial magnetic stimulation in Alzheimer's disease. J Neurol Neurosurg Psychiatry. 2004;75(4):555–9.
26. Grundey J, Freznosa S, Klinker F, Lang N, Paulus W, Nitsche MA. Cortical excitability in smoking and not smoking individuals with and without nicotine. Psychopharmacology. 2013;229(4):653–64.
27. Koch G, Di Lorenzo F, Bonnì S, Ponzo V, Caltagirone C, Martorana A. Impaired LTP-but not LTD-like cortical plasticity in Alzheimer's disease patients. J Alzheimers Dis. 2012;31(3):593–9.
28. Huang YZ, Chen RS, Rothwell JC, Wen HY. The after-effect of human theta burst stimulation is NMDA receptor dependent. Clin Neurophysiol. 2007;118(5):1028–32.
29. Hallett M. Transcranial magnetic stimulation: a primer. Neuron. 2007;55(2):187–99.
30. Miniussi C, Thut G. Combining TMS and EEG offers new prospects in cognitive neuroscience. Brain Topogr. 2010;22(4):249.

31. Benussi A, Alberici A, Ferrari C, Cantoni V, Dell'Era V, Turrone R, Cotelli MS, Binetti G, Paghera B, Koch G, Padovani A. The impact of transcranial magnetic stimulation on diagnostic confidence in patients with Alzheimer disease. Alzheimers Res Ther. 2018;10(1):94.
32. Klyubin I, Betts V, Welzel AT, Blennow K, Zetterberg H, Wallin A, Lemere CA, Cullen WK, Peng Y, Wisniewski T, Selkoe DJ. Amyloid β protein dimer-containing human CSF disrupts synaptic plasticity: prevention by systemic passive immunization. J Neurosci. 2008;28(16):4231–7.
33. Palop JJ, Mucke L. Amyloid-β–induced neuronal dysfunction in Alzheimer's disease: from synapses toward neural networks. Nat Neurosci. 2010;13(7):812.
34. Li S, Hong S, Shepardson NE, Walsh DM, Shankar GM, Selkoe D. Soluble oligomers of amyloid β protein facilitate hippocampal long-term depression by disrupting neuronal glutamate uptake. Neuron. 2009;62(6):788–801.
35. Battaglia F, Wang HY, Ghilardi MF, Gashi E, Quartarone A, Friedman E, Nixon RA. Cortical plasticity in Alzheimer's disease in humans and rodents. Biol Psychiatry. 2007;62(12):1405–12.
36. Di Lorenzo F, Motta C, Bonnì S, Mercuri NB, Caltagirone C, Martorana A, Koch G. LTP-like cortical plasticity is associated with verbal memory impairment in Alzheimer's disease patients. Brain Stimul. 2019;12(1):148–51.
37. Motta C, Di Lorenzo F, Ponzo V, Pellicciari MC, Bonnì S, Picazio S, Mercuri NB, Caltagirone C, Martorana A, Koch G. Transcranial magnetic stimulation predicts cognitive decline in patients with Alzheimer's disease. J Neurol Neurosurg Psychiatry. 2018;89(12):1237–42.
38. Koch G, Di Lorenzo F, Loizzo S, Motta C, Travaglione S, Baiula M, Rimondini R, Ponzo V, Bonnì S, Toniolo S. Sallustio F. CSF tau is associated with impaired cortical plasticity, cognitive decline and astrocyte survival only in APOE4-positive Alzheimer's disease. Sci Rep. 2017;7(1):13728.
39. Ferreri F, Vecchio F, Vollero L, Guerra A, Petrichella S, Ponzo D, Määtta S, Mervaala E, Könönen M, Ursini F, Pasqualetti P. Sensorimotor cortex excitability and connectivity in Alzheimer's disease: a TMS-EEG co-registration study. Hum Brain Mapp. 2016;37(6):2083–96.
40. Koch G, Bonnì S, Pellicciari MC, Casula EP, Mancini M, Esposito R, Ponzo V, Picazio S, Di Lorenzo F, Serra L, Motta C. Transcranial magnetic stimulation of the precuneus enhances memory and neural activity in prodromal Alzheimer's disease. NeuroImage. 2018;169:302–11.
41. Lefaucheur JP, André-Obadia N, Antal A, Ayache SS, Baeken C, Benninger DH, Cantello RM, Cincotta M, de Carvalho M, De Ridder D, Devanne H. Evidence-based guidelines on the therapeutic use of repetitive transcranial magnetic stimulation (rTMS). Clin Neurophysiol. 2014;125(11):2150–206.
42. Rutherford G, Lithgow B, Moussavi Z. Short and long-term effects of rTMS treatment on Alzheimer's disease at different stages: a pilot study. J Exp Neurosci. 2015;9:JEN-S24004.
43. Cotelli M, Manenti R, Cappa SF, Geroldi C, Zanetti O, Rossini PM, Miniussi C. Effect of transcranial magnetic stimulation on action naming in patients with Alzheimer disease. Arch Neurol. 2006;63(11):1602–4.
44. Ferrucci R, Mameli F, Guidi I, Mrakic-Sposta S, Vergari M, Marceglia SE, Cogiamanian F, Barbieri S, Scarpini E, Priori A. Transcranial direct current stimulation improves recognition memory in Alzheimer disease. Neurology. 2008;71(7):493–8.
45. Turriziani P. Enhancing memory performance with rTMS in healthy subjects and individuals with mild cognitive impairment: the role of the right dorsolateral prefrontal cortex. Front Hum Neurosci. 2012;6:62.
46. Buckner RL, Andrews-Hanna JR, Schacter DL. The brain's default network: anatomy, function, and relevance to disease. Ann N Y Acad Sci. 2008;1124:1–38.
47. Rabey JM, Dobronevsky E, Aichenbaum S, Gonen O, Marton RG, Khaigrekht M. Repetitive transcranial magnetic stimulation combined with cognitive training is a safe and effective modality for the treatment of Alzheimer's disease: a randomized, double-blind study. J Neural Transm. 2013;120(5):813–9.

48. Gili T, Cercignani M, Serra L, Perri R, Giove F, Maraviglia B, Caltagirone C, Bozzali M. Regional brain atrophy and functional disconnection across Alzheimer's disease evolution. J Neurol Neurosurg Psychiatry. 2011;82(1):58–66.
49. Lundstrom BN, Ingvar M, Petersson KM. The role of precuneus and left inferior frontal cortex during source memory episodic retrieval. NeuroImage. 2005;27(4):824–34.
50. Bonnì S, Veniero D, Mastropasqua C, Ponzo V, Caltagirone C, Bozzali M, Koch G. TMS evidence for a selective role of the precuneus in source memory retrieval. Behav Brain Res. 2015;282:70–5.

Transcranial Magnetic Stimulation in the Treatment of Anxiety Disorders

13

Giorgio Di Lorenzo, Tommaso B. Jannini, Lucia Longo, Rodolfo Rossi, Alberto Siracusano, and Bernardo Dell'Osso

13.1 Introduction

Anxiety disorders are invalidating conditions, highly prevalent and commonly distributed worldwide [1, 2]. The Diagnostic and Statistical Manual of Mental Disorders 5 (DSM-5) describes anxiety disorders as conditions that feature excessive fear and anxiety responses. Fear can be summarized as a complex series of physiological mechanisms that starts in response to a real or perceived threat (also known as *fight or flight* response), whereas anxiety can be defined as an emotional response to a vague or potential threat [3]; apprehension, sustained

G. Di Lorenzo (✉)
Department of Systems Medicine, University of Rome Tor Vergata, Rome, Italy

Psychiatry and Clinical Psychology Unit, Fondazione Policlinico Tor Vergata, Rome, Italy

IRCCS Fondazione Santa Lucia, Rome, Italy
e-mail: di.lorenzo@med.uniroma2.it

T. B. Jannini · A. Siracusano
Department of Systems Medicine, University of Rome Tor Vergata, Rome, Italy

Psychiatry and Clinical Psychology Unit, Fondazione Policlinico Tor Vergata, Rome, Italy

L. Longo · R. Rossi
Department of Systems Medicine, University of Rome Tor Vergata, Rome, Italy

B. Dell'Osso
Department of Biomedical and Clinical Sciences Luigi Sacco, University of Milan, Milan, Italy

Ospedale Luigi Sacco-Polo Universitario, ASST Fatebenefratelli Sacco, Milan, Italy

Department of Psychiatry and Behavioural Sciences, Bipolar Disorders Clinic, Stanford University, Stanford, CA, USA

CRC "Aldo Ravelli" for Neuro-technology and Experimental Brain Therapeutics, University of Milan, Milan, Italy

© Springer Nature Switzerland AG 2020
B. Dell'Osso, G. Di Lorenzo (eds.), *Non Invasive Brain Stimulation in Psychiatry and Clinical Neurosciences*,
https://doi.org/10.1007/978-3-030-43356-7_13

arousal and vigilance are paired with an autonomic response, leading to specific patterns of defensive behaviour. Anxiety disorders comprise Generalized Anxiety Disorder (GAD), Panic Disorder (PD), Social Anxiety Disorder (SAD), Specific Phobia (SP) and Agoraphobia. Overall, they represent the most common mental disorders in western societies, with a prevalence of 14% of the general population [1]. Nevertheless, anxiety disorders are, unfortunately, under-diagnosed and under-treated. Most anxiety disorders start developing during early ages, with SP and SAD showing a very early onset (7 years) [4, 5]. However, in some anxiety disorders, such as GAD, anxiety can arise in the later years of adulthood [6–8].

Several risk factors are associated with anxiety disorders, including female sex and family history of anxiety or depressive disorders. Furthermore, many stressful life events (such as family divorce, socioeconomical status including poverty and the presence of illness) may be decisive in generating these disorders during childhood [9, 10].

Therapeutic strategies for managing acute anxiety symptoms (mainly benzodiazepines) and the whole anxiety syndrome (with psychopharmacological therapy, mainly drugs modulating serotonin transmission, and/or psychotherapy, mainly cognitive behavioral therapy) are frequently effective. Increasingly specific treatments for anxiety disorders are necessary not only to increase the efficacy and the effectiveness but also, if not above all, for better management of the side effects of the drugs, in particular in special populations (e.g., childhood and adolescence, women in peripartum period, the elderly people) and in those patients with comorbid conditions for other psychiatric and medical diseases. Non-invasive brain stimulation (NIBS) techniques provide an alternative treatment, directed at the stimulation and modulation of the activity of a specific brain area implicated in the circuitry sustaining anxiety. In this chapter, after a brief overview of the main cortical neural circuits implicated in anxiety disorders, we will present the state of the art of the clinical use of Transcranial Magnetic Stimulation (TMS) protocols[1] in the treatment of anxiety disorders, through the description (and the summary in the Table 13.1) of the main findings of studies in which TMS was used to treat the different types of anxiety disorders.

13.2   Cortical Neural Circuits in the Pathophysiology of Anxiety

The central neural mechanisms underlying fear and anxiety share many common features, although the exact cortical neural circuitries of anxiety are still to be elucidated. Recent studies have highlighted what could be called an "anxiety network", i.e. a complex system of brain structures that are mutually co-activated during anxiety processes [11] (see Fig. 13.1). An important role in this

---

[1] See Chap. 1 for details about the general technical bases of TMS and its several therapeutic protocols.

Table 13.1 Main descriptive, technical and clinical features of the studies in which TMS was used as a treatment for anxiety disorders

Authors	Year	Disorder	Study type	N	M/F	Psychiatric comorbidities	Drug therapy	Stimulation site	Stimulation site identification	TMS coil	Stimulation type	Frequency/Intensity	Pulses per session	Session number and duration	Main outcomes (changes in)	Main findings
Notzon et al.	2015	SP (spiders)	RCT	81	9/72	No	No	Left DLPFC	No	8-figure	iTBS	15 Hz/80% RMT	600	1 × 3'	SPQ, FSQ, ASI	No symptom changes
Herman et al.	2017	SP (heights)	RCT	39	13/26	No	No	vmPFC	Fpz	8-figure	aHF rTMS	10 Hz/100% RMT	1560	2 × 20'	AQ, BAT	Symptom improvement
Paes et al.	2013	SAD	CS	1	1/0	No	No	Right vmPFC	No	8-figure	LF rTMS	1 Hz/120% MT	1500	1 × 25'	SSI, BDI, BAI	Symptom improvement
Paes et al.	2013	SAD	SSD	2	1/1	MDD	SSRI	Right vmPFC	No	8-figure	LF rTMS	1 Hz/120% MT	1500	12 × 25'	LSAS, BDI, BAI	Symptom improvement
Zwanzger et al.	2002	PD	CS	1	0/1	No	No	Right DLPFC	No	8-figure	LF rTMS	1 Hz/110% MT	1200	10 × N.A.	ACI, PSS, HAS, PAS	Symptom improvement
Guaiana et al.	2005	PD	CS	1	0/1	No	No	Right and left PFC	No	8-figure	LF and HF rTMS	1 Hz/100% MT 20 Hz/100% MT	600	9 × N.A. 20 × N.A.	PDSS	Symptom improvement only after HF rTMS
Dresler et al.	2009	PD	CS	1	1/0	MDD	TCA	Left DLPFC	No	8-figure	HF rTMS	10 Hz/110% MT	2400	15 × 20'	HDS, Stroop accuracy	No changes in task performance
Machado et al.	2014	PD	CS	1	0/1	No	No	Right and left DLPFC	No	8-figure	LF and HF rTMS	1 Hz/120% MT 10 Hz/120 MT	1000 (right)/ N.A. (left)	12 × 15'	BAI, PDSS	Symptom improvement
Mantovani et al.	2007	PD	OLT	6	3/3	MDD	SSRI, NaSSA, BZD, AED	Right DLPFC	No	8-figure	LF rTMS	1 Hz/100% RMT	1200	10 × 28'	PDSS, SCRAS, HAS	Symptom improvement
Prasko et al.	2007	PD	RCT	15	4/11	No	SSRI	Right DLPFC	No	8-figure	LF rTMS	1 Hz/110% MT	1800	10 × 30'	PDSS, BAI, HAMA	Symptom improvement

(continued)

Table 13.1 (continued)

Authors	Year	Disorder	Study type	N	M/F	Psychiatric comorbidities	Drug therapy	Stimulation site	Stimulation site identification	TMS coil	Stimulation type	Frequency/Intensity	Pulses per session	Session number and duration	Main outcomes (changes in)	Main findings
Mantovani et al.	2013	PD	RCT	25	12/13	MDD	SSRI, SNRI, NaSSA, BZD, AED, AAP, SARI, LDX, Li	Right DLPFC	No	8-figure	LF rTMS	1 Hz/110% RMT	1800	40 × 30′	PDSS, HDRS	Symptom improvement
Kumar et al.	2018	PD	OLT	13	NS	MDD	Yes (N.A.)	Left DLPFC	No	8-figure	HF rTMS	20 Hz/110% RMT	1000	20 × 4′	PDSS, HDRS	Symptom improvement
Bystritsky et al.	2008	GAD	OLT	10	5/5	No	SSRI, BZD	Right DLPFC	MRI-guided	8-figure	LF rTMS	1 Hz/90% RMT	900	6 × 15′	HAM-A, CGI-I	Symptom improvement
White et al.	2015	GAD	OLT	13	5/8	MDD	No	Right and left DLPFC	No	8-figure	LF and HF rTMS	1 Hz/N.A. 10 Hz/N.A.	1000	24–36 × N.A.	GAD-7, HDRS-21	Symptom improvement
Diefenbach et al.	2016	GAD	RCT	25′	6/19	No	Yes (N.A.)	Right DLPFC	MRI-guided	8-figure	LF rTMS	1 Hz/90 RMT	900	30 × 15′	HRS-A	Symptom improvement
Dilkov et al.	2017	GAD	RCT	40	21/19	No	SSRI, SNRI, SARI, NaSSA, BZD, NBZD, APD, AAP, APK, AED	Right DLPFC	No	8-figure	HF rTMS	20 Hz/110 RMT	1600	25 × 20′	HRS-A, CGI-I	Symptom improvement

Assaf et al.	2018	GAD	RCT	16	7/24	No	Yes (N.A.)	Right DLPFC	No	8-figure	LF rTMS	1 Hz/90% RMT	900	30 × 15′	PSWQ	Symptom improvement
Huang et al.	2018	GAD	RCT	36	18/18	Insomnia	SSRI, BZD	Right PC	No	8-figure	LF rTMS	1 Hz/90% RMT	1500	10 × 36′	HRS-A	Symptom improvement
Deppermann et al.	2017	AGO	RCT	44	17/27	PD, depression	Yes (N.A.)	Left DLPFC	No	8-figure	iTBS	15 Hz/80% RMT	600	15 × 3′	PAS, HAMA, CAQ, ES-fNIRS	No verum iTBS effect on symptoms; Verum iTBS increased bilateral PFC activity

AAP atypical antipsychotic, *AED* antiepileptic drugs, *AGO* agoraphobia, *APD* antipsychotic drugs, *APK* antiparkinsonian drugs, *AQ* acrophobia questionnaire, *ASI* anxiety sensitivity index, *BAI* Beck Anxiety Inventory, *BAT* behavioral avoidance test, *BDI* Beck Depression Inventory, *BZD* benzodiazepines, *CAQ* cardiac anxiety questionnaire, *CGI-I* clinical global impression—improvement scale, *CS* case study, *DLPFC* dorsolateral prefrontal cortex, *ES-fNIRS* emotional stroop test during recordings of functional near infrareds spectroscopy, *FSQ* fear of spiders questionnaire, *HAMA* Hamilton rating scale for anxiety, *HAS* Hamilton anxiety scale, *HDRS* Hamilton depression rating scale, *HDS* Hamilton depression scale, *HF* high frequency, *iTBS* intermittent theta-burst stimulation, *LDX* lisdexamfetamine, *LF* low frequency, *Li* lithium, *LSAS* Liebowitz social anxiety scale, *MDD* major depressive disorder, *MRI* magnetic resonance imaging, *N.A.* not applicable, *NaSSA* noradrenergic and specific serotoninergic antidepressant, *NBDZ* nonbenzodiazepine drugs, *OLT* open label trial, *PAS* panic and agoraphobia scale, *PC* parietal cortex, *PD* panic disorder, *PDSS* panic disorder severity scale, *PSS* panic symptom scale, *PSWQ* Penn State Worry Questionnaire, *RMT* resting motor threshold, *rTMS* repetitive transcranial magnetic stimulation, *SAD* social anxiety disorder, *SARI* serotonin agonist and reuptake inhibitor, *SCRAS* Sheehan clinician rated anxiety scale, *SNRI* serotonin noradrenalin reuptake inhibitor, *SP* specific phobia, *SPQ* spider phobia questionnaire, *SSD* single subject design, *SSI* social skill inventory, *SSRI* selective serotonin reuptake inhibitor, *TCA* tricyclic antidepressant, *vmPFC* ventromedial prefrontal cortex

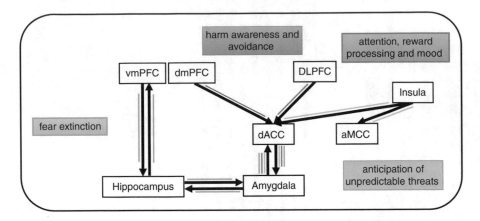

Fig. 13.1 A schematic representation of main brain structures involved in the so-called "anxiety network". *aMCC* anterior midcingulate cortex, *dACC* dorsal anterior cingulate cortex, *DLPFC* dorsolateral prefrontal cortex, *dmPFC* dorsomedial prefrontal cortex, *vmPFC* ventromedial prefrontal cortex

network is played by the prefrontal cortex (PFC), which deeply interacts with the dorsal anterior cingulate cortex (dACC). Based on functional magnetic resonance imaging (fMRI) studies, the complex dorsomedial PFC (dmPFC)/dACC shows elevated activity in most anxiety disorders, reflecting its fundamental function of harm awareness and avoidance [12]. Moreover, the limbic system seems to be deeply implicated in the pathogenesis of anxiety. Besides dACC, in fact, the subgenual anterior cingulate cortex (sgACC), situated under the *genu* of the *corpus callosum*, plays a key role in processing autonomic responses to emotional stimuli (visceral feedback), such as fear or stress [13]. Indeed, Jaworska and colleagues found an inverse relation between sgACC volumes and anxiety symptoms, highlighting its role in the pathophysiology of anxiety and mood disorders [14].

Other important pathological alterations associated with anxiety include the hypoactivity of the left dorsolateral prefrontal cortex (left DLPFC) and the hyperactivity of the right DLPFC, both observed in patients with PD [15–17]. The DLPFC shows intimate connections with several structures of the meso-cortico-limbic reward circuit, e.g. the ACC, typically associated with attention, reward processing and mood, and the amygdala [18]. Amygdala, a cluster of nuclei deeply implicated in fear generalization [19], seems to work together with the aforementioned complex dmPFC/dACC in the pathophysiology of anxiety. This connectivity, in fact, is straightened when individuals with higher dispositional anxiety are exposed to the threat of unpredictable shock [20].

Failure and delay in fear extinction are intensely implicated in anxiety disorders. The process of constructing new memories involves the extinction of the old ones and, thus, the inhibition of original condition trace that may lead to a dysfunctional state [21]. To this regard, the hippocampus seems to work together with the amygdala in fear extinction, being activated jointly with the vmPFC [22, 23].

Furthermore, also the insula and the bed nucleus of the stria terminalis (BNST) are commonly implicated in the generation of anxiety in humans. Both are broadly involved in the anticipation of unpredictable threats, being heightened either in post-traumatic stress disorder (PTSD) or in PD [24, 25]. In particular, functional neuroimaging studies showed that the anterior insular cortex may be vastly involved in the anticipation of unpredictable aversive events (e.g. stimuli given with a temporal unpredictability, occurring at any time) [26, 27]. As many of these anxiety-related structures seem to work in concert with other regions of the brain, the anterior insula shows intrinsic connections with the anterior midcingulate cortex (aMCC) and the dACC. This complex is thought to be part of the so-called salience network, a brain system involved in the detection of behaviourally relevant stimuli and the coordination of adaptive responses [28–30].

13.3   TMS in the Treatment of Specific Phobias

Specific phobias (SPs) represent anxiety disorders in which fear, anxiety and avoidance are elicited by a particular situation or object (i.e. heights, spiders, etc.) [31].

To date, in the literature, only two studies that use repetitive TMS (rTMS) in SP patients are available. Although preliminary, these results show that excitatory TMS sessions on PFC have some beneficial effects on patients. Nevertheless, an important heterogeneity in terms of the protocol used, specific cortical targets and symptoms can be observed in these studies. This does not allow drawing any specific conclusion yet, but, on the other hand, it could pave the way for future and more standardized trials.

The first TMS study on patients with SP used virtual reality scenarios and was conducted on 41 participants with spider phobia versus 40 healthy adult controls [16]. Authors used several measurements to assess symptoms, such as the Specific Phobia Questionnaire (SPQ) [32] and the Fear of Spiders Questionnaire (FSQ) [33]. Anxiety and disgust were considered as well through the Questionnaire for the Assessment of Disgust Sensitivity [34], the Subjective Units of Discomfort Scale [35] and the Anxiety Sensitivity Index [36]. Autonomic responses were recorded by monitoring the heart rate (HR) and skin conductance. The protocol consisted of one session of intermittent Theta Burst Stimulation (iTBS) over the left DLPFC. Authors found that iTBS did not impact on self-report measures, but only on heart rate variability, a marker of mental well-being [37], increasing its levels in the active group. No difference was reported in the sham group.

On the other hand, Herrmann et al. used rTMS over the vmPFC on acrophobic patients [38]. This protocol consisted of two sessions of 10 Hz rTMS conducted on 20 participants and 19 controls (average age 44.9, standard deviation 13.1), followed by virtual reality exposure therapy (VRET). Results on self-reported measurements showed that high-frequency rTMS improved the VRET response of acrophobia symptoms, providing the first proof of concept of its efficacy in specific phobias.

13.4   TMS in the Treatment of Social Anxiety Disorder

Social anxiety disorder (SAD) is a common and debilitating condition that features fear of scrutiny by other people and avoidance of social situations, associated with high vegetative responses [31]. The application of rTMS in people with SAD is now preliminary and at early stages. The lack of standardized, double-blinded, sham-controlled protocols has led to inconclusive results about the efficacy of this treatment. However, results from the only two trials conducted so far using low-frequency stimulation seem to be encouraging.

The first study that used rTMS to treat SAD was a case report done by Paes et al. on a 38-year-old male patient [39]. This patient received a single session of 1 Hz (low frequency) rTMS applied over the right vmPFC. Symptoms were evaluated using the Beck Anxiety Inventory (BAI) and the Social Skills Inventory (SSI) [40, 41]. Scores on BAI and symptoms were significantly decreased compared to pre-TMS treatment and, after 2 months, the patient showed only a mild increase of anxiety. The same authors extended their clinical trial to 2 additional patients: a 23-year-old male and a 45-year-old female [42]. Both were diagnosed with SAD and comorbid depression. They were treated with a similar protocol to that in a previous study, using low-frequency rTMS (1 Hz) over the right vmPFC, 3 times per week, for 4 weeks (12 stimulations in total). Anxiety symptoms were evaluated using BAI and Liebowitz Social Anxiety Scale (LSAS) [43] at baseline, 2 and 4 weeks of TMS and after 2 weeks of follow-up. Both patients showed a significant decrease of BAI and LSAS scores, maintaining the same trend at the follow-up examination. These improvements were also observed for depressive symptoms, assessed with the Beck Depression Inventory [44].

13.5   TMS in the Treatment of Panic Disorder

Panic disorder (PD) is described in DSM-5 as a condition in which patients experience recurrent and unexpected panic attacks followed by anticipatory anxiety and phobic avoidance. A panic attack is characterized by intense fear or discomfort associated with a powerful vegetative response that reaches the peak in a very short time [31].

Most studies with rTMS in patients with PD—eight, taken as a whole—were found to be single case reports, providing a wide range of clinical scenarios. In particular, only two randomized, double-blind, sham-controlled studies are available in the literature, whereas the remaining ones are open-label reports. Even though these data have to be considered as preliminary, the results of single case studies seem to be consistent with those from more standardized protocols, supporting the effectiveness of rTMS in the treatment of PD. However, more trials with a sufficient number of stimulating sessions and larger samples are required to make consistent conclusions.

The first trial was a single case study conducted on a 52-year-old woman who had been suffering from PD with six panic attacks per week for 13 months [45]. This patient was treated with low-frequency rTMS (1 Hz) over the right DLPFC for 2 weeks. Symptoms were assessed using the Panic and Agoraphobia Scale (PAS) [46], the Hamilton Anxiety Scale (HAS) [47] and by determining cortisol and adrenocorticotropic hormone (ACTH) blood levels during a cholecystokinin (CCK)-4 challenge. After 2 weeks of treatment, the patient scored significantly better both on PAS and on HAS. Moreover, a marked reduction in her cortisol levels during CCK-4 challenge was observed.

Guaiana and colleagues treated a 34-year-old female with 9 sessions of low-frequency rTMS (1 Hz) over the right PFC, without observing any clinically relevant result. However, after switching to 20 sessions of a high-frequency protocol (20 Hz) over the left PFC, a significant improvement in PD symptoms was observed [48].

Dresler and co-workers conducted a single case study on a 44-year-old man who was suffering from PD and comorbid depression [49]. The patient was treated with a high-frequency rTMS (10 Hz) over the left DLPFC, once a day, five times per week over 3 weeks. A Stroop task, involving 12-panic-related and 12 neutral words displayed on a screen in three different colours, was presented to test the therapeutic effect. Although rTMS did not impact on the Stroop task, the authors reported no further panic attack that occurred during the treatment.

The last single case study was conducted by Machado et al. on a 34-year-old patient, refractory to cognitive behaviour therapy [50]. The protocol consisted of a sequential stimulation of the right DLPFC (1 Hz) and left DLPFC (10 Hz), 3 times per week for 4 weeks, resulting in a significant improvement of PD symptoms assessed with BAI and Panic Disorder Severity Scale (PDSS).

Mantovani and co-authors assessed rTMS treatment in six patients with PD and comorbid depression, using a protocol of 1 Hz stimulation over the right DLPFC for 2 weeks in an open-label trial [51]. Patients scored significantly better than baseline in the Sheehan Clinician Rated Anxiety Scale (SCRAS) [52], the HAS and the Hamilton Depression Scale (HDS) in the first and the second week of treatment. The same authors conducted a randomized, double-blinded, sham-controlled clinical trial extending the same clinical population up to 25 patients [53]. The treatment consisted of low-frequency stimulation (1 Hz) over the right DLPFC, once a day for 5 consecutive days, for 4 weeks. With regard to panic symptoms, half of the participants from the active group demonstrated a full response of the treatment, whereas in the sham group, the percentage of responders was only 8%.

Prasko et al. recruited 15 patients suffering from PD and resistant to selective serotonin reuptake inhibitor (SSRI) therapy and randomly assigned them to either active treatment with 10 sessions of 1 Hz rTMS over the right DLPFC or the sham group [54]. In both cases, the patients were taking SSRI therapy. The aim was to compare the efficacy at the second and fourth week. The results showed that treatment effect did not differ between groups, since both of them improved during the study period. This negative finding, as suggested by the authors, could be due to small sample size.

The last study was performed by Kumar et al. on 13 drug-resistant patients who were suffering from PD in comorbidity with a major depressive disorder (MDD) [55]. The protocol was structured as 20 sessions of 20 Hz (high frequency) rTMS over the left DLPFC, 5 days per week, over a period of 4 weeks. The symptoms were assessed via PDSS and HDS, showing a significant reduction of scores in both scales.

13.6 TMS as Treatment of Generalized Anxiety Disorder

Generalized anxiety disorder (GAD) is a prevalent condition affecting the 2.9% of the adult population in the U.S. Patients with GAD experience excessive anxiety and feeling of apprehensive expectation, being unable to control the worry. This clinical picture is often associated with restlessness, irritably, muscle tension, sleep disturbance and somatization [31].

The application of rTMS in patients diagnosed with GAD seems to be one of the more promising NIBS treatment among the various anxiety disorders. Four randomized, sham-controlled, double-blinded clinical trials have shown positive outcomes in treating this condition, with low-frequency stimulation over the right DLPFC being the most used protocol. However, the sample sizes of these trials (13–36 patients) allow to draw only some preliminary conclusions. This means that future studies with larger populations will be required to draw more consistent conclusions.

Bystrisky and colleagues were the first to use rTMS to treat GAD, stimulating ten participants over the right DLPFC with 1 Hz (low frequency) [56]. They completed 6 sessions over a period of 3 weeks. Patients first underwent an fMRI task to identify the most active location of the prefrontal cortex. The symptoms were monitored using HAM-A [47] and CGI-I, defining the treatment response as a $\geq 50\%$ score reduction of these scales. Overall, rTMS was associated with a significant decrease of both HAM-A and CGI-I in 6 participants (60%).

Another open-label trial was conducted by White and Tavakoli on 13 patients with GAD and comorbid MDD [57]. The protocol they used consisted of the application of low-frequency rTMS (1 Hz) over the right DLPFC followed by a high-frequency rTMS (10 Hz) over the left DLPFC. The number of stimulations ranged from 24 to 36 over 5 to 6 weeks. At the end of the treatment period, 11 out of 13 patients (84.6%) reported symptom remission, scoring less than 5 on the GAD Scale (GAD-7) [58], and 10 out of 13 patients (79.9%) did the same on the Hamilton Rating Scale for Depression (HAM-D-21), scoring less than 8.

The first randomized, double-blind, sham-controlled clinical trial was performed by Diefenbach et al. on 25 patients (13 active vs. 12 sham) diagnosed with GAD [59]. The active group was treated using a low-frequency rTMS delivered over the right DLPFC for 15 min, for 30 sessions (5 days/week for 6 weeks). Patients were also asked to undergo a decision gambling task with fMRI to localize the area to stimulate. Symptoms were assessed via HARS and the Penn State Worry Questionnaire (PSWQ) [60]. At post-treatment, significantly more patients met the responder and the remitter status in the active versus sham group, showing this trend even at 3-month follow-up. The same authors published additional material on the same cohort of patients, showing that patients treated with rTMS had significant improvements in self-reported emotion regulation difficulties at 3-month follow up [61].

Dilikov et al. recruited 40 patients with GAD, randomly assigning them to active [15] and sham groups [25, 62]. Authors used high-frequency-stimulation (20 Hz) rTMS applied over the right DLPFC. The active group received 5 sessions per week for the first 4 weeks. During the fifth week, the sessions were reduced to 3 times per week, whereas at the sixth and final week, the patients received 2 sessions of rTMS. The symptoms were evaluated using the HARS. By the end of 25 rTMS treatments, the patients in the active group scored significantly less compared to those in the sham group. Moreover, HARS scores remained stable at the 4-week follow-up, corroborating the efficacy of the treatment.

Assaf and colleagues first explored the neural architecture of GAD patients through fMRI. Then they treated 16 patients (9 = active; 7 = sham) with 30 sessions (5 days/week for 6 weeks) of low-frequency (1 Hz) rTMS over the right DLPFC [63], monitoring symptoms with PSQW and the Intolerance of Uncertainty Scale [64]. The results showed the "normalization" of functional connectivity of the dorsal anterior and the subgenual cingulate cortex, associated with an improvement in worry symptoms in patients treated with active rTMS.

Finally, Huang and co-workers conducted a randomized, double-blind, sham-controlled study on patients affected by GAD and comorbid insomnia [65]. Eighteen participants in the active group (out of a total of 36) were treated with 1 Hz rTMS over the right parietal cortex (PC), administering 6 sessions twice a week for 3 weeks. At the endpoint, 60% of the patients met the criteria for remission, defined as a HARS score less than 8. These results largely remained stable at 6-month follow-up.

13.7 TMS as Treatment of Agoraphobia

Agoraphobia is an anxiety disorder in which individuals develop marked anxiety or fear in situations like open spaces, public transportation or being outside of home alone. These patients tend to avoid these circumstances because of thoughts that escape might be difficult or even impossible [31].

To date, literature offers only a single study, where the selectd sample was mainly affected by PD and comorbid agoraphobia. This means that only limited conclusions can be drawn with regard to rTMS as a treatment for agoraphobia.

Deppermann et al. randomized 44 patients to the sham or active group, treating them with 15 sessions of iTBS over the left DLPFC in addition to 9 weeks of Cognitive Behavioral Therapy (CBT). Main outcome measures were evaluated with the PAS [46], the HARS and the Cardiac Anxiety Questionnaire (CAQ) [66]. Cortical activity was monitored through functional near-infrared spectroscopy (fNIRS) during an Emotional Stroop task, at baseline and post-iTBS. Clinical ratings significantly improved and remained stable at follow-up. However, no clinical differences between the active and the sham group were identified, except for a more stable reduction of agoraphobic avoidance during follow-up in the group treated with active iTBS.

13.8 Future Perspectives

TMS showed many significant and encouraging results for the treatment of patients with anxiety disorders. To date, except for conditions like agoraphobia or specific phobias, rTMS over the prefrontal cortex, with excitatory stimulation at the left side and/or inhibitory stimulation at the right side, can be considered effective to reduce anxiety symptoms in PD and GAD. However, the level of evidence available is considered low.

Several clinical features are implicated as possible confounding factors: limited sample size, the presence of psychiatric comorbidities (including mainly major depression) and heterogeneous psychotropic and psychotherapeutic concomitant treatments. On the other hand, some methodological improvements must be taken into account to reach higher quality of evidence, including larger samples and extended periods of observation. One of the reasons for limited efficacy may be the reliance on a scalp-based method rather than neuronavigation based on individual MRI for targeting brain regions. Moving from anatomical to functional imaging positioning (e.g. fMRI, fNIRS) could allow achieving a greater efficacy for targeting TMS coils. Finally, coupling functional imaging with physiological parameters, such as skin conductance or heart rate variability, would allow better elucidation of the biological mechanisms underlying rTMS treatment.

Another methodological issue is the coil positioning site in the rTMS stimulation protocol. Looking at the "anxiety network" (Fig. 13.1), the sites of stimulation target of TMS therapeutic protocols are indeed limited mainly to PFC. In fact, areas such as the dmPFC or deeper areas such as those of cingulate cortices (dACC and aMCC) are not the targets of stimulation in TMS protocols to treat anxiety disorders (see Fig. 13.2). The use of the Double-Cone Coil or the H-coil in TMS therapeutic protocols for anxiety disorder treatment may extend the number of stimulation sites of "anxiety network", different from the "classical" DLPFC, allowing the modulation of deeper areas as dmPFC, anterior cingulate cortices and insulae.

To extend the field of TMS treatment for anxiety disorders, it would be interesting to investigate the clinical efficacy of TMS in special populations with anxiety disorders, such as elderly people, pregnant women, adolescents or drug abusers with comorbid anxiety, as well as all those comorbid medical conditions in which the treatment of anxiety with current therapeutic strategies is limited or contraindicated due to drug interactions. To date, only one case study has been conducted to investigate the role of rTMS in treating panic attacks during pregnancy: even though the results seem to be promising, it is premature to speculate about the efficacy of this protocol on such delicate patients [67]. Of note, Segev and colleagues tested rTMS on a 17-year-old adolescent who was admitted in the psychiatric ward due to intensified suicidal intention in comorbid MDD [68]. Interestingly, anxiety measures showed significant improvements, paving the way for future double-blind, sham-controlled clinical trials.

13.9   Conclusions

According to the literature reviewed in this chapter, therapeutic protocols using TMS were applied in approximately 370 subjects affected by, at least, one anxiety disorder. Consequently, until now, the level of evidence in the current guidelines is relatively low in relation to the clinical use of TMS therapeutic protocols in anxiety disorders, even though the clinical efficacy of rTMS in reducing anxiety symptom severity was consistently observed in PD and GAD. Future research, with refined methodological issues and study designs, is expected to reveal the real usefulness of TMS therapeutic protocols in the treatment of anxiety disorders.

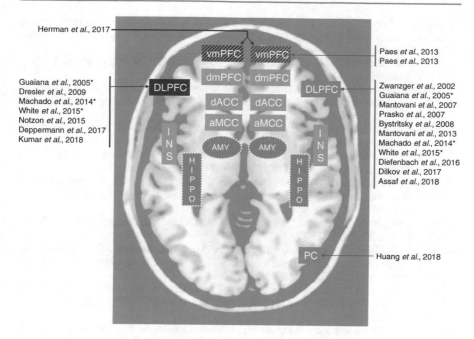

Fig. 13.2 Target brain areas for therapeutic TMS protocols in anxiety disorders. Red colour indicates those cortical areas where TMS coils were placed for implementing excitatory TMS protocols; blue colour indicates those areas where inhibitory TMS protocols were used; mixed colours indicate those areas where both excitatory and inhibitory TMS protocols were implemented. Green colour indicates brain structures involved in the "anxiety network" and potential sites of direct stimulation but not yet targeted by TMS protocols. Grey colour indicates the deepest areas of the "anxiety network" that cannot be directly stimulated by TMS protocols. *aMCC* anterior midcingulate cortex, *AMY* amygdala, *dACC* dorsal anterior cingulate cortex, *DLPFC* dorsolateral prefrontal cortex, *dmPFC* dorsomedial prefrontal cortex, *HIPPO* hippocampus, *INS* insula, *vmPFC* ventromedial prefrontal cortex

References

1. Baxter AJ, Scott KM, Vos T, Whiteford HA. Global prevalence of anxiety disorders: a systematic review and meta-regression. Psychol Med. 2013;43(5):897–910.
2. Baxter AJ, Vos T, Scott KM, Ferrari AJ, Whiteford HA. The global burden of anxiety disorders in 2010. Psychol Med. 2014;44(11):2363–74.
3. American Psychiatric Association. Diagnostic and statistical manual of mental disorders. 5th ed. Washington, DC: American Psychiatric Association; 2013.
4. Kessler RC, Angermeyer M, Anthony JC, De Graaf R, Demyttenaere K, Gasquet I, et al. Lifetime prevalence and age-of-onset distributions of mental disorders in the World Health Organization's World Mental Health Survey Initiative. World Psychiatry. 2007;6(3):168–76.
5. Beesdo K, Knappe S, Pine DS. Anxiety and anxiety disorders in children and adolescents: developmental issues and implications for DSM-V. Psychiatr Clin North Am. 2009;32(3):483–524.
6. Silove D, Alonso J, Bromet E, Gruber M, Sampson N, Scott K, et al. Pediatric-onset and adult-onset separation anxiety disorder across countries in the world mental health survey. Am J Psychiatry. 2015;172(7):647–56.

7. Zhang X, Norton J, Carriere I, Ritchie K, Chaudieu I, Ancelin ML. Generalized anxiety in community-dwelling elderly: prevalence and clinical characteristics. J Affect Disord. 2015;172:24–9.
8. Kessler RC, Ruscio AM, Shear K, Wittchen HU. Epidemiology of anxiety disorders. Curr Top Behav Neurosci. 2010;2:21–35.
9. McLean CP, Asnaani A, Litz BT, Hofmann SG. Gender differences in anxiety disorders: prevalence, course of illness, comorbidity and burden of illness. J Psychiatr Res. 2011;45(8): 1027–35.
10. Beesdo-Baum K, Knappe S. Developmental epidemiology of anxiety disorders. Child Adolesc Psychiatr Clin N Am. 2012;21(3):457–78.
11. Robinson OJ, Pike AC, Cornwell B, Grillon C. The translational neural circuitry of anxiety. J Neurol Neurosurg Psychiatry. 2019;90(12):1353–60.
12. McTeague LM, Huemer J, Carreon DM, Jiang Y, Eickhoff SB, Etkin A. Identification of common neural circuit disruptions in cognitive control across psychiatric disorders. Am J Psychiatry. 2017;174(7):676–85.
13. Drevets WC, Savitz J, Trimble M. The subgenual anterior cingulate cortex in mood disorders. CNS Spectr. 2008;13(8):663–81.
14. Jaworska N, Yucel K, Courtright A, MacMaster FP, Sembo M, MacQueen G. Subgenual anterior cingulate cortex and hippocampal volumes in depressed youth: the role of comorbidity and age. J Affect Disord. 2016;190:726–32.
15. Etkin A, Wager TD. Functional neuroimaging of anxiety: a meta-analysis of emotional processing in PTSD, social anxiety disorder, and specific phobia. Am J Psychiatry. 2007;164(10):1476–88.
16. Notzon S, Deppermann S, Fallgatter A, Diemer J, Kroczek A, Domschke K, et al. Psychophysiological effects of an iTBS modulated virtual reality challenge including participants with spider phobia. Biol Psychol. 2015;112:66–76.
17. Prasko J, Horacek J, Zalesky R, Kopecek M, Novak T, Paskova B, et al. The change of regional brain metabolism (18FDG PET) in panic disorder during the treatment with cognitive behavioral therapy or antidepressants. Neuro Endocrinol Lett. 2004;25(5):340–8.
18. Duval ER, Javanbakht A, Liberzon I. Neural circuits in anxiety and stress disorders: a focused review. Ther Clin Risk Manag. 2015;11:115–26.
19. Asok A, Kandel ER, Rayman JB. The neurobiology of fear generalization. Front Behav Neurosci. 2018;12:329.
20. Vytal KE, Overstreet C, Charney DR, Robinson OJ, Grillon C. Sustained anxiety increases amygdala-dorsomedial prefrontal coupling: a mechanism for maintaining an anxious state in healthy adults. J Psychiatry Neurosci. 2014;39(5):321–9.
21. Myers KM, Davis M. Mechanisms of fear extinction. Mol Psychiatry. 2007;12(2):120–50.
22. Lang S, Kroll A, Lipinski SJ, Wessa M, Ridder S, Christmann C, et al. Context conditioning and extinction in humans: differential contribution of the hippocampus, amygdala and prefrontal cortex. Eur J Neurosci. 2009;29(4):823–32.
23. Milad MR, Quirk GJ. Fear extinction as a model for translational neuroscience: ten years of progress. Annu Rev Psychol. 2012;63:129–51.
24. Alvarez RP, Chen G, Bodurka J, Kaplan R, Grillon C. Phasic and sustained fear in humans elicits distinct patterns of brain activity. Neuroimage. 2011;55(1):389–400.
25. Brinkmann L, Buff C, Feldker K, Tupak SV, Becker MPI, Herrmann MJ, et al. Distinct phasic and sustained brain responses and connectivity of amygdala and bed nucleus of the stria terminalis during threat anticipation in panic disorder. Psychol Med. 2017;47(15): 2675–88.
26. Carlsson K, Andersson J, Petrovic P, Petersson KM, Ohman A, Ingvar M. Predictability modulates the affective and sensory-discriminative neural processing of pain. Neuroimage. 2006;32(4):1804–14.
27. Shankman SA, Gorka SM, Nelson BD, Fitzgerald DA, Phan KL, O'Daly O. Anterior insula responds to temporally unpredictable aversiveness: an fMRI study. Neuroreport. 2014;25(8):596–600.

28. Seeley WW, Menon V, Schatzberg AF, Keller J, Glover GH, Kenna H, et al. Dissociable intrinsic connectivity networks for salience processing and executive control. J Neurosci. 2007;27(9):2349–56.
29. Shackman AJ, Salomons TV, Slagter HA, Fox AS, Winter JJ, Davidson RJ. The integration of negative affect, pain and cognitive control in the cingulate cortex. Nat Rev Neurosci. 2011;12(3):154–67.
30. Uddin LQ. Salience processing and insular cortical function and dysfunction. Nat Rev Neurosci. 2015;16(1):55–61.
31. American Psychiatric Association. DSM-5 Task Force. Diagnostic and statistical manual of mental disorders: DSM-5. 5th ed. Washington, DC: American Psychiatric Association; 2013. xliv, 947 p.
32. Olatunji BO, Woods CM, de Jong PJ, Teachman BA, Sawchuk CN, David B. Development and initial validation of an abbreviated Spider Phobia Questionnaire using item response theory. Behav Ther. 2009;40(2):114–30.
33. Szymanski J, O'Donohue W. Fear of Spiders Questionnaire. J Behav Ther Exp Psychiatry. 1995;26(1):31–4.
34. Haidt J, McCauley C, Rozin P. Individual differences in sensitivity to disgust: a scale sampling seven domains of disgust elicitors. Pers Individ Differ. 1994;16(5):701–13.
35. Wolpe J. The practice of behavior therapy. 2nd ed. Oxford: Pergamon; 1973. xvi, 318-xvi, p.
36. Reiss S, Peterson RA, Gursky DM, McNally RJ. Anxiety sensitivity, anxiety frequency and the prediction of fearfulness. Behav Res Ther. 1986;24(1):1–8.
37. Perna G, Riva A, Defillo A, Sangiorgio E, Nobile M, Caldirola D. Heart rate variability: can it serve as a marker of mental health resilience? J Affect Disord. 2020;263:754–61.
38. Herrmann MJ, Katzorke A, Busch Y, Gromer D, Polak T, Pauli P, et al. Medial prefrontal cortex stimulation accelerates therapy response of exposure therapy in acrophobia. Brain Stimul. 2017;10(2):291–7.
39. Paes F, Machado S, Arias-Carrion O, Silva AC, Nardi AE. rTMS to treat social anxiety disorder: a case report. Braz J Psychiatry. 2013;35(1):99–100.
40. Beck A, Emery G. Anxiety disorders and phobias: a cognitive perspective. New York: Basic Books; 1985. p. 368.
41. Riggio RE. Assessment of basic social skills. J Pers Soc Psychol. 1986;51(3):649–60.
42. Paes F, Baczynski T, Novaes F, Marinho T, Arias-Carrion O, Budde H, et al. Repetitive transcranial magnetic stimulation (rTMS) to treat social anxiety disorder: case reports and a review of the literature. Clin Pract Epidemiol Ment Health. 2013;9:180–8.
43. Liebowitz MR. Social phobia. Mod Probl Pharmacopsychiatry. 1987;22:141–73.
44. Beck AT, Ward CH, Mendelson M, Mock J, Erbaugh J. An inventory for measuring depression. Arch Gen Psychiatry. 1961;4:561–71.
45. Zwanzger P, Minov C, Ella R, Schule C, Baghai T, Moller HJ, et al. Transcranial magnetic stimulation for panic. Am J Psychiatry. 2002;159(2):315–6.
46. Bandelow B, Brunner E, Beinroth D, Pralle L, Broocks A, Hajak G, et al. Application of a new statistical approach to evaluate a clinical trial with panic disorder patients. Eur Arch Psychiatry Clin Neurosci. 1999;249(1):21–7.
47. Hamilton M. The assessment of anxiety states by rating. Br J Med Psychol. 1959;32(1):50–5.
48. Guaiana G, Mortimer AM, Robertson C. Efficacy of transcranial magnetic stimulation in panic disorder: a case report. Aust N Z J Psychiatry. 2005;39(11–12):1047.
49. Dresler T, Ehlis AC, Plichta MM, Richter MM, Jabs B, Lesch KP, et al. Panic disorder and a possible treatment approach by means of high-frequency rTMS: a case report. World J Biol Psychiatry. 2009;10(4 Pt 3):991–7.
50. Machado S, Santos V, Paes F, Arias-Carrion O, Carta MG, Silva AC, et al. Repetitive transcranial magnetic stimulation (rTMS) to treat refractory panic disorder patient: a case report. CNS Neurol Disord Drug Targets. 2014;13(6):1075–8.
51. Mantovani A, Lisanby SH, Pieraccini F, Ulivelli M, Castrogiovanni P, Rossi S. Repetitive transcranial magnetic stimulation (rTMS) in the treatment of panic disorder (PD) with comorbid major depression. J Affect Disord. 2007;102(1–3):277–80.

52. Sheenan DV. The anxiety disease. New York: Charles Scribner & Sons; 1983. 151 p.
53. Mantovani A, Aly M, Dagan Y, Allart A, Lisanby SH. Randomized sham controlled trial of repetitive transcranial magnetic stimulation to the dorsolateral prefrontal cortex for the treatment of panic disorder with comorbid major depression. J Affect Disord. 2013;144(1–2):153–9.
54. Prasko J, Zalesky R, Bares M, Horacek J, Kopecek M, Novak T, et al. The effect of repetitive transcranial magnetic stimulation (rTMS) add on serotonin reuptake inhibitors in patients with panic disorder: a randomized, double blind sham controlled study. Neuro Endocrinol Lett. 2007;28(1):33–8.
55. Kumar S, Singh S, Parmar A, Verma R, Kumar N. Effect of high-frequency repetitive transcranial magnetic stimulation (rTMS) in patients with comorbid panic disorder and major depression. Australas Psychiatry. 2018;26(4):398–400.
56. Bystritsky A, Kaplan JT, Feusner JD, Kerwin LE, Wadekar M, Burock M, et al. A preliminary study of fMRI-guided rTMS in the treatment of generalized anxiety disorder. J Clin Psychiatry. 2008;69(7):1092–8.
57. White D, Tavakoli S. Repetitive transcranial magnetic stimulation for treatment of major depressive disorder with comorbid generalized anxiety disorder. Ann Clin Psychiatry. 2015;27(3):192–6.
58. Spitzer RL, Kroenke K, Williams JB, Lowe B. A brief measure for assessing generalized anxiety disorder: the GAD-7. Arch Intern Med. 2006;166(10):1092–7.
59. Diefenbach GJ, Bragdon LB, Zertuche L, Hyatt CJ, Hallion LS, Tolin DF, et al. Repetitive transcranial magnetic stimulation for generalised anxiety disorder: a pilot randomised, double-blind, sham-controlled trial. Br J Psychiatry. 2016;209(3):222–8.
60. Meyer TJ, Miller ML, Metzger RL, Borkovec TD. Development and validation of the Penn State Worry Questionnaire. Behav Res Ther. 1990;28(6):487–95.
61. Diefenbach GJ, Assaf M, Goethe JW, Gueorguieva R, Tolin DF. Improvements in emotion regulation following repetitive transcranial magnetic stimulation for generalized anxiety disorder. J Anxiety Disord. 2016;43:1–7.
62. Dilkov D, Hawken ER, Kaludiev E, Milev R. Repetitive transcranial magnetic stimulation of the right dorsal lateral prefrontal cortex in the treatment of generalized anxiety disorder: a randomized, double-blind sham controlled clinical trial. Prog Neuropsychopharmacol Biol Psychiatry. 2017;78:61–5.
63. Assaf M, Rabany L, Zertuche L, Bragdon L, Tolin D, Goethe J, et al. Neural functional architecture and modulation during decision making under uncertainty in individuals with generalized anxiety disorder. Brain Behav. 2018;8(8):e01015.
64. Freeston MH, Rhéaume J, Letarte H, Dugas MJ, Ladouceur R. Why do people worry? Pers Individ Differ. 1994;17(6):791–802.
65. Huang Z, Li Y, Bianchi MT, Zhan S, Jiang F, Li N, et al. Repetitive transcranial magnetic stimulation of the right parietal cortex for comorbid generalized anxiety disorder and insomnia: a randomized, double-blind, sham-controlled pilot study. Brain Stimul. 2018;11(5):1103–9.
66. Eifert GH, Thompson RN, Zvolensky MJ, Edwards K, Frazer NL, Haddad JW, et al. The cardiac anxiety questionnaire: development and preliminary validity. Behav Res Ther. 2000;38(10):1039–53.
67. Nahas Z, Bohning DE, Molloy MA, Oustz JA, Risch SC, George MS. Safety and feasibility of repetitive transcranial magnetic stimulation in the treatment of anxious depression in pregnancy: a case report. J Clin Psychiatry. 1999;60(1):50–2.
68. Segev A, Spellun J, Bloch Y. Anxiety as a central outcome measure in an adolescent with major depressive disorder treated with repetitive transcranial magnetic stimulation. J ECT. 2014;30(4):e54–5.

Transcranial Magnetic Stimulation for Cognitive Neurosciences: Applications and Open Questions

14

Michela Balconi and Davide Crivelli

This chapter focuses on the last 15 years of basic cognitive-affective neuroscience research using Transcranial Magnetic Stimulation (TMS) as the non-invasive brain stimulation (NIBS) technique to investigate neural bases of cognitive and affective functions in healthy people. Besides helping to critically revise traditional models of cognitive functions, the notable amount of empirical evidence coming from such basic research tradition often provided, together with clinical observations, relevant background information for the definition of novel intervention protocols targeted at cognitive impairments that connote many neuropsychiatric disorders.

Next paragraphs represent an overall introduction to the most consistent outcomes of TMS-based research with regard to attention and executive functions, memory, language, emotion processing, and social perception and behaviour, with a specific focus on critical issues and open questions (Fig. 14.1).

14.1 Attention and Executive Functions

Basic neuroscience research on human cognitive functions and higher cognitive processes is probably one of the first areas of investigation that benefitted from the explanatory potential of TMS techniques. In particular, most of the magnetic stimulation studies focused on the domains of attention regulation and executive control, working memory, and decision-making.

Indeed, the ability to orient, focus, maintain, and disengage attention when performing specific tasks as well as everyday activities and when exposed to exogenous

M. Balconi (✉) · D. Crivelli
Research Unit in Affective and Social Neuroscience,
Catholic University of the Sacred Heart, Milan, Italy

Department of Psychology, Catholic University of the Sacred Heart, Milan, Italy
e-mail: michela.balconi@unicatt.it

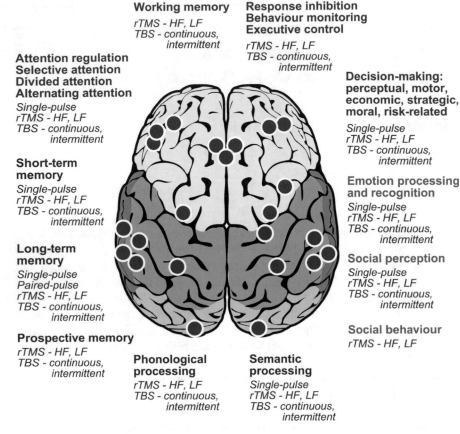

Working memory
rTMS - HF, LF
TBS - continuous,
*   intermittent*

Response inhibition
Behaviour monitoring
Executive control
rTMS - HF, LF
TBS - continuous,
*   intermittent*

Attention regulation
Selective attention
Divided attention
Alternating attention
Single-pulse
rTMS - HF, LF
TBS - continuous,
*   intermittent*

Decision-making:
perceptual, motor,
economic, strategic,
moral, risk-related
Single-pulse
rTMS - HF, LF
TBS - continuous,
*   intermittent*

Short-term
memory
Single-pulse
rTMS - HF, LF
TBS - continuous,
*   intermittent*

Emotion processing
and recognition
Single-pulse
rTMS - HF, LF
TBS - continuous,
*   intermittent*

Long-term
memory
Single-pulse
Paired-pulse
rTMS - HF, LF
TBS - continuous,
*   intermittent*

Social perception
Single-pulse
rTMS - HF, LF
TBS - continuous,
*   intermittent*

Prospective memory
rTMS - HF, LF
TBS - continuous,
*   intermittent*

Social behaviour
rTMS - HF, LF

Phonological
processing
rTMS - HF, LF
TBS - continuous,
*   intermittent*

Semantic
processing
Single-pulse
rTMS - HF, LF
TBS - continuous,
*   intermittent*

Fig. 14.1 Synoptic schema of higher processes and functions that have been most consistently explored via TMS in the last 15 years of cognitive and affective neuroscience research, with a focus on main stimulation targets and methods. *rTMS* repetitive transcranial magnetic stimulation, *HF* high frequency, *LF* low frequency, *TBS* theta burst stimulation

or endogenous stimuli lies at the core of human cognition and plays an essential role in the efficiency of every other cognitive process. A traditional cognitive model of attention processes distinguishes between different facets of the attention function—i.e. focused, sustained, selective, alternating, and divided attention—and a very vast electrophysiological and neuroimaging literature helped to outline associations between specific attention processes and partly distinct cortical areas. Both single-pulse and repetitive (simple or patterned, i.e. theta burst stimulation—TBS) TMS protocols have been used, across the years, to probe the actual causal role of structures that constitute the broad frontal-parietal attention and executive network.

Specifically, left dorsolateral prefrontal cortex (dlPFC) has been found to consistently contribute to selective attention, top-down endogenous orientation of attention resources, and even divided attention [1–3], while prolonged attention regulation—i.e. sustained attention—has also been associated with the contribution of frontal eye-fields (FEF) [4]. In addition, TMS-induced perturbation of ongoing neural activity has been used to verify that alternating attention and, especially, disengagement from distractors and re-orientation mechanisms rely on the contribution of cortical structures within the right FEF, right temporoparietal junction (TPJ), left intraparietal sulcus (IPS), and bilateral posterior parietal cortices (PPC), which encompass the dorsal and ventral attention networks [5–7].

TMS served as a probing technique even with regard to the neural underpinnings of response inhibition, monitoring, and executive control processes. In particular, non-invasive magnetic stimulation allowed us to trace back the ability to inhibit, stop or restrain behavioural responses to the interconnected activity of the right inferior and superior frontal gyrus (IFG, SFG) and pre-supplementary motor areas (pre-SMA) [8, 9], even if the investigation of the role of pre-SMA regions via TMS also led to contrasting results [8, 10]. As for behaviour monitoring mechanisms, the perturbation of dorsolateral and dorsal-medial prefrontal regions highlighted their critical role with regard to the ability to keep track of own behaviours and their consequences in order to efficiently adapt to the context and properly develop an agentive stance [11–13]. Finally, TMS investigation further underlined the causal contribution of dlPFC to the ability to flexibly change the mindset and behaviour when switching between different tasks [14, 15].

Working memory (WM)—intended as the ability to temporarily maintain information accessible for conscious processing and manipulation—has been the functional target of many TMS-based investigations. Overall, one of the most consistent conclusions from TMS studies on anatomical-functional correlates of WM is the posterior localization of WM buffers and the role of dlPFC as a superordinated amodal central executive hub [16]. More specifically, the majority of NIBS stimulation studies on WM concluded that, besides partly contrasting pieces of evidence in favour of a left-sided dlPFC dominance in verbal WM tasks, the right dlPFC is crucially involved in regulating bottom-up information flow from sensory buffers, information maintenance, and WM executive processes with the possible support of the medial prefrontal cortex [16–18].

TMS literature exploring cognitive and neural processing underlying decision-making focused on both basic mechanisms explaining evidence accumulation and speed-accuracy trade-off in simple perceptual decision-making tasks and on more complex processes guiding and shaping higher decision-making, e.g. moral and economic strategic tasks.

A few TMS studies focused, besides dlPFC and pre-SMA [19], on the role of motor regions during simple decision-making tasks. In particular, it was shown that implicit decisional rules conveyed by biased rewarding can not only covertly modulate behavioural responses (thus increasing the selection of facilitated responses) but also consistently modulate pre-decisional corticospinal excitability, as measured via TMS-induced motor evoked potentials—MEPs [20]. In addition, it has been reported that both corticospinal excitability and reaction times can vary during decision-making as a function of the value that is subjectively attributed to different response alternatives [21]. This suggests that subjectively defined values that guide the decision-making process might even modulate the competition between different representations of alternative responses in the motor cortex while the decisional process is still ongoing, consistent with a form of parallel processing of decision and response selection.

Moving to complex decision-making processes, prefrontal areas still remain the primary targets of NIBS studies. Higher strategic decision-making processes have been typically explored by using economic decision tasks—such as the Ultimatum Game—or cooperative/competitive tasks—such as the Prisoner's Dilemma. In particular, it was shown that perturbation of prefrontal activity via TMS alters the tendency to adopt cooperative choices when individuals have to choose between a mutual or a selfish strategy, the appraisal and higher processes concerning values that guide our decisions, the propensity to accept unfair offers, and the efficiency of strategic planning [22–24]. Furthermore, dlPFC proved to be involved in impulsivity and cognitive control against cognitive biases during decision-making [25], as well as in risky decision-making and risk tolerance. In particular, the inhibition of the right dlPFC resulted in increased risky behaviour and significantly riskier decision-making strategies during risk-tolerance and gambling tasks [26, 27], even if contrasting data have been reported too [28]. Notably, even inferior parietal areas seem to play a role in the decision-making process by modulating risk-taking and propensity towards safer behaviours [29]. Finally, TMS-based research on moral decision making rather equally underlined the involvement of prefrontal and inferior parietal areas—namely, the TPJ. Specifically, the integration of moral, economic, and contextual information to guide moral decisions seems to be primarily mediated by the right TPJ [30], while the right dlPFC seems to primarily modulate the propensity towards emotional vs. utilitarian decisions when presented with moral dilemmas [31].

Overall, it may be concluded that TMS-based research on decision-making processes—as well as on attention, executive control, and working memory ones—has been recently characterized by a global tendency towards replication more than innovation. Therefore, one of the next relevant challenges should be the systematic commitment to devise and validate efficacious intervention protocols to empower those essential cognitive abilities and, therefore, reduce the detrimental effect of common cognitive implications of psychiatric disorders.

14.2 Memory

Taking into consideration the last few years of basic TMS research on memory functions in humans, the most relevant research trends are actually focused on the interplay of cortical structures mediating memory-related processes and, in particular, on the specific contribution of lateralized prefrontal regions to encoding and retrieval of information and memories, as well as on neural underpinnings of modality-specific short-term memory and of memories concerning doing things in the future, i.e. prospective memory. Furthermore, a few recent studies also tried to answer relevant questions about specific aspects of metacognition in memory, such as confidence and awareness of the mnestic process.

14.2.1 Short-Term Memory: A Distributed Network

Short-term memory is the ability to retain relatively small amounts of information active and readily available for short periods of time. It has been traditionally modelled as a first stage memory store, where information are temporarily but necessarily kept before passing them to long-term memory stores. Available empirical evidence suggests that short-term memory is supported by a network of modality-specific stores and that basic stimulus features are retained in sensory areas that are primarily involved in processing such features. TMS has been used as a probing technique to test those predictions and verify correlational findings on anatomical-functional associations for short-term memory processes.

Consistent with previous evidence, as an example, perturbation of cortical hotspots involved in processing speech sounds and word stimuli reduces the efficiency of short-term memory for verbal material, while perturbation of hotspots involved in visual and spatial processing reduces short-term memory performance for visual material. Indeed, it was shown that inhibiting left Broca's area, left anterior middle temporal gyrus (MTG), and the left anterior supramarginal gyrus (SMG) impairs short-term recall of words and non-words [32]. Again, the administration of TMS pulses in correspondence to primary visual areas during retention decreases short-term memory performance for stimuli presented in the contralateral (but not ipsilateral) visual hemifield to the non-invasive stimulation [33], thus suggesting a retinotopic organization even for stored visual information. In addition, perturbation of the left FEF results in altered storage of information on spatial positions [34]. On top of such modality-specific stores, TMS investigation also allowed us to identify modality-aspecific structures within the short-term memory network, and to identify their role. In particular, it has been recently proposed that the left SMG [35] and the right cerebellum [36] are involved in retaining information concerning the serial order of previously presented stimuli.

14.2.2 Long-Term Memory: Encoding Vs. Retrieval

Experimental, clinical and neuroimaging findings contributed to the definition of a functional model of encoding and retrieval processes that mainly focuses on the role of dorsal and lateral prefrontal regions, i.e. the Hemispheric Encoding-Retrieval Asymmetry (HERA) model [37]. According to such a model, the left dlPFC would primarily be associated with encoding of information to begin with the creation of the memory trace, while the right dlPFC would primarily be associated with retrieval of stored information for recognition or proper recall of past events, experiences, or notions.

In order to further test the consistency of such a model and to investigate the actual causal role of left vs. right dlPFC in different steps of the memory formation process, TMS was primarily used as an online interference tool. Going down to specifics, both paired-pulse [38] and rapid high-frequency [39] stimulation protocols were applied. TMS proved to be able to affect ongoing memory processes in the direction suggested by the HERA functional model. Indeed, during the encoding phase, non-invasive stimulation of the left dlPFC—but not of the right dlPFC—modulates memory performance in terms of reaction times, accuracy or discrimination. Conversely, memory performance is modulated by stimulation of the right (but not left) dlPFC, when TMS is applied during the retrieval phase. Nonetheless, even contrasting findings have been reported, with enhanced recognition memory performance following inhibition of the right dlPFC via rTMS [40] and with reduced recollection performance following perturbation of the right dlPFC via online high-frequency rTMS during the encoding phase [41].

Interestingly, such lateralized effects were also reported regardless of the verbal vs. visual-spatial nature of the material [38], in partial contrast with previous neuro-imaging and NIBS works, suggesting a differential contribution of the left and right prefrontal cortex in encoding verbal and visual-spatial materials, respectively [42]. While such a discrepancy might be explained on the basis of differences in methods and stimulation sites across studies, it also opens potentially valuable questions on fine-grained functional segregation within prefrontal areas and connectivity between its subregions.

A second interesting point concerns, instead, the investigation on age-related changes of functional lateralization postulated by the HERA model. Indeed, a broad set of neuroimaging findings suggested that the lateralization of memory-related processes within prefrontal areas tends to reduce during ageing, named the Hemispheric Asymmetry Reduction for Older Adults (HAROLD) model [43]. TMS was used as a tool to test whether such changes mirrored a progressive de-differentiation process or a compensatory mechanism. Progressive reduction of prefrontal asymmetry was initially deemed as a marker of positive compensation along ageing especially with regard to memory retrieval [44]. It was later reported that even encoding processes present a reduction of functional lateralization along ageing, though its manifestation depends on individuals' memory performance [45]. Again, it was suggested that TMS effects on encoding processes in ageing could be state-dependent. Indeed, it was shown that intermittent TBS applied to the left IFG of elderly participants resulted in an increase of left prefrontal and posterior-cerebellar areas, but only during deep vs. shallow encoding of information [46]. Findings concerning the mediatory role of individual performance and strategies once more highlight the relevance of properly accounting for or of investigating the interaction between individual factors, inter-individual differences, and the outcomes of NIBS.

14.2.3 Prospective Memory

Prospective memory is the ability to remember to perform a pre-planned behaviour in response to a future event or at some future point in time. Such an ability is crucial for most of the everyday activities and is at the core of our ability to adapt to and to act within a complex context. TMS research helped to better define the contribution of anterior and posterior cortical structures to the prospective memory function. In particular, while the early components of the prospective memory process, such as target checking, proved to be supported by the right dlPFC, later components, such as the retrieval of planned action and related, proved to be mediated by left PPC [47, 48].

In parallel with previous research on long-term memory, one of the most relevant research challenges in elderly age lies in the field of neurocognitive empowerment and likely is the qualification of neural underpinning of the difficulty to recall planned intentions and effectively enact intended behaviours when needed. The first pieces of evidence suggest that excitatory stimulation (intermittent TBS) of fronto-polar cortices of healthy elderly people might improve their performance at event-based prospective memory tasks, i.e. remembering to do something when a specific event happens [49]. Evidence for efficacy, short-term effects and long-term effects of NIBS training for prospective memory is still lacking. A better understanding of cognitive and neural processes supporting such an ability would help designing novel effective empowerment programs.

14.3   Language

The ability to create, learn, produce and understand language is probably among the most investigated functions of the human mind. The relevance of our ability to exchange information, convey meaning, and share thoughts, intentions and emotions—together with the typically devastating consequences of language impairments following brain lesions or degeneration—have pushed onward research on neural correlates of human language and related processes in healthy and damaged brains, via both neuroimaging and NIBS techniques.

Following a historical perspective, TMS studies with healthy participants initially focused on verifying the actual boundaries of the functional role of core language areas—i.e. Broca's and Wernicke's areas—so to refine and corroborate evidence coming from clinical observations on neurological patients [50, 51], as well as on trying to replicate fine-graded dissociations emerging from peculiar clinical cases—such as dissociations between the processing of abstract and concrete words and comprehension of idioms [52, 53].

Then, a first main research trend was focused on exploring specificities and interactions between cortical networks that support phonological and semantic processing of language, according to cognitive and psycholinguistic models of central processing of verbal material. Finally, a second core trend was mainly guided by a methodological purpose and was focused on the use of TMS as a probing tool to map language-eloquent cortex non-invasively.

14.3.1   Phonological and Semantic Processing

Converging psycholinguistic, clinical, and neuroimaging evidence contributed to define a global model of language processing that highlighted the distinct contribution of frontal and parietal regions to phonological and semantic levels of analysis.

Moving from such an evidence base and theoretical model, TMS allowed us to further test the neural underpinnings of processes that are activated while comprehending language and the causal contribution of specific cortical structures. TMS investigation consistently confirmed that language processing grounds on a quite broad network and that different processing steps rely on distinct frontal-parietal networks.

In particular, first-level phonological processing is reliably supported by both cortical structures within the posterior portion of the left IFG and by the left SMG in the inferior parietal lobule—IPL [54–56]. Conversely, it has been systematically reported that higher-level semantic processing of language—understood as the analysis of the meaning of language and words—is mediated by cortical structures within the anterior portion of the left IFG, by left MTG, and, within the IPL, by the left angular gyrus—AG [54, 57]. Such parcelling of left frontal and temporal-parietal language areas pointed out the fine organization of the network of cortical structures that allow us to comprehend language. It is worth reporting that, besides the contribution of higher cortical regions, a few TMS studies also focused on the supplementary role of the cerebellum in processing verbal material and suggested that the cerebellar vermis might support higher-level lexical decision-making [58].

As an additional note, it has to be acknowledged that while left-lateralized effects are generally and systematically reported when investigating phonological and semantic processing, evidence in favour of the contribution of right homologue areas has also been found [55, 56], which open relevant questions on the actual interaction between the right and left frontal-parietal language areas, on their potentially reciprocal compensation in the case of virtual as well as actual impairments, and on implications of inter-hemispheric interactions for the design of effective neuromodulation empowerment protocols.

Moreover, a few interesting TMS studies complemented previously available neuroimaging and behavioural evidence on the interface between language and motor functions and helped to better define the causal contribution of cortical motor regions to semantic processing of action- and movement-related words. Indeed, in line with the action-perception theory of language and embodied semantics models [59], it has been reported that perturbing the primary motor cortex (MI) and the SMA affects the processing time of action language [60, 61] and, vice versa, that specific linguistic factors—such as reading action verbs conjugated in the future with respect to past tense—can trigger implicit activation of motor regions with a consequent increase of TMS-induced MEPs [62]. While available pieces of evidence already helped to answer a few questions on the interdependence and interaction between sensorimotor and linguistic processes, the explanatory potential of the TMS technique is reasonably yet to be fully exerted. Sketching a clearer picture of functional connections and causal links between the sensorimotor and language systems would serve both to try and answer core questions on the foundations of human language and its development and to define novel intervention protocols to help patients to recover from language and sensorimotor impairment by building also on, respectively, residual motor and linguistic functions.

Finally, despite the presence of few studies, one of the most interesting and promising developments of TMS-based language research has to do with neural correlates of language in use, moving from the investigation of basic language functions to higher levels of analysis, such as pragmatics and communication skills. In this vein, it was reported that modulation of the dorsal anterior portion of the left IFG, but not the right one, reduces the lexical informativeness and global coherence of narratives in healthy people [63]. And again, it was shown that interfering with the activity of left IFG and of the left posterior MTG impairs the integration of speech and gesture, not allowing a proper combination of semantic information coming from verbal and non-verbal communication channels [64]. As for language comprehension, repetitive stimulation of the AG highlighted the critical role of this inferior parietal region in supporting speech understanding even when the acoustic signal is degraded [65], as it may happen in many real listening contexts. Although studies like those mentioned above have the merit of being among the first TMS-based studies complementing the broader correlational evidence base on neural signatures and bases of communication skills, much still has to be done.

14.3.2 Mapping Language Processes

While direct current stimulation is still regarded as the gold standard in terms of language mapping, the use of TMS as a mapping tool for language-eloquent cortical regions has become in the last few years a growing research trend. The non-invasive nature of the technique, indeed, allows us to easily create functional maps of cortex portions that are crucial for language-related processes in both the healthy and the dysfunctional brain, to directly compare such maps, and to easily replicate the examination. Because of this, TMS has become increasingly used for preoperative cortical mapping, at first with regard to the cortical substrate of motor functions and then even to cortical correlates of language functions. Notwithstanding the methodological and practical purpose of such a research line, its implications with respect to theoretical and functional models of language have still been valuable. Indeed, starting from the first applications based on repetitive TMS protocols to the most recent ones based on online neuronavigated stimulations, language mapping studies allowed us to define standardized stimulation protocols (in terms of intensity, frequency, and coil orientation) in order to maximize the observable stimulation effects depending on the stimulated region and shared procedures to report TMS-induced alterations of language processing, i.e. errors classifications and mapping [66, 67]. Different mapping studies focused alternatively on the left vs. right hemisphere or on both of them, but systematically reported the involvement of inferior and middle frontal regions, superior temporal areas, AG, and SMG in processing language. Conversely, evidence becomes scanter if we focus on cortical mapping of verbal and written production of language [68, 69] or on peculiar organization of language processing in bilinguals [70], which highlight how many core questions on the organization of language functions and on neural correlates of language skills are still left open.

14.4 Emotional and Social Processes

Although neuroscience research tradition has initially focused mainly on the core elements of cognition besides sensory, perceptual and motor functions, between the 90s and the early 2000s the interest in neural correlates of the human ability to feel and understand affective states as well as to interact and create social bonds grew more and more, leading to the formal definition of the social neuroscience discipline.

In that field, the TMS technique has been first and most systematically used to complement clinical, psychophysiological, electrophysiological, and neuroimaging research and investigate the contribution of specific cortical structures as primary hubs or as elements of broad networks mediating the ability to recognize and regulate emotions and affective states. Then, a second trend implied the use of such magnetic NIBS technique to explore the neural circuitry that supports human ability to perceive and process social signals, as well as to interact and exert prosocial behaviours.

14.4.1 Emotion Processing and Recognition

One of the most influential neurofunctional models in research on emotion recognition and regulation processes is the dual system model [71], which postulates the distinct contribution of a left-lateralized vs. right-lateralized prefrontal neural system to differently valenced emotional experiences. In particular, according to such model, left prefrontal structures would mediate positive emotional experience and approach behaviours, thus defining a behavioural activation system. Conversely, right prefrontal structures would mediate negative emotional experience and avoidance behaviours, thus contributing to a behavioural inhibition system. The model has also clinical implications both in terms of assessment and intervention practice, with a primary focus on mood disorders and deficits in emotional regulation.

The assumptions of the model have been tested via TMS by looking at the effect of induced perturbations with regard to the processing of different emotion-laden stimuli, both vocal and visual. In particular, it was shown that right and left prefrontal structures play the expected roles while processing emotional prosody or vocalizations [72], although even evidence in favour of an undifferentiated contribution of the right and left IFG to processing of emotional prosody has been reported [73]. Similarly, TMS investigation totally or partly corroborated model's assumptions even for visual emotion-laden stimuli, such as words and complex pictures [74, 75], and in particular for facial expressions [76], although—even in the case of visual stimuli—negative results concerning valence-related lateralization of prefrontal areas have also been reported [77]. Remarkably, a consistent lateralized prefrontal contribution was reported even concerning emotional memory and retrieval of affectively connoted material. Indeed, even if contrasting findings have also been reported [78], a quite systematic set of studies suggested that left- and right-sided prefrontal cortices play peculiar roles in encoding and retrieval processes for positive vs. negative words [79–81]. Conversely, with regard to emotion regulation processes in healthy individuals, TMS-based investigations seem not to corroborate model assumptions, with unexpected reports of lack of mood improvement or even stronger mood decline in healthy participants after high-frequency modulation of the left dlPFC [82].

In addition to the above-mentioned investigations on frontal asymmetries, TMS studies also helped to outline the global organization of the frontal-temporal-parietal network mediating emotion perception and recognition. By using emotionally con- noted pictures of scenes and, in the vast majority of studies, facial expressions, it was shown that proper emotional appraisal in terms of valence and arousal and efficient emotion recognition overall ground on the interaction between cortical structures within the IFG, dorsal-medial prefrontal area, pre-SMA, anterior insula, posterior superior temporal sulcus (STS), somatosensory cortex, TPJ, and even cer- ebellum [83–87].

As a final note, it is important to underline that, in view of the notable amount of studies on the role and interaction between different cortical structures supporting emotion processing skills, only a few of such studies actually took into consider- ation additional individual factors—such as personality traits or measures of empa- thy—that have a strong connection with the development of investigated affective processes and that might account for partly unexpected empirical findings. As an example, Paracampo and colleagues [84] showed that people that present high vs. low proficiency in emotion perception rely on distinct cortical structures to infer emotional states from facial expressions. As for personality factors, instead, Balconi and colleagues highlighted the mediatory role of individual empathy trait on the medial PFC contribution to emotion recognition processes [83], as well as the medi- atory role of anxiety trait and motivational mechanisms on the contribution of later- alized prefrontal areas to recognition and retrieval of emotion-laden verbal material [79, 80].

By taking into account the complexity of individual and contextual influences that actually mediate emotion appraisal and perception in real life and keeping in mind the original rationale of social neuroscience as a discipline interested in both how our brains support affective-social processes and how individual, affective, and social factors shape the way our brain works, those examples help to highlight that many relevant questions on the interaction between social-affective processes and individual/contextual characteristics still deserve further investigation.

14.4.2 Social Perception and Behaviour

Moving to TMS-based investigation of social perception and behaviour, the most explored topic likely concerns the detection and processing of social signals. In particular, such social skill has been typically investigated via both explicit and implicit measures, by presenting participants with neutral, threatening, and (in a few cases) joyful body stimuli and asking them to classify them or measuring covert indices of corticospinal excitability (e.g. amplitude of MEPs or intracortical facilitation, ICF). Overall, such set of studies highlighted that processing of social threat is mediated by the combined contribution of the left dlPFC, right ventral premotor cortex, right posterior STS, right anterior IPS, and right IPL [88–90].

Besides exploring such basic social perception skill, TMS has also been used to probe the neural underpinnings of higher social cognition skills and demonstrate the distinct role of cortical structures within the medial prefrontal cortex and right TPJ with regard to agency-attribution, self-other-distinction and perspective-taking [12, 91, 92], mentalization (understood as the ability to create theories about others' thought, intentions, and beliefs) [91], social judgement [93], and overcoming of self-centeredness and self-enhancement [94].

Finally, a third main research trend in TMS-based research on social skills focused on social behaviour and, in particular, on prosocial attitudes. In line with the vast neuroimaging and electrophysiological literature on the preferential involvement of frontal lobe cortices in higher social processes—such as social reasoning, moral decision-making, and interpersonal fairness—NIBS findings showed a remarkable consistency in confirming the causal role of dlPFC regions—especially right-sided structures—in controlling selfish behaviour and exercising forgiveness, as well as in empathic resonance and in fostering supportive behaviour [95, 96].

To conclude, the present collection of research data has the merit of having complemented available correlational evidence and of having further confirmed the causal role of specific cortical structures within the neural networks that support some of the basic social perception, cognition, and behaviour skills. It has nonetheless to be acknowledged that—notwithstanding the progressive tendency towards a greater and greater attention to the ecological value of stimuli, tasks, and experimental settings—ecological validity of laboratory-based research in social neuroscience is still a critical issue. And this point becomes even more critical when the focuses of analysis are processes and functions that support and shape interpersonal interactions and everyday social dynamics. Given the overall consistency of available evidence base, it might be now the right time to step forward and begin to focus also on complex interaction skills and to move towards a systematic investigation of neural underpinnings of social processes when they are put in play during actual social exchanges, following a new recent trend that is influencing neuroimaging, electrophysiological and psychophysiological research in social neuroscience.

14.5 Conclusions

The present work aimed at identifying and introducing main research trends in basic TMS research on the neural underpinnings of cognitive and affective processes, with a focus on the last 15 years. Based on a reasoned recognition of available relevant literature, we have summarized the most consistent findings concerning TMS studies on attention and executive functions, memory, language, emotion processing, and social perception and behaviour. Without claiming to be exhaustive, this tentative systematization also allowed to point out specific open questions and to outline novel research topics to be better explored via TMS techniques.

As a final remark, the analysis of the evidence base concerning TMS basic research in cognitive and affective neuroscience highlighted even a few global critical issues.

Firstly, it has to be acknowledged that research in cognitive-affective and, in particular, social neuroscience typically targets complex and highly interdependent processes. It is often rather difficult, then, to model and parcel out mechanisms or processing steps that clearly and solely identify a specific cognitive function. As a consequence, implementing TMS-based investigation of higher cognitive-affective-social processes—given the fine-grained spatial, temporal, and cognitive resolution of the technique and its potential for probing structurally and functionally distinct modules—requires strict and reasoned theoretical and methodological assumptions. Remarkably, implications of such first point could be accounted for by assuming a multi-method investigation approach, i.e. by integrating behavioural outcome measures with hemodynamic and electrophysiological measures to better outline the effects of TMS-induced perturbations on global neural dynamics and functional connections within the network of structures supporting the investigated functions. An additional critical issue is the well-known limitation concerning the depth of TMS-induced perturbations. It is, indeed, impossible to selectively reach and modulate the activity of deep structures by using such a technique, at least in its traditional variants. It is then not possible to exploit the explanatory potential of the technique to investigate the causal role of many relevant subcortical nodes of networks mediating higher functions, especially affective and social ones. Finally, much still needs to be done to properly devise and implement valid NIBS intervention protocols targeting many higher cognitive, affective and social skills. Further basic research on long-term behavioural and functional effects induced by TMS protocols in both healthy participants and neurology-psychiatry patients are indeed needed to accurately assess the potential of non-invasive magnetic stimulation as a supportive tool for early intervention at prodromic or initial clinical phases and, in particular, for neurocognitive empowerment, besides neurorehabilitation. A last critical point is, then, represented by the ethical implications of using TMS—and, more generally, NIBS—as a tool to pre-emptively induce the modulation of neural activity and of the individual cognitive-affective-social profile, especially in healthy individuals. Possible implications in terms of undesired secondary effects of NIBS protocols, as well as of threats to the core concepts of human authenticity and inter-individual equity (which might be affected by differences in the opportunity to access such techniques) are to date fuelling the neuroethics debate and are yet to be fully explored.

References

1. Vanderhasselt M-A, De Raedt R, Leyman L, Baeken C. Role of the left DLPFC in endogenous task preparation: experimental repetitive transcranial magnetic stimulation study. Neuropsychobiology. 2010;61(3):162–8.
2. Vanderhasselt M-A, De Raedt R, Baeken C, Leyman L, Clerinx P, D'Haenen H. The influence of rTMS over the right dorsolateral prefrontal cortex on top-down attentional processes. Brain Res. 2007;1137(1):111–6.

3. Wagner M, Rihs TA, Mosimann UP, Fisch HU, Schlaepfer TE. Repetitive transcranial magnetic stimulation of the dorsolateral prefrontal cortex affects divided attention immediately after cessation of stimulation. J Psychiatr Res. 2006;40(4):315–21.
4. Esterman M, Liu G, Okabe H, Reagan A, Thai M, DeGutis J. Frontal eye field involvement in sustaining visual attention: evidence from transcranial magnetic stimulation. Neuroimage. 2015;111:542–8.
5. Heinen K, Feredoes E, Ruff CC, Driver J. Functional connectivity between prefrontal and parietal cortex drives visuo-spatial attention shifts. Neuropsychologia. 2017;99:81–91.
6. Kiyonaga A, Korb FM, Lucas J, Soto D, Egner T. Dissociable causal roles for left and right parietal cortex in controlling attentional biases from the contents of working memory. Neuroimage. 2014;100:200–5.
7. Mevorach C, Hodsoll J, Allen H, Shalev L, Humphreys G. Ignoring the elephant in the room: a neural circuit to downregulate salience. J Neurosci. 2010;30(17):6072–9.
8. Dambacher F, Sack AT, Lobbestael J, Arntz A, Brugmann S, Schuhmann T. The role of right prefrontal and medial cortex in response inhibition: interfering with action restraint and action cancellation using transcranial magnetic brain stimulation. J Cogn Neurosci. 2014;26(8):1775–84.
9. Lee HW, Lu M-S, Chen C-Y, Muggleton NG, Hsu T-Y, Juan C-H. Roles of the pre-SMA and rIFG in conditional stopping revealed by transcranial magnetic stimulation. Behav Brain Res. 2016;296:459–67.
10. Parmigiani S, Cattaneo L. Stimulation of the dorsal premotor cortex, but not of the supplementary motor area proper, impairs the stop function in a STOP signal task. Neuroscience. 2018;394:14–22.
11. Balconi M. Dorsolateral prefrontal cortex, working memory and episodic memory processes: insight through transcranial magnetic stimulation techniques. Neurosci Bull. 2013;29(3):381–9.
12. Crivelli D, Balconi M. The agent brain: a review of non-invasive brain stimulation studies on sensing agency. Front Behav Neurosci. 2017;11(November):229.
13. Ko JH, Monchi O, Ptito A, Petrides M, Strafella AP. Repetitive transcranial magnetic stimulation of dorsolateral prefrontal cortex affects performance of the Wisconsin Card Sorting Task during provision of feedback. Int J Biomed Imaging. 2008;2008:143238.
14. Bahlmann J, Beckmann I, Kuhlemann I, Schweikard A, Münte TF. Transcranial magnetic stimulation reveals complex cognitive control representations in the rostral frontal cortex. Neuroscience. 2015;300:425–31.
15. Ko JH, Monchi O, Ptito A, Bloomfield P, Houle S, Strafella AP. Theta burst stimulation-induced inhibition of dorsolateral prefrontal cortex reveals hemispheric asymmetry in striatal dopamine release during a set-shifting task: a TMS-[(11)C]raclopride PET study. Eur J Neurosci. 2008;28(10):2147–55.
16. Mottaghy FM. Interfering with working memory in humans. Neuroscience. 2006;139(1):85–90.
17. Aleman A, van't Wout M. Repetitive transcranial magnetic stimulation over the right dorsolateral prefrontal cortex disrupts digit span task performance. Neuropsychobiology. 2008;57(1–2):44–8.
18. Miyauchi E, Kitajo K, Kawasaki M. TMS-induced theta phase synchrony reveals a bottom-up network in working memory. Neurosci Lett. 2016;622:10–4.
19. Georgiev D, Rocchi L, Tocco P, Speekenbrink M, Rothwell JC, Jahanshahi M. Continuous theta burst stimulation over the dorsolateral prefrontal cortex and the pre-SMA alter drift rate and response thresholds respectively during perceptual decision-making. Brain Stimul. 2016;9(4):601–8.
20. Klein P-A, Olivier E, Duque J. Influence of reward on corticospinal excitability during movement preparation. J Neurosci. 2012;32(50):18124–36.
21. Klein-Flügge MC, Bestmann S. Time-dependent changes in human corticospinal excitability reveal value-based competition for action during decision processing. J Neurosci. 2012;32(24):8373–82.
22. De Dreu CKW, Kret ME, Sligte IG. Modulating prefrontal control in humans reveals distinct pathways to competitive success and collective waste. Soc Cogn Affect Neurosci. 2016;11(8):1236–44.

23. Knoch D, Pascual-Leone A, Meyer K, Treyer V, Fehr E. Diminishing reciprocal fairness by disrupting the right prefrontal cortex. Science (80-). 2006;314(5800):829–32.
24. Soutschek A, Sauter M, Schubert T. The importance of the lateral prefrontal cortex for strategic decision making in the prisoner's dilemma. Cogn Affect Behav Neurosci. 2015;15(4):854–60.
25. Ballard IC, Aydogan G, Kim B, McClure SM. Causal evidence for the dependence of the magnitude effect on dorsolateral prefrontal cortex. Sci Rep. 2018;8(1):16545.
26. Knoch D, Gianotti LRR, Pascual-Leone A, Treyer V, Regard M, Hohmann M, et al. Disruption of right prefrontal cortex by low-frequency repetitive transcranial magnetic stimulation induces risk-taking behavior. J Neurosci. 2006;26(24):6469–72.
27. Tulviste J, Bachmann T. Diminished risk-aversion after right DLPFC stimulation: effects of rTMS on a risky ball throwing task. J Int Neuropsychol Soc. 2019;25(1):72–8.
28. Cho SS, Ko JH, Pellecchia G, Van Eimeren T, Cilia R, Strafella AP. Continuous theta burst stimulation of right dorsolateral prefrontal cortex induces changes in impulsivity level. Brain Stimul. 2010;3(3):170–6.
29. Coutlee CG, Kiyonaga A, Korb FM, Huettel SA, Egner T. Reduced risk-taking following disruption of the intraparietal sulcus. Front Neurosci. 2016;10:588.
30. Obeso I, Moisa M, Ruff CC, Dreher J-C. A causal role for right temporo-parietal junction in signaling moral conflict. Elife. 2018;7:e40671.
31. Tassy S, Oullier O, Duclos Y, Coulon O, Mancini J, Deruelle C, et al. Disrupting the right prefrontal cortex alters moral judgement. Soc Cogn Affect Neurosci. 2012;7(3):282–8.
32. Savill NJ, Cornelissen P, Pahor A, Jefferies E. rTMS evidence for a dissociation in short-term memory for spoken words and nonwords. Cortex. 2019;112:5–22.
33. van de Ven V, Jacobs C, Sack AT. Topographic contribution of early visual cortex to short-term memory consolidation: a transcranial magnetic stimulation study. J Neurosci. 2012;32(1):4–11.
34. Campana G, Cowey A, Casco C, Oudsen I, Walsh V. Left frontal eye field remembers "where" but not "what". Neuropsychologia. 2007;45(10):2340–5.
35. Guidali G, Pisoni A, Bolognini N, Papagno C. Keeping order in the brain: the supramarginal gyrus and serial order in short-term memory. Cortex. 2019;119:89–99.
36. Ferrari C, Cattaneo Z, Oldrati V, Casiraghi L, Castelli F, D'Angelo E, et al. TMS over the cerebellum interferes with short-term memory of visual sequences. Sci Rep. 2018;8(1): 6722.
37. Tulving E, Kapur S, Craik FI, Moscovitch M, Houle S. Hemispheric encoding/retrieval asymmetry in episodic memory: positron emission tomography findings. Proc Natl Acad Sci. 1994;91(6):2016–20.
38. Gagnon G, Blanchet S, Grondin S, Schneider C. Paired-pulse transcranial magnetic stimulation over the dorsolateral prefrontal cortex interferes with episodic encoding and retrieval for both verbal and non-verbal materials. Brain Res. 2010;1344:148–58.
39. Rossi S, Innocenti I, Polizzotto NR, Feurra M, De Capua A, Ulivelli M, et al. Temporal dynamics of memory trace formation in the human prefrontal cortex. Cereb Cortex. 2011;21(2):368–73.
40. Turriziani P, Smirni D, Zappalà G, Mangano GR, Oliveri M, Cipolotti L. Enhancing memory performance with rTMS in healthy subjects and individuals with mild cognitive impairment: the role of the right dorsolateral prefrontal cortex. Front Hum Neurosci. 2012;6:62.
41. Turriziani P, Oliveri M, Salerno S, Costanzo F, Koch G, Caltagirone C, et al. Recognition memory and prefrontal cortex: dissociating recollection and familiarity processes using rTMS. Behav Neurol. 2008;19(1–2):23–7.
42. Floel A, Poeppel D, Buffalo EA, Braun A, CW-H W, Seo H-J, et al. Prefrontal cortex asymmetry for memory encoding of words and abstract shapes. Cereb Cortex. 2004;14(4):404–9.
43. Cabeza R. Hemispheric asymmetry reduction in older adults: the HAROLD model. Psychol Aging. 2002;17(1):85–100.
44. Rossi S, Miniussi C, Pasqualetti P, Babiloni C, Rossini PM, Cappa SF. Age-related functional changes of prefrontal cortex in long-term memory: a repetitive transcranial magnetic stimulation study. J Neurosci. 2004;24(36):7939–44.
45. Manenti R, Cotelli M, Miniussi C. Successful physiological aging and episodic memory: a brain stimulation study. Behav Brain Res. 2011;216(1):153–8.

46. Vidal-Piñeiro D, Martin-Trias P, Arenaza-Urquijo EM, Sala-Llonch R, Clemente IC, Mena-Sánchez I, et al. Task-dependent activity and connectivity predict episodic memory network-based responses to brain stimulation in healthy aging. Brain Stimul. 2014;7(2): 287–96.
47. Bisiacchi PS, Cona G, Schiff SJ, Basso D. Modulation of a fronto-parietal network in event-based prospective memory: an rTMS study. Neuropsychologia. 2011;49(8): 2225–32.
48. Cona G, Marino G, Bisiacchi PS. Superior parietal cortex and the attention to delayed intention: an rTMS study. Neuropsychologia. 2017;95:130–5.
49. Debarnot U, Crépon B, Orriols E, Abram M, Charron S, Lion S, et al. Intermittent theta burst stimulation over left BA10 enhances virtual reality-based prospective memory in healthy aged subjects. Neurobiol Aging. 2015;36(8):2360–9.
50. Hartwigsen G, Saur D, Price CJ, Ulmer S, Baumgaertner A, Siebner HR. Perturbation of the left inferior frontal gyrus triggers adaptive plasticity in the right homologous area during speech production. Proc Natl Acad Sci U S A. 2013;110(41):16402–7.
51. Smirni D, Turriziani P, Mangano GR, Bracco M, Oliveri M, Cipolotti L. Modulating phonemic fluency performance in healthy subjects with transcranial magnetic stimulation over the left or right lateral frontal cortex. Neuropsychologia. 2017;102:109–15.
52. Papagno C, Fogliata A, Catricalà E, Miniussi C. The lexical processing of abstract and concrete nouns. Brain Res. 2009;1263:78–86.
53. Oliveri M, Romero L, Papagno C. Left but not right temporal involvement in opaque idiom comprehension: a repetitive transcranial magnetic stimulation study. J Cogn Neurosci. 2004;16(5):848–55.
54. Hartwigsen G, Weigel A, Schuschan P, Siebner HR, Weise D, Classen J, et al. Dissociating parieto-frontal networks for phonological and semantic word decisions: a condition-and-perturb TMS study. Cereb Cortex. 2016;26(6):2590–601.
55. Hartwigsen G, Baumgaertner A, Price CJ, Koehnke M, Ulmer S, Siebner HR. Phonological decisions require both the left and right supramarginal gyri. Proc Natl Acad Sci U S A. 2010;107(38):16494–9.
56. Hartwigsen G, Price CJ, Baumgaertner A, Geiss G, Koehnke M, Ulmer S, et al. The right posterior inferior frontal gyrus contributes to phonological word decisions in the healthy brain: evidence from dual-site TMS. Neuropsychologia. 2010;48(10):3155–63.
57. Zhu Z, Gold BT, Chang C-F, Wang S, Juan C-H. Left middle temporal and inferior frontal regions contribute to speed of lexical decision: a TMS study. Brain Cogn. 2015;93:11–7.
58. Argyropoulos GP. Cerebellar theta-burst stimulation selectively enhances lexical associative priming. Cerebellum. 2011;10(3):540–50.
59. Buccino G, Colagè I, Gobbi N, Bonaccorso G. Grounding meaning in experience: a broad perspective on embodied language. Neurosci Biobehav Rev. 2016;69:69–78.
60. Courson M, Macoir J, Tremblay P. Role of medial premotor areas in action language processing in relation to motor skills. Cortex. 2017;95:77–91.
61. Vukovic N, Feurra M, Shpektor A, Myachykov A, Shtyrov Y. Primary motor cortex functionally contributes to language comprehension: an online rTMS study. Neuropsychologia. 2017;96:222–9.
62. Candidi M, Leone-Fernandez B, Barber HA, Carreiras M, Aglioti SM. Hands on the future: facilitation of cortico-spinal hand-representation when reading the future tense of hand-related action verbs. Eur J Neurosci. 2010;32(4):677–83.
63. Marini A, Urgesi C. Please get to the point! A cortical correlate of linguistic informativeness. J Cogn Neurosci. 2012;24(11):2211–22.
64. Zhao W, Riggs K, Schindler I, Holle H. Transcranial magnetic stimulation over left inferior frontal and posterior temporal cortex disrupts gesture-speech integration. J Neurosci. 2018;38(8):1891–900.
65. Hartwigsen G, Golombek T, Obleser J. Repetitive transcranial magnetic stimulation over left angular gyrus modulates the predictability gain in degraded speech comprehension. Cortex. 2015;68:100–10.

66. Sollmann N, Fuss-Ruppenthal S, Zimmer C, Meyer B, Krieg SM. Investigating stimulation protocols for language mapping by repetitive navigated transcranial magnetic stimulation. Front Behav Neurosci. 2018;12:197.
67. Krieg SM, Lioumis P, Mäkelä JP, Wilenius J, Karhu J, Hannula H, et al. Protocol for motor and language mapping by navigated TMS in patients and healthy volunteers; workshop report. Acta Neurochir. 2017;159(7):1187–95.
68. Könönen M, Tamsi N, Säisänen L, Kemppainen S, Määttä S, Julkunen P, et al. Non-invasive mapping of bilateral motor speech areas using navigated transcranial magnetic stimulation and functional magnetic resonance imaging. J Neurosci Methods. 2015;248:32–40.
69. Rogić Vidaković M, Gabelica D, Vujović I, Šoda J, Batarelo N, Džimbeg A, et al. A novel approach for monitoring writing interferences during navigated transcranial magnetic stimulation mappings of writing related cortical areas. J Neurosci Methods. 2015;255: 139–50.
70. Tussis L, Sollmann N, Boeckh-Behrens T, Meyer B, Krieg SM. Identifying cortical first and second language sites via navigated transcranial magnetic stimulation of the left hemisphere in bilinguals. Brain Lang. 2017;168:106–16.
71. Harmon-Jones E. Asymmetrical frontal cortical activity, affective valence, and motivation direction. In: Harmon-Jones E, Winkielman P, editors. Social neuroscience integrating biological and psychological explanations of social behavior. New York: The Guildford Press; 2007. p. 137–56.
72. Donhauser PW, Belin P, Grosbras M-H. Biasing the perception of ambiguous vocal affect: a TMS study on frontal asymmetry. Soc Cogn Affect Neurosci. 2014;9(7):1046–51.
73. Hoekert M, Vingerhoets G, Aleman A. Results of a pilot study on the involvement of bilateral inferior frontal gyri in emotional prosody perception: an rTMS study. BMC Neurosci. 2010;11:93.
74. Berger C, Domes G, Balschat J, Thome J, Höppner J. Effects of prefrontal rTMS on autonomic reactions to affective pictures. J Neural Transm. 2017;124(Suppl 1):139–52.
75. Roesmann K, Dellert T, Junghoefer M, Kissler J, Zwitserlood P, Zwanger P, et al. The causal role of prefrontal hemispheric asymmetry in valence processing of words—insights from a combined cTBS-MEG study. Neuroimage. 2019;191:367–79.
76. Notzon S, Steinberg C, Zwanger P, Junghöfer M. Modulating emotion perception: opposing effects of inhibitory and excitatory prefrontal cortex stimulation. Biol Psychiatry Cogn Neurosci Neuroimaging. 2018;3(4):329–36.
77. Ferrari C, Gamond L, Gallucci M, Vecchi T, Cattaneo Z. An exploratory TMS study on prefrontal lateralization in valence categorization of facial expressions. Exp Psychol. 2017;64(4):282–9.
78. Schutter DJLG, van Honk J. Increased positive emotional memory after repetitive transcranial magnetic stimulation over the orbitofrontal cortex. J Psychiatry Neurosci. 2006;31(2):101–4.
79. Balconi M, Cobelli C. Motivational mechanisms (BAS) and prefrontal cortical activation contribute to recognition memory for emotional words. rTMS effect on performance and EEG (alpha band) measures. Brain Lang. 2014;137:77–85.
80. Balconi M, Ferrari C. Repeated transcranial magnetic stimulation on dorsolateral prefrontal cortex improves performance in emotional memory retrieval as a function of level of anxiety and stimulus valence. Psychiatry Clin Neurosci. 2013;67(4): 210–8.
81. Balconi M, Ferrari C. rTMS stimulation on left DLPFC increases the correct recognition of memories for emotional target and distractor words. Cogn Affect Behav Neurosci. 2012;12(3):589–98.
82. Möbius M, Lacomblé L, Meyer T, Schutter DJLG, Gielkens T, Becker ES, et al. Repetitive transcranial magnetic stimulation modulates the impact of a negative mood induction. Soc Cogn Affect Neurosci. 2017;12(4):526–33.
83. Balconi M, Bortolotti A. Emotional face recognition, empathic trait (BEES), and cortical contribution in response to positive and negative cues. The effect of rTMS on dorsal medial prefrontal cortex. Cogn Neurodyn. 2013;7(1):13–21.

84. Paracampo R, Pirruccio M, Costa M, Borgomaneri S, Avenanti A. Visual, sensorimotor and cognitive routes to understanding others' enjoyment: an individual differences rTMS approach to empathic accuracy. Neuropsychologia. 2018;116:86–98.
85. Balconi M, Canavesio Y. High-frequency rTMS improves facial mimicry and detection responses in an empathic emotional task. Neuroscience. 2013;236:12–20.
86. Ferrari C, Oldrati V, Gallucci M, Vecchi T, Cattaneo Z. The role of the cerebellum in explicit and incidental processing of facial emotional expressions: a study with transcranial magnetic stimulation. Neuroimage. 2018;169:256–64.
87. Sliwinska MW, Pitcher D. TMS demonstrates that both right and left superior temporal sulci are important for facial expression recognition. Neuroimage. 2018;183:394–400.
88. Candidi M, Stienen BMC, Aglioti SM, de Gelder B. Event-related repetitive transcranial magnetic stimulation of posterior superior temporal sulcus improves the detection of threatening postural changes in human bodies. J Neurosci. 2011;31(48):17547–54.
89. Mazzoni N, Jacobs C, Venuti P, Silvanto J, Cattaneo L. State-dependent TMS reveals representation of affective body movements in the anterior intraparietal cortex. J Neurosci. 2017;37(30):7231–9.
90. Sagliano L, D'Olimpio F, Panico F, Gagliardi S, Trojano L. The role of the dorsolateral prefrontal cortex in early threat processing: a TMS study. Soc Cogn Affect Neurosci. 2016;11(12):1992–8.
91. Hill CA, Suzuki S, Polania R, Moisa M, O'Doherty JP, Ruff CC. A causal account of the brain network computations underlying strategic social behavior. Nat Neurosci. 2017;20(8):1142–9.
92. Heinisch C, Krüger MC, Brüne M. Repetitive transcranial magnetic stimulation over the temporoparietal junction influences distinction of self from famous but not unfamiliar others. Behav Neurosci. 2012;126(6):792–6.
93. Ferrari C, Nadal M, Schiavi S, Vecchi T, Cela-Conde CJ, Cattaneo Z. The dorsomedial prefrontal cortex mediates the interaction between moral and aesthetic valuation: a TMS study on the beauty-is-good stereotype. Soc Cogn Affect Neurosci. 2017;12(5):707–17.
94. Soutschek A, Ruff CC, Strombach T, Kalenscher T, Tobler PN. Brain stimulation reveals crucial role of overcoming self-centeredness in self-control. Sci Adv. 2016;2(10):e1600992.
95. Balconi M, Canavesio Y. High-frequency rTMS on DLPFC increases prosocial attitude in case of decision to support people. Soc Neurosci. 2014;9(1):82–93.
96. Müller-Leinß J-M, Enzi B, Flasbeck V, Brüne M. Retaliation or selfishness? An rTMS investigation of the role of the dorsolateral prefrontal cortex in prosocial motives. Soc Neurosci. 2018;13(6):701–9.

Cortical Excitability, Plasticity and Oscillations in Major Psychiatric Disorders: A Neuronavigated TMS-EEG Based Approach

15

Mario Rosanova, Simone Sarasso, Marcello Massimini, and Silvia Casarotto

15.1 Corticothalamic Oscillations and Psychiatric Disorders

Brain functions critically depend on the interactions between functionally specialized neural structures, encompassing cortical areas and thalamic nuclei [1]. In this framework, information processing within local circuits and communication at distance are thought to be reflected by rhythmic and coordinated fluctuations of excitability [2]. These oscillations emerge from the interactions between local intrinsic neuronal properties and structural connectivity, and play a key role in perceptual, motor and cognitive functions [3]. For instance, oscillations of neural circuits distributed over frontal and parietal cortices have been related to working memory functions [4, 5]. During working memory tasks, fronto-parietal circuits generate electrical oscillations at different frequency bands, each playing a specific role. As such, gamma-band oscillations seem specifically involved in active retaining of information while theta-band oscillations may specifically be involved in ordering items over time, with alpha-band oscillations being mostly involved in the inhibition of task-irrelevant information [6].

M. Rosanova (✉)
Department of Biomedical and Clinical Sciences "L. Sacco", University of Milan, Milan, Italy

Fondazione Europea per la Ricerca Biomedica Onlus, Milan, Italy
e-mail: mario.rosanova@unimi.it

S. Sarasso · S. Casarotto
Department of Biomedical and Clinical Sciences "L. Sacco", University of Milan, Milan, Italy

M. Massimini
Department of Biomedical and Clinical Sciences "L. Sacco", University of Milan, Milan, Italy

IRCCS Fondazione Don Gnocchi, Milan, Italy

© Springer Nature Switzerland AG 2020
B. Dell'Osso, G. Di Lorenzo (eds.), *Non Invasive Brain Stimulation in Psychiatry and Clinical Neurosciences*,
https://doi.org/10.1007/978-3-030-43356-7_15

Oscillatory properties of cortical circuits have been classically studied by means of non-invasive techniques, such as EEG. Since its introduction by Hans Berger almost a century ago [7], the EEG has become an essential tool for investigating the relationships between brain rhythms and neuropsychiatric disorders. In psychiatry research, EEG recordings are traditionally performed either at rest or when subjects are engaged by sensory stimuli (Event-Related Potentials—ERPs), motor or cognitive tasks ("cognitive probes").

Such EEG and ERP approaches have revealed abnormal cortical oscillatory patterns in many psychiatric disorders [8, 9] and some of them have been linked with specific cognitive deficits [10, 11]. For example, working memory deficits in schizophrenic patients were found to be associated with reduced prefrontal cortical gamma-band oscillations [12], whereas patients affected by major depressive disorder (MDD) showed left/right asymmetries in the topographical distribution of the alpha-band oscillations [13].

Recording of the ongoing EEG provides valuable information about the oscillatory properties of cortical circuits under different conditions. However, spontaneous brain rhythms are difficult to control even in standardized conditions, and may radically change depending on the experimental conditions, such as fluctuation in the state of vigilance and the level of attention. A classic example is represented by the drastic changes in EEG topography and power that rapidly occur upon eye closing. In relation to psychiatric patients, all these factors are even more difficult to control.

A more reliable assessment of the intrinsic oscillatory properties of cortical circuits can be obtained by measuring steady-state-evoked responses. In this case, visual flashes, or auditory tones, are presented at different rates, and the stimulation frequency that results in the largest EEG or the magnetoencephalography output, the resonance frequency, is detected. This standardized approach yielded consistent results and demonstrated the existence of clear-cut resonance frequencies in specific parts of the human corticothalamic system, around 10 Hz in the visual cortex and around 40 Hz in the auditory cortex. However, steady-state responses, as other responses evoked by the stimulation of peripheral receptors, can only probe a limited set of primary sensory cortices [14–18].

In the following, we will focus on an alternative electrophysiological method to study the oscillatory properties of cortical circuits, i.e. the combination of TMS and EEG. Aided by neuronavigation, TMS-EEG allows to directly perturbate a wide range of cortical areas (including frontal and posterior association cortices) and to record the ensuing electrical oscillations. This technique may thus offer a standardized way of mapping the oscillatory properties of the cerebral cortex in a way that is not dependent on the level of the subject's engagement, and not, restricted to the exploration of sensory areas, two features that seem particularly valuable in the case of psychiatric patients.

15.2   A Short Introduction to TMS-EEG

TMS is based on the physical principle of electromagnetic induction, which was discovered by Faraday in 1831. In the case of TMS, when a strong and short-lasting electric current passes through a TMS coil applied over the scalp, a brief but strong magnetic field (duration: 1 ms; intensity: 1–2 T) is generated. This magnetic pulse locally depolarizes axonal membranes, leading cortical neurons under the TMS coil to fire action potentials [19, 20]. Then, the synchronous volley of action potentials triggered in the target area by the TMS pulse is conducted down the existing anatomical pathways, such as the corticospinal tract, the activation of which results in a motor evoked potential that can be recorded by combining TMS with electromyography (TMS-EMG) [21, 22]. A similar mechanism leads to the activation of corticocortical and corticothalamic tracts, resulting in local and remote cortical electrical waves and oscillations that can be captured by employing TMS-EEG. Thus, TMS-EEG allows observing the electrical oscillations generated by the thalamocortical circuits activated upon a direct perturbation of a given cortical area.

Due to the large electric field generated by the TMS pulse, its combination with EEG required the development of dedicated TMS-compatible EEG amplifiers. The earliest attempts in this direction trace back to 1989, when Cracco and colleagues measured transcallosal responses by targeting TMS over the primary motor cortex [23]. A few years later, the same group recorded the response of the cerebral cortex to cerebellar magnetic stimulation [24]. However, since a traditional EEG amplifier was employed, these pioneering studies were still strongly limited by large artifacts related to the TMS pulse, and that did not allow to record the immediate responses at the EEG leads under the coil. The first fully TMS-compatible EEG amplifiers were implemented almost 20 years ago [25, 26] and, by obliterating the large and long-lasting electromagnetic artifact induced by the TMS coil discharge, allowed the reliable recording of artifact-free TMS-evoked potentials (TEPs) under the coil a few milliseconds after the TMS pulse [25, 27, 28]. More recently, DC-amplifiers provided with a wide dynamic range and high sampling rates ($\geq$5 KHz) have been employed to successfully record TEPs devoid of long-lasting pulse artifacts [29].

Besides the electromagnetic artifact, spurious and unspecific biological activations may still contaminate the EEG response to TMS. A major challenge is represented by the high-amplitude scalp muscle artifacts that can be triggered by the TMS pulse when areas below cranial muscles are targeted [30]. Second, the sound (TMS "click") and the vibrations produced by the TMS discharge can evoke sensory evoked potentials, which can be effectively abolished by employing a masking noise reproducing the time-varying frequency components of the TMS "click" [28] and by placing a layer of foam between the TMS coil and the subject's head [31]. In order to control these confounding factors, one can follow different approaches, such as performing control experiments that employ sham conditions [32, 33] or removing the artifacts by means of off-line data preprocessing procedures [34]. A third and more dependable approach relies on a real-time quality check of the TMS-EEG signals. Crucially, after choosing a cortical target based on the neuronavigation system and before starting the measurement session, the operator must apply all the available procedures to minimize the possible confounding factors due to the sensory co-stimulation and to maximize the effectiveness of the TMS pulse on the cerebral cortex [35]. First, the parameters of the masking noise, such as the volume of the audio output, should be adjusted in order to effectively mask the TMS "click". In the same vein, the very large early biphasic deflections due to the direct activation of scalp muscles can be reduced or abolished by changing the orientation of the coil [30]. Finally, the stimulation parameters (coil rotation and stimulator output) should be fine-tuned in order to record TEPs with a good signal to noise ratio and characterized by stimulation site-specific topographies [36]. The employment of a neuronavigation system can help in keeping the selected stimulation parameters constant within and across sessions in the case of longitudinal studies [37].

Once the electromagnetic artifacts evoked by the discharge of the TMS coil are properly managed [36, 38] and generating spurious and unspecific cortical responses to TMS, namely the ones associated with auditory or somatosensory stimulations that are appropriately reduced or abolished, TEPs reflect genuine responses of cortical circuits to TMS [39]. In this way, TEPs can be used to reliably keep track of cortical excitability and intrinsic oscillatory properties of human thalamocortical circuits in both research and clinical settings [40, 41].

The very early components (waves) of TEPs reflect the immediate neural responses of the circuits that are underneath the stimulator and hence are directly excited by the TMS pulse. Therefore, measuring the slope and amplitude of those very early waves of TEPs (10–30 ms) is a dependable way to assess cortical excitability and its changes, i.e. cortical plasticity. This approach, which closely matches the one used in animal studies of cortical plasticity [42, 43], allowed the observation of plastic changes of cortical circuits during wakefulness [44, 45], after a protocol of induction of cortical plasticity via rTMS [46], to compare the effects of single and paired-pulse TMS [47], during and after anodic stimulation with Transcranial Direct Current Stimulation [48, 49], and after the administration of L-DOPA in patients suffering from Parkinson's disease [50] (Fig. 15.1).

To measure cortical excitability and plasticity through TMS one should focus on single components of TEPs, such as the waves that immediately follow the TMS pulse. On the other hand, analyzing the sustained EEG oscillations triggered by TMS can help to better understand the intrinsic oscillatory properties of corticothalamic circuits in healthy and diseased brains. For instance, a TMS-EEG study conducted in healthy subjects showed that different corticothalamic modules oscillate at a preferred "natural" frequency when perturbed by TMS. Specifically, TEPs were consistently dominated by EEG oscillations in the alpha band (8–12 Hz) after stimulation of the occipital cortex (Brodmann area 19), in the beta-band (13–20 Hz) after stimulation of the parietal cortex (Brodmann area 7), and in the fast beta/gamma-band (21–50 Hz) after stimulation of the premotor cortex (Brodmann area 6) [51]. Interestingly, the study also showed that each cortical area tends to oscillate at its own natural frequency, even when it is indirectly activated after the discharge of a TMS pulse over a remote, yet connected cortical area (Fig. 15.2). A further modeling study suggested that the connectivity pattern of each cortical area is a key factor in determining its natural frequency [52]. Along with the evidence that the lesion of thalamic nuclei specifically disrupts TMS-EEG oscillations [53], these studies suggest that the natural frequency is a measure of the intrinsic properties of corticocortical and corticothalamic connections.

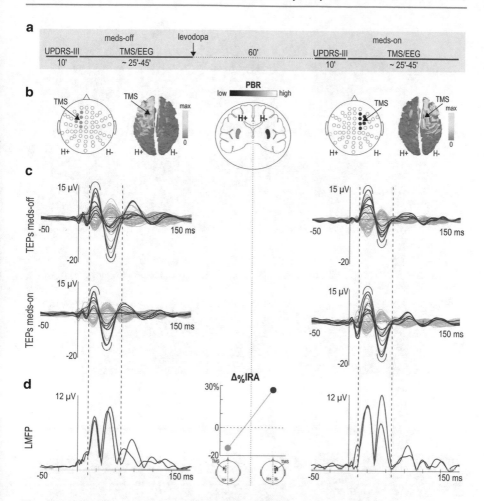

Fig. 15.1 TEPs recorded in patients affected by Parkinson's disease. L-DOPA intake (meds-on) induces a significant increase of the amplitude of the very early components of TEPs in the hemisphere more affected by the degeneration of the basal ganglia circuits (H+), greater than in the less affected hemisphere (H−). Panel **a** shows the overall EEG channel layout with the selected clusters of channels close to the targeted frontal area (cyan contours on the brain maps). Panel **b** shows the butterfly plots of the TEPs recorded at all 60 EEG channels (blue traces in the meds-off condition; red traces in the meds-on condition). U-shaped traces indicate the positive and negative early components of TEPs. Panel **c** shows the Local Mean Field Power (LMFP) and the percentage values of the area under the curve (between the two local minima and encompassing the early consecutive positive and negative waves triggered by TMS; Immediate Response Area: IRA) in the meds-on and meds-off conditions. (Modified from [50])

15.3 TMS-EEG Studies of Major Psychiatric Disorders

Cortical excitability and plasticity in psychiatric disorders have been studied mainly by employing TMS-EMG [54]. This technique has also been employed to assess changes

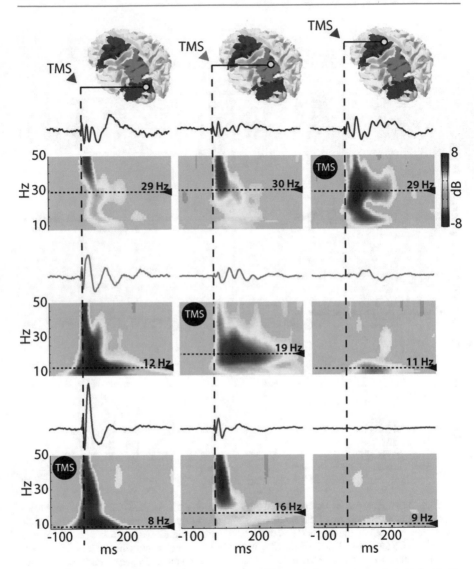

Fig. 15.2 The natural frequency is a local property of individual corticothalamic modules. In the top row, the colored patches on the cortical surface mark the areas from which cortical currents are recorded after the reconstruction of the cortical source activations. Below, time series and Event-Related Spectral Perturbation (ERSP) plots of local cortical currents are displayed for the premotor cortex (first row, blue traces, Brodmann area 6), the posterior parietal cortex (second row, green traces, Brodmann area 7), and the occipital cortex (third row, red traces, Brodmann area 19), when the occipital cortex is stimulated (first column), the posterior parietal cortex is stimulated (second column) and the premotor cortex is stimulated (third column). The dotted lines highlight the peak frequency for each plot. The comparison of the ERSP plots on the diagonal line (marked by the TMS icon) reveals that each cortical area responds with a distinctive natural frequency when directly stimulated. Comparing the plots on the horizontal and on the vertical lines reveals that the natural frequency is a local, intrinsic property that is partially preserved also when its cortical generator is not directly stimulated. (Modified from [51])

due to pharmacological treatments in psychiatric patients [55]. However, TMS-EMG provides indirect measures of cortical excitability and plasticity, as it measures responses to TMS of the corticospinal tract rather than direct responses of the corticocortical and corticothalamic circuits. Most importantly, the use of TMS-EMG is by definition limited to the primary motor cortex, whereas pathophysiological underpinnings of psychiatric disorders mostly involve non-motor cortical regions, such as the prefrontal cortex.

At odds with TMS-EMG, neuronavigated TMS-EEG allows the direct measurement of cortical excitability and plasticity of virtually any cortical area. Moreover, TMS-EEG can provide a read-out of the oscillatory properties of corticothalamic modules without necessarily relying on cognitive probes, i.e. without engaging the subject in a cognitive task. By virtue of these technical advantages, in recent years, neuronavigated TMS-EEG has been employed in psychiatric research to identify possible electrophysiological biomarkers and to study the neurophysiological underpinnings of psychiatric disorders (for recent reviews on the use of TMS-EEG in psychiatry research, see [56–58]).

In a series of TMS-EEG studies conducted in schizophrenic patients, Ferrarelli and coworkers measured the early components of TEPs, and observed a significant reduction of excitability of the primary motor cortex [59] and of the premotor and prefrontal cortical areas [60, 61] in patients compared to healthy controls, whereas parietal cortical areas showed preserved levels of excitability. On the other hand, applying some of the methods used in the studies cited above to measure cortical excitability by means of TMS-EEG, a recent study observed plastic changes in the cortex of patients affected by drug-resistant MDD after treatment [62]. Specifically, in this study, the slope and amplitude of early TEP components, recorded over the premotor cortex, increased after the application of Electroconvulsive Therapy (ECT) in MDD patients compared to baseline (Fig. 15.3). In a similar study, by measuring the slope and amplitude of early TEP waves, an increase of cortical excitability was observed after light therapy and sleep deprivation in the prefrontal cortex of MDD patients [63].

Other research groups focused on specific cortical areas and used TMS-EEG to study the electrophysiological properties of those areas. One relevant example is the dorsolateral prefrontal cortex (DLPFC), which underpins high cognitive functions and plays a key role in the pathophysiology of major psychiatric disorders [64]. In a recent paper, Daskalakis and his coworkers performed TMS-EEG measurements by targeting DLPFC in MDD patients and, compared to healthy controls, observed a larger early TEP negative component named N45, whose amplitude was reliably predicting the state of the patients [65]. In another study, the same group found an altered modulation of the TEP positive component named P60 that correlated with the cognitive impairments in schizophrenic patients [66]. Notably, as both N45 and P60 are thought to be markers of the excitation-inhibition balance in the targeted cortical area, these studies suggest that TMS-EEG measurements can provide further insight into the pathophysiology of MDD and schizophrenia.

TMS-EEG has also been employed to investigate the oscillatory properties of corticothalamic circuits in major psychiatric disorders. In a TMS-EEG study on schizophrenia [59], TEPs were recorded by targeting different cortical sites, such as parietal, motor, premotor, and prefrontal areas in schizophrenic patients and healthy

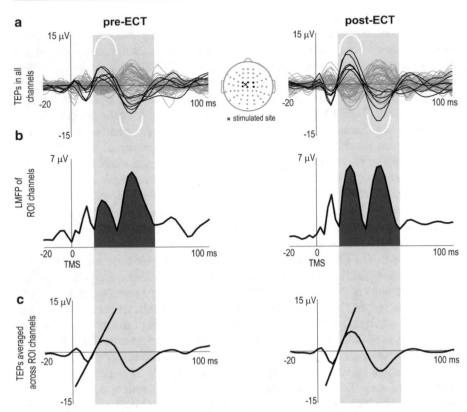

Fig. 15.3 Estimation of cortical excitability after Electroconvulsive Therapy (ECT) by means of TMS-EEG. Panel **a** represents the butterfly plots of the TEPs recorded at all EEG channels before (pre-) and after (post-) ECT. The central map depicts the EEG electrode layout (black and gray dots) on the scalp. Black traces correspond to selected channels (channels from the Region Of Interest; ROI), located nearby the stimulated site (black cross) and containing a large, early TEP component, consisting of a positive wave (white reversed U-shaped trace), followed by a negative wave (white U-shaped trace). Panel **b** reports the LMFP computed considering the channels in the ROI. Cortical excitability was measured by calculating the area (dark gray shadow) between the two local minima (light gray shadow) and encompassing the early consecutive positive and negative waves triggered by TMS (Immediate Response Area: IRA). Panel **c** shows the TEPs averaged across the ROI channels in the two conditions. Slanting lines highlight the slope of the rising side of the early large positive wave evoked by TMS (Immediate Response Slope: IRS). (Modified from [62])

controls. TEPs were then analyzed in the time-frequency domain in order to measure the natural frequency [51] for each cortical site in the two populations. These results further supported the idea that in healthy subjects, more posterior cortical areas, such as the parietal and the primary motor ones, oscillate in a lower frequency range (low beta range) compared to premotor and prefrontal cortices (high beta/ gamma range). On the contrary, in comparison to healthy subjects, schizophrenic patients showed reduced natural frequency with significant lower values for the primary motor cortex and highly significant lower values for the premotor and the prefrontal cortex (Fig. 15.4). These findings confirmed the impairment of the oscillatory

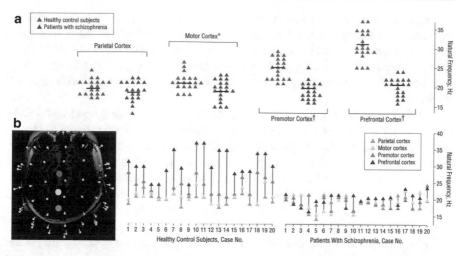

Fig. 15.4 The natural frequency of TEP oscillations is a sensitive parameter for discriminating patients with schizophrenia and healthy control subjects. In panel **a**, the individual natural frequency values of healthy control subjects and patients with schizophrenia are plotted for 4 cortical areas. Horizontal lines indicate mean natural frequency values of each group for each cortical area ($*P < 0.05$; $†P < 0.001$). Panel **b** shows the natural frequency values of targeted parietal, motor, premotor and prefrontal cortical areas (red, orange, yellow, green dots on the 3D reconstruction of the cortical surface), for each study participant. (Modified from [59])

properties of the frontal thalamocortical circuits, which had been already suggested by the same research group in a previous TMS-EEG study [60] and it has been recently reproduced in patients with acute, first-episode schizophrenia [67]. Moreover, the study suggested a pathophysiological link between oscillatory deficits in the frontal lobe and clinical features of schizophrenia. Indeed, it has been observed that the prefrontal natural frequency values in patients with schizophrenia are negatively correlated with positive symptoms and that the strongest correlation was with delusion Positive and Negative Syndrome Scale (PANSS) subscores. A further TMS-EEG study conducted in psychiatric patients not only confirmed the reduction of natural frequency in schizophrenia, but also observed a similar deficit in bipolar disorder and MDD [68]. Overall, these results suggest that abnormal oscillations could be a common feature of different psychiatric disorders. Most importantly, they strengthen the hypothesis that dysfunctions in the generation of neural oscillations play a key role in the pathophysiology of major psychiatric disorders [8, 69, 70].

15.4 Future Directions for TMS-EEG in Psychiatric Research

TMS-EEG offers the possibility to directly and non-invasively measure cortical excitability and oscillatory properties, which are often altered in major psychiatric disorders. In this context, the analysis of TEPs has revealed a specific decrease or altered excitability of frontal cortical areas in MDD and schizophrenic patients compared to healthy controls. Moreover, measuring TEPs allowed to keep track of plastic modifications of the cortical circuits in MDD

patients due to invasive or non-invasive treatments, such as ECT, sleep deprivation and light therapy. Most importantly, the assessment of the intrinsic oscillatory properties of corticothalamic modules by means of TMS-EEG, i.e.
natural frequency, showed that frontal circuits in major psychiatric disorders
are characterized by abnormal intrinsic oscillations in comparison with healthy
controls.

The few examples reported above suggest that TMS-EEG may represent a useful tool to explore the electrophysiological properties of cortical circuits in major
psychiatric disorders. In this perspective, future studies may consider and further
develop at least two interesting applications. First, as direct and non-invasive
measures of cortical excitability, TEPs could be systematically used to assess and
titrate the cortical effects of different stimulation protocols toward an individualized approach. Second, the study of TMS-evoked oscillations should be extended
to other clinical populations, such as first-episode, drug-naïve patients as well as
to siblings to define novel early markers of schizophrenia and to shed light on its
electrophysiological underpinnings.

References

1. Park HJ, Friston K. Structural and functional brain networks: from connections to cognition.
   Science. 2013;342(6158):1238411. https://doi.org/10.1126/science.1238411.
2. Buzsáki G, Draguhn A. Neuronal oscillations in cortical networks. Science.
   2004;304(5679):1926–9.
3. Wang XJ. Neurophysiological and computational principles of cortical rhythms in cognition.
   Physiol Rev. 2010;90(3):1195–268. https://doi.org/10.1152/physrev.00035.2008.
4. Wang XJ. Synaptic reverberation underlying mnemonic persistent activity. Trends Neurosci.
   2001;24(8):455–63.
5. Constantinidis C, Klingberg T. The neuroscience of working memory capacity and training. Nat Rev Neurosci. 2016;17(7):438–49. Epub 2016 May 26. https://doi.org/10.1038/
   nrn.2016.43.
6. Roux F, Uhlhaas PJ. Working memory and neural oscillations: α-γ versus θ-γ codes for distinct WM information? Trends Cogn Sci. 2014;18(1):16–25. Epub 2013 Nov 19. https://doi.
   org/10.1016/j.tics.2013.10.010.
7. Millett D. Hans Berger: from psychic energy to the EEG. Perspect Biol Med. 2001;44(4):522–42.
8. Buzsáki G, Watson BO. Brain rhythms and neural syntax: implications for efficient coding of
   cognitive content and neuropsychiatric disease. Dialogues Clin Neurosci. 2012;14(4):345–67.
9. Leuchter AF, Cook IA, Jin Y, Phillips B. The relationship between brain oscillatory activity and
   therapeutic effectiveness of transcranial magnetic stimulation in the treatment of major depressive disorder. Front Hum Neurosci. 2013;7:37. https://doi.org/10.3389/fnhum.2013.00037.
   eCollection.2013.
10. Uhlhaas PJ, Singer W. Neural synchrony in brain disorders: relevance for cognitive dysfunc-
    tions and pathophysiology. Neuron. 2006;52(1):155–68.
11. Bruder GE, Stewart JW, McGrath PJ. Right brain, left brain in depressive disorders: clini-
    cal and theoretical implications of behavioral, electrophysiological and neuroimaging find-
    ings. Neurosci Biobehav Rev. 2017;78:178–91. Epub 2017 Apr 23. https://doi.org/10.1016/j.
    neubiorev.2017.04.021.
12. Senkowski D, Gallinat J. Dysfunctional prefrontal gamma-band oscillations reflect working
    memory and other cognitive deficits in schizophrenia. Biol Psychiatry. 2015;77(12):1010–9.
    Epub 2015 Mar 4. https://doi.org/10.1016/j.biopsych.2015.02.034.

13. Smart OL, Tiruvadi VR, Mayberg HS. Multimodal approaches to define network oscillations in depression. Biol Psychiatry. 2015;77(12):1061–70. Epub 2015 Jan 28. https://doi.org/10.1016/j.biopsych.2015.01.002.
14. Narici L, Romani GL. Neuromagnetic investigation of synchronized spontaneous activity. Brain Topogr. 1989;2(1–2):19–30.
15. Regan D. Human brain electrophysiology: evoked potentials and evoked magnetic fields in science and medicine. New York: Elsevier; 1989.
16. Silberstein S. Steady-state visually evoked potentials, brain resonances and cognitive processes. In: Nunez P, editor. Neocortical dynamics and human EEG rhythms. New York: Oxford UP; 1995.
17. Rager G, Singer W. The response of cat visual cortex to flicker stimuli of variable frequency. Eur J Neurosci. 1998;10:1856–77.
18. Herrmann CS. Human EEG responses to 1–100 Hz flicker: resonance phenomena in visual cortex and their potential correlation to cognitive phenomena. Exp Brain Res. 2001;137:346–53.
19. Mueller JK, Grigsby EM, Prevosto V, Petraglia FW, Rao H, Deng ZD, Peterchev AV, Sommer MA, Egner T, Platt ML, Grill WM. Simultaneous transcranial magnetic stimulation and single-neuron recording in alert non-human primates. Nat Neurosci. 2014;17(8):1130–6. Epub 2014 Jun 29. https://doi.org/10.1038/nn.3751.
20. Romero MC, Davare M, Armendariz M, Janssen P. Neural effects of transcranial magnetic stimulation at the single-cell level. Nat Commun. 2019;10(1):2642. https://doi.org/10.1038/s41467-019-10638-7.
21. Barker AT, Jalinous R, Freeston IL. Non-invasive magnetic stimulation of human motor cortex. Lancet. 1985;1(8437):1106–7.
22. Hallett M. Transcranial magnetic stimulation: a primer. Neuron. 2007;55(2):187–99.
23. Cracco RQ, Amassian VE, Maccabee PJ, Cracco JB. Comparison of human transcallosal responses evoked by magnetic coil and electrical stimulation. Electroencephalogr Clin Neurophysiol. 1989;74(6):417–24.
24. Amassian VE, Cracco RQ, Maccabee PJ, Cracco JB. Cerebello-frontal cortical projections in humans studied with the magnetic coil. Electroencephalogr Clin Neurophysiol. 1992;85(4):265–72.
25. Ilmoniemi RJ, Virtanen J, Ruohonen J, Karhu J, Aronen HJ, Näätänen R, Katila T. Neuronal responses to magnetic stimulation reveal cortical reactivity and connectivity. Neuroreport. 1997;8(16):3537–40.
26. Virtanen J, Ruohonen J, Näätänen R, Ilmoniemi RJ. Instrumentation for the measurement of electric brain responses to transcranial magnetic stimulation. Med Biol Eng Comput. 1999;37(3):322–6.
27. Paus T, Sipila PK, Strafella AP. Synchronization of neuronal activity in the human primary motor cortex by transcranial magnetic stimulation: an EEG study. J Neurophysiol. 2001;86(4):1983–90.
28. Massimini M, Ferrarelli F, Huber R, Esser SK, Singh H, Tononi G. Breakdown of cortical effective connectivity during sleep. Science. 2005;309(5744):2228–32.
29. Bonato C, Miniussi C, Rossini PM. Transcranial magnetic stimulation and cortical evoked potentials: a TMS/EEG co-registration study. Clin Neurophysiol. 2006;117(8):1699–707. Epub 2006 Jun 22.
30. Mutanen T, Mäki H, Ilmoniemi RJ. The effect of stimulus parameters on TMS-EEG muscle artifacts. Brain Stimul. 2013;6(3):371–6. Epub 2012 Aug 10. https://doi.org/10.1016/j.brs.2012.07.005.
31. ter Braack EM, de Vos CC, van Putten MJ. Masking the auditory evoked potential in TMS-EEG: a comparison of various methods. Brain Topogr. 2015;28(3):520–8. Epub 2013 Sep 1. https://doi.org/10.1007/s10548-013-0312-z.
32. Conde V, Tomasevic L, Akopian I, Stanek K, Saturnino GB, Thielscher A, Bergmann TO, Siebner HR. The non-transcranial TMS-evoked potential is an inherent source of ambiguity in TMS-EEG studies. Neuroimage. 2019;185:300–12. Epub 2018 Oct 19. https://doi.org/10.1016/j.neuroimage.2018.10.052.

33. Gordon PC, Desideri D, Belardinelli P, Zrenner C, Ziemann U. Comparison of cortical EEG responses to realistic sham versus real TMS of human motor cortex. Brain Stimul. 2018;11(6):1322–30. Epub 2018 Aug 16. https://doi.org/10.1016/j.brs.2018.08.003.

34. Rogasch NC, Thomson RH, Farzan F, Fitzgibbon BM, Bailey NW, Hernandez-Pavon JC, Daskalakis ZJ, Fitzgerald PB. Removing artefacts from TMS-EEG recordings using independent component analysis: importance for assessing prefrontal and motor cortex network properties. Neuroimage. 2014;101:425–39. Epub 2014 Jul 25. https://doi.org/10.1016/j.neuroimage.2014.07.037.

35. Belardinelli P, Biabani M, Blumberger DM, Bortoletto M, Casarotto S, David O, Desideri D, Etkin A, Ferrarelli F, Fitzgerald PB, Fornito A, Gordon PC, Gosseries O, Harquel S, Julkunen P, Keller CJ, Kimiskidis VK, Lioumis P, Miniussi C, Rosanova M, Rossi S, Sarasso S, Wu W, Zrenner C, Daskalakis ZJ, Rogasch NC, Massimini M, Ziemann U, Ilmoniemi RJ. Reproducibility in TMS-EEG studies: a call for data sharing, standard procedures and effective experimental control. Brain Stimul. 2019;12(3):787–90. Epub 2019 Jan 19. https://doi.org/10.1016/j.brs.2019.01.010.

36. Rosanova M, Casarotto S, Pigorini A, Canali P, Casali AG, Massimini M. Combining transcranial magnetic stimulation with electroencephalography to study human cortical excitability and effective connectivity. In: Fellin T, Halassa M, editors. Neuronal network analysis. Berlin: Springer; 2012, XIII, 490 p. 118. Springer.

37. Casarotto S, Romero Lauro LJ, Bellina V, Casali AG, Rosanova M, Pigorini A, Defendi S, Mariotti M, Massimini M. EEG responses to TMS are sensitive to changes in the perturbation parameters and repeatable over time. PLoS One. 2010;5(4):e10281. https://doi.org/10.1371/journal.pone.0010281.

38. Ilmoniemi RJ, Kicić D. Methodology for combined TMS and EEG. Brain Topogr. 2010;22(4):233–48. Epub 2009 Dec 10. https://doi.org/10.1007/s10548-009-0123-4.

39. Gosseries O, Sarasso S, Casarotto S, Boly M, Schnakers C, Napolitani M, Bruno MA, Ledoux D, Tshibanda JF, Massimini M, Laureys S, Rosanova M. On the cerebral origin of EEG responses to TMS: insights from severe cortical lesions. Brain Stimul. 2015;8(1):142–9. Epub 2014 Oct 18. https://doi.org/10.1016/j.brs.2014.10.008.

40. Ziemann U. Transcranial magnetic stimulation at the interface with other techniques: a powerful tool for studying the human cortex. Neuroscientist. 2011;17(4):368–81. Epub 2011 Feb 10. https://doi.org/10.1177/1073858410390225.

41. Rossini PM, Burke D, Chen R, Cohen LG, Daskalakis Z, Di Iorio R, Di Lazzaro V, Ferreri F, Fitzgerald PB, George MS, Hallett M, Lefaucheur JP, Langguth B, Matsumoto H, Miniussi C, Nitsche MA, Pascual-Leone A, Paulus W, Rossi S, Rothwell JC, Siebner HR, Ugawa Y, Walsh V, Ziemann U. Non-invasive electrical and magnetic stimulation of the brain, spinal cord, roots and peripheral nerves: basic principles and procedures for routine clinical and research application. An updated report from an I.F.C.N. Committee. Clin Neurophysiol. 2015;126(6):1071–107. Epub 2015 Feb 10. https://doi.org/10.1016/j.clinph.2015.02.001.

42. Bliss TV, Lomo T. Long-lasting potentiation of synaptic transmission in the dentate area of the anaesthetized rabbit following stimulation of the perforant path. J Physiol. 1973;232(2):331–56.

43. Vyazovskiy VV, Cirelli C, Pfister-Genskow M, Faraguna U, Tononi G. Molecular and electrophysiological evidence for net synaptic potentiation in wake and depression in sleep. Nat Neurosci. 2008;11(2):200–8. Epub 2008 Jan 20. https://doi.org/10.1038/nn2035.

44. Huber R, Mäki H, Rosanova M, Casarotto S, Canali P, Casali AG, Tononi G, Massimini M. Human cortical excitability increases with time awake. Cereb Cortex. 2013;23(2):332–8. Epub 2012 Feb 7. https://doi.org/10.1093/cercor/bhs014.

45. Ly JQM, Gaggioni G, Chellappa SL, Papachilleos S, Brzozowski A, Borsu C, Rosanova M, Sarasso S, Middleton B, Luxen A, Archer SN, Phillips C, Dijk DJ, Maquet P, Massimini M, Vandewalle G. Circadian regulation of human cortical excitability. Nat Commun. 2016;7:11828. https://doi.org/10.1038/ncomms11828.

46. Esser SK, Huber R, Massimini M, Peterson MJ, Ferrarelli F, Tononi G. A direct demonstration of cortical LTP in humans: a combined TMS/EEG study. Brain Res Bull. 2006;69(1):86–94. Epub 2005 Dec 1.

47. Ferreri F, Pasqualetti P, Määttä S, Ponzo D, Ferrarelli F, Tononi G, Mervaala E, Miniussi C, Rossini PM. Human brain connectivity during single and paired pulse transcranial magnetic stimulation. Neuroimage. 2011;54(1):90–102. Epub 2010 Aug 1. https://doi.org/10.1016/j.neuroimage.2010.07.056.

48. Romero Lauro LJ, Rosanova M, Mattavelli G, Convento S, Pisoni A, Opitz A, Bolognini N, Vallar G. DCS increases cortical excitability: direct evidence from TMS-EEG. Cortex. 2014;58:99–111. Epub 2014 Jun 6. https://doi.org/10.1016/j.cortex.2014.05.003.

49. Pisoni A, Mattavelli G, Papagno C, Rosanova M, Casali AG, Romero Lauro LJ. Cognitive enhancement induced by anodal tDCS drives circuit-specific cortical plasticity. Cereb Cortex. 2018;28(4):1132–40. https://doi.org/10.1093/cercor/bhx021.

50. Casarotto S, Turco F, Comanducci A, Perretti A, Marotta G, Pezzoli G, Rosanova M, Isaias IU. Excitability of the supplementary motor area in Parkinson's disease depends on subcortical damage. Brain Stimul. 2019;12(1):152–60. Epub 2018 Oct 23. https://doi.org/10.1016/j.brs.2018.10.011.

51. Rosanova M, Casali A, Bellina V, Resta F, Mariotti M, Massimini M. Natural frequencies of human corticothalamic circuits. J Neurosci. 2009;29(24):7679–85. https://doi.org/10.1523/JNEUROSCI.0445-09.2009.

52. Cona F, Zavaglia M, Massimini M, Rosanova M, Ursino M. A neural mass model of interconnected regions simulates rhythm propagation observed via TMS-EEG. Neuroimage. 2011;57(3):1045–58. Epub 2011 May 11. https://doi.org/10.1016/j.neuroimage.2011.05.007.

53. Van Der Werf YD, Sadikot AF, Strafella AP, Paus T. The neural response to transcranial magnetic stimulation of the human motor cortex. II Thalamocortical contributions. Exp Brain Res. 2006;175(2):246–55. Epub 2006 Jul 11.

54. Bunse T, Wobrock T, Strube W, Padberg F, Palm U, Falkai P, Hasan A. Motor cortical excitability assessed by transcranial magnetic stimulation in psychiatric disorders: a systematic review. Brain Stimul. 2014;7(2):158–69. Epub 2013 Dec 14. https://doi.org/10.1016/j.brs.2013.08.009.

55. Minzenberg MJ, Leuchter AF. The effect of psychotropic drugs on cortical excitability and plasticity measured with transcranial magnetic stimulation: implications for psychiatric treatment. J Affect Disord. 2019;253:126–40. Epub 2019 Apr 10. https://doi.org/10.1016/j.jad.2019.04.067.

56. Kaskie RE, Ferrarelli F. Investigating the neurobiology of schizophrenia and other major psychiatric disorders with transcranial magnetic stimulation. Schizophr Res. 2018;192:30–8. Epub 2017 May 3. https://doi.org/10.1016/j.schres.2017.04.045.

57. Tremblay S, Rogasch NC, Premoli I, Blumberger DM, Casarotto S, Chen R, Di Lazzaro V, Farzan F, Ferrarelli F, Fitzgerald PB, Hui J, Ilmoniemi RJ, Kimiskidis VK, Kugiumtzis D, Lioumis P, Pascual-Leone A, Pellicciari MC, Rajji T, Thut G, Zomorrodi R, Ziemann U, Daskalakis ZJ. Clinical utility and prospective of TMS-EEG. Clin Neurophysiol. 2019;130(5):802–44. Epub 2019 Jan 19. https://doi.org/10.1016/j.clinph.2019.01.001.

58. Hui J, Tremblay S, Daskalakis ZJ. The current and future potential of transcranial magnetic stimulation with electroencephalography in psychiatry. Clin Pharmacol Ther. 2019;106(4):734–46. Epub 2019 Aug 30. https://doi.org/10.1002/cpt.1541.

59. Ferrarelli F, Sarasso S, Guller Y, Riedner BA, Peterson MJ, Bellesi M, Massimini M, Postle BR, Tononi G. Reduced natural oscillatory frequency of frontal thalamocortical circuits in schizophrenia. Arch Gen Psychiatry. 2012;69(8):766–74.

60. Ferrarelli F, Massimini M, Peterson MJ, Riedner BA, Lazar M, Murphy MJ, Huber R, Rosanova M, Alexander AL, Kalin N, Tononi G. Reduced evoked gamma oscillations in the frontal cortex in schizophrenia patients: a TMS/EEG study. Am J Psychiatry. 2008;165(8):996–1005. Epub 2008 May 15. https://doi.org/10.1176/appi.ajp.2008.07111733.

61. Ferrarelli F, Riedner BA, Peterson MJ, Tononi G. Altered prefrontal activity and connectivity predict different cognitive deficits in schizophrenia. Hum Brain Mapp. 2015;36(11):4539–52. Epub 2015 Aug 19. https://doi.org/10.1002/hbm.22935.

62. Casarotto S, Canali P, Rosanova M, Pigorini A, Fecchio M, Mariotti M, Lucca A, Colombo C, Benedetti F, Massimini M. Assessing the effects of electroconvulsive therapy on cortical

excitability by means of transcranial magnetic stimulation and electroencephalography. Brain Topogr. 2013;26(2):326–37. Epub 2012 Oct 9. https://doi.org/10.1007/s10548-012-0256-8.

63. Canali P, Sferrazza Papa G, Casali AG, Schiena G, Fecchio M, Pigorini A, Smeraldi E, Colombo C, Benedetti F. Changes of cortical excitability as markers of antidepressant response in bipolar depression: preliminary data obtained by combining transcranial magnetic stimulation (TMS) and electroencephalography (EEG). Bipolar Disord. 2014;16(8):809–19. Epub 2014 Sep 15. https://doi.org/10.1111/bdi.12249.

64. Arnsten AF, Rubia K. Neurobiological circuits regulating attention, cognitive control, motivation, and emotion: disruptions in neurodevelopmental psychiatric disorders. J Am Acad Child Adolesc Psychiatry. 2012;51(4):356–67. Epub 2012 Mar 3. https://doi.org/10.1016/j.jaac.2012.01.008.

65. Voineskos D, Blumberger DM, Zomorrodi R, Rogasch NC, Farzan F, Foussias G, Rajji TK, Daskalakis ZJ. Altered transcranial magnetic stimulation-electroencephalographic markers of inhibition and excitation in the dorsolateral prefrontal cortex in major depressive disorder. Biol Psychiatry. 2019;85(6):477–86. Epub 2018 Oct 18. https://doi.org/10.1016/j.biopsych.2018.09.032.

66. Noda Y, Barr MS, Zomorrodi R, Cash RFH, Farzan F, Rajji TK, Chen R, Daskalakis ZJ, Blumberger DM. Evaluation of short interval cortical inhibition and intracortical facilitation from the dorsolateral prefrontal cortex in patients with schizophrenia. Sci Rep. 2017;7(1):17106. https://doi.org/10.1038/s41598-017-17052-3.

67. Ferrarelli F, Kaskie RE, Graziano B, Reis CC, Casali AG. Abnormalities in the evoked frontal oscillatory activity of first-episode psychosis: a TMS/EEG study. Schizophr Res. 2019;206:436–9. Epub 2018 Nov 23. https://doi.org/10.1016/j.schres.2018.11.008.

68. Canali P, Sarasso S, Rosanova M, Casarotto S, Sferrazza-Papa G, Gosseries O, Fecchio M, Massimini M, Mariotti M, Cavallaro R, Smeraldi E, Colombo C, Benedetti F. Shared reduction of oscillatory natural frequencies in bipolar disorder, major depressive disorder and schizophrenia. J Affect Disord. 2015;184:111–5. Epub 2015 Jun 3. https://doi.org/10.1016/j.jad.2015.05.043.

69. Mathalon DH, Sohal VS. Neural oscillations and synchrony in brain dysfunction and neuropsychiatric disorders: it's about time. JAMA Psychiat. 2015;72(8):840–4. https://doi.org/10.1001/jamapsychiatry.2015.0483.

70. Vinogradov S, Herman A. Psychiatric illnesses as oscillatory connectomopathies. Neuropsychopharmacology. 2016;41(1):387–8. https://doi.org/10.1038/npp.2015.308.

Part III

tDCS and Its Applications in Neuropsychiatry and Clinical Neuroscience

tDCS in Depressive Disorders

16

Andre R. Brunoni and Lucas Borrione

16.1 Introduction

Depression is estimated to affect more than 300 million people worldwide, showing a 1-year prevalence of 6.6%, and a lifetime prevalence of 16.2% [1]. It is the third most important global cause of years lived with disability (YLD) [2], and is associated with suicidal ideation and suicide attempts (the rate of suicide in its most severe forms can reach 15%) [3].

According to the fifth edition of the Diagnostic and Statistical Manual of Mental Disorders (DSM-5) of the American Psychiatric Association (APA), major depressive disorder (MDD) consists of either depressed mood and/or diminished pleasure and/or interest, for at least 2 weeks, associated with somatic, psychomotor, and neurocognitive symptoms [4] (Table 16.1). The illness causes significant functional impairment in multiple areas of a patient's life.

Nowadays, first-line treatments for MDD are the diverse antidepressant medications and/or cognitive-behavioral therapy. However, results from a large and multicentric study, the STAR*D trial, have shown that less than one-third of depressed patients achieve remission after one medication, and another third do not achieve

A. R. Brunoni
Interdisciplinary Service of Neuromodulation, Laboratory of Neurosciences (LIM-27),
Department and Institute of Psychiatry, Hospital das Clínicas, University of São Paulo,
São Paulo, Brazil

Department and Institute of Psychiatry, National Institute of Biomarkers in Psychiatry
(InBioN), Hospital das Clínicas, University of São Paulo, São Paulo, Brazil

University Hospital, University of São Paulo, São Paulo, Brazil
e-mail: brunowsky@gmail.com

L. Borrione (✉)
Interdisciplinary Service of Neuromodulation, Laboratory of Neurosciences (LIM-27),
Department and Institute of Psychiatry, Hospital das Clínicas, University of São Paulo,
São Paulo, Brazil
e-mail: lucas.borrione@hc.fm.usp.br

© Springer Nature Switzerland AG 2020
B. Dell'Osso, G. Di Lorenzo (eds.), *Non Invasive Brain Stimulation
in Psychiatry and Clinical Neurosciences*,
https://doi.org/10.1007/978-3-030-43356-7_16

Table 16.1 Diagnostic criteria for major depressive disorder according to DSM-5 (APA)

Depressed mood most of the day and/or markedly diminished interest of pleasure for at least 2 weeks, associated with 5 or more of the following symptoms:
Significant weight loss or weight gain (or increased or decreased appetite)
Insomnia or hypersomnia
Psychomotor agitation or retardation
Fatigue or loss of energy
Diminished ability to think or concentrate or indecisiveness
Recurrent thoughts of death and/or suicidal ideation

remission after four or more adequate antidepressant trials [5]. Furthermore, as higher dosages of antidepressants are used, intolerable adverse effects become more frequent. Psychotherapy, on the other hand, albeit free of medication adverse effects, is costly and time-consuming.

In this scenario, noninvasive brain stimulation (NIBS) techniques, like transcranial direct current stimulation (tDCS), are being considered as treatment alternatives for depressive disorders.

16.2 The Traditional tDCS Montage

tDCS consists of a low-intensity, continuous electrical current (usually ≤3 mA) that is generated between two electrodes placed over the scalp: the anode (positive electrode) and the cathode (negative electrode), with the current flowing in a radial direction from the former to the latter [6]. However, only 10% of the total current effectively reaches the nervous tissue, because the intermediate layers (skin, subcutaneous tissue, skull, and cerebrospinal fluid) exhibit high impedance [7].

The current is generated through a low-voltage source, generally consisting of 9-Volt rechargeable batteries. The International 10/20 EEG system is a traditional reference for electrode positioning (i.e., most recent trials have positioned the anode over the F3 and the cathode over the F4) [8] (Fig. 16.1). Due to the spatial characteristics of this montage, the elicited current flow is perpendicular to the axons, thereby polarizing the synapses and influencing deeper brain areas other than the cortex [9]. Since the electrode surface area is large (25–35 cm^2), tDCS is considered to be nonfocal [7].

16.3 tDCS in Depression: Neurobiological Rationale

In depressive episodes, there is evidence of interhemispheric functional asymmetry: the left dorsolateral prefrontal cortex (DLPFC) is observed to be hypoactive, and the right DLPFC is observed to be hyperactive [10]. The DLPFC establishes connections with the frontoparietal network (FPN), which is implicated in decision-making, working memory and attention, and it has been found to be hypoactive in depression [11]. Hypoactivity of the FPN is associated, in its turn, with

Fig. 16.1 The figure depicts the traditional tDCS montage for the treatment of depression. The anode (in yellow) is placed over F3, and the cathode (in blue) placed is over F4 (areas corresponding to the left and right dorsolateral prefrontal cortices, respectively)

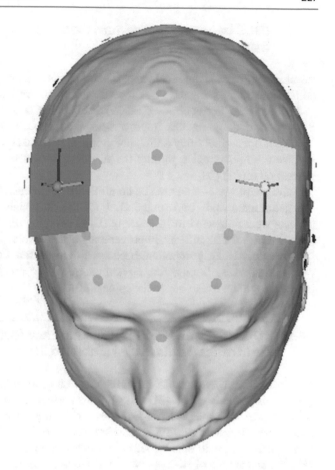

hyperactivity of the default mode network (DMN), composed by the anterior medial prefrontal cortex, posterior cingulate cortex, and angular gyrus [12]. The hyperfunctional DMN has been related to depressive behaviors, such as negative ruminations [13].

The net effect of tDCS on the underlying brain regions depends on the direction of current flow: the anode depolarizes and the cathode hyperpolarizes the neurons [14]. For this reason, traditional tDCS montages use anodal stimulation over the left DLPFC, thereby aiming to counterbalance the hypoactivity of this brain area and the subsequent hyperactivity of the DMN [14]. The placement of the cathode has been variable, as shall be discussed throughout this chapter.

Furthermore, tDCS induces long-lasting changes in neuronal plasticity, through N-methyl-D-aspartate receptor-dependent mechanisms, similar to long-term potentiation and long-term depression processes [15].

tDCS has also been associated with effects on ion channels in the cell membrane resulting in neurochemical redistribution, changes in neurotransmitter concentrations (like serotonin and dopamine) and in the functioning of blood vessels and astrocytes [16].

16.4   tDCS in Acute Depression: Evidence from Open-Label Trials

Results from early open-label trials involving tDCS in depressive disorders were quite promising, paving the way for randomized, controlled trials (RCTs).

For instance, Ferrucci et al. (2009) studied tDCS in 14 patients with severe depression, obtaining a 30% improvement in depressive symptoms [17], and later, in another open-label study (2009) involving 32 patients, the authors observed tDCS to have a larger effect regarding the response in severe (50%) versus moderate depression (10%) [18].

Subsequent open-label studies continued to demonstrate positive effects [19]. The naturalistic study by Brunoni et al. (2013), in which 82 unipolar and bipolar patients were subjected to twice-daily tDCS sessions for 5 days (totaling 10 sessions), showed a significant improvement in the levels of depression [20]. This study was particularly important because it demonstrated that the effects of tDCS were potentialized through the co-administration of antidepressants, and diminished through the use of benzodiazepines [20].

16.5   tDCS in Acute Depression: Evidence from Randomized, Controlled Trials (RCTs) (Table 16.2)

The first RCT involving tDCS in depressed adults was published in 2006 by Fregni et al., with positive results [21]. The authors further investigated the pro-cognitive effects of tDCS in major depression, also achieving positive outcomes [22]. Both trials were pilot studies with small samples ($n = 10$ and $n = 18$, respectively). Subsequently, Boggio et al. (2008) also observed clinical improvement with tDCS in a larger sample of 40 depressed individuals, without the use of antidepressants [23].

Although these initial studies showed positive findings, two ensuing RCTs with medicated and treatment-resistant patient samples presented negative outcomes [24, 25]. The reasons that might explain such negative findings include the negative impact of mood stabilizers/anticonvulsants in tDCS efficacy in the RCT by Blumberger et al. (2012) [26], and the high treatment resistance in the sample recruited by Palm et al. (2012) [24].

Later, two larger RCTs by Brunoni et al. (2013 and 2017), which specifically incorporated pharmacotherapy as an independent variable in their designs, have shown that the combination of tDCS with a conventional antidepressant (sertraline 50 mg/day) is superior to isolated treatment alone [27], and that even though tDCS is inferior to another antidepressant (escitalopram 20 mg/day), it is still superior to the sham alternative [28].

Aiming to optimize tDCS efficacy, two RCTs have combined it with cognitive control therapy (CCT), a procedure consisting of cognitive tasks associated with DLPFC activity, like working memory and sustained attention training. Seagrave et al. (2014) [29] observed a sustained antidepressant response at follow-up only in

Table 16.2 Randomized controlled trials (RCT) involving transcranial direct current stimulation (tDCS) in acute depression

Authors (year)	Sample number (n)	Medication	Arm types and number of arms	Anode/cathode/current density (A/cm²)	Protocol	Results
Fregni et al. (2006)	18	No antidepressants in the last 3 months	tDCS and Sham (2)	F3/RSO/0.03	20 min; 5 sessions in 1 week	Positive
Boggio et al. (2008)	40	No antidepressants in the last 2 months	tDCS DLPFC, tDCS occipital and Sham (3)	F3 or occipital/RSO/0.06	20 min; 10 sessions in 2 weeks	Positive
Palm et al. (2012)	22	With antidepressant medication, stable dose >3 week	tDCS → sham and Sham → tDCS (2)	F3/RSO/0.03–0.06	20 min; 20 sessions in 4 weeks	Negative
Blumberger et al. (2012)	24	With antidepressant medication, stable dose >4 weeks	tDCS and Sham (2)	F3/F4/0.06	20 min; 15 sessions in 3 weeks	Negative
Brunoni et al. (2013)	120	Sertraline 50 mg and benzodiazepines	tDCS, sertraline, tDCS + sertraline, Sham + placebo (4)	F3/F4/0.08	30 min; 12 sessions in 4 weeks	Positive: Sertraline + tDCS superior to the other 3 arms
Segrave et al. (2014)	27	With antidepressant medication, stable dose >4 weeks	CCT + tDCS, Sham CCT + tDCS, CCT + Sham tDCS (3)	F3/F8/0.06	24 min; 5 sessions in 5 days	Positive
Brunoni et al. (2014)	37	With antidepressant medication, stable dose >6 weeks and benzodiazepines	CCT + tDCS and CCT + Sham tDCS (2)	F3/F4/0.08	30 min; 10 sessions in 2 weeks	Negative
Brunoni et al. (2017)	245	Escitalopram 10–20 mg and benzodiazepines	tDCS + placebo, Sham + escitalopram, Sham + placebo (3)	F3/F4/0.08	30 min; 22 sessions in 10 weeks	Negative (noninferiority design: tDCS inferior to escitalopram, but superior to sham)

(continued)

Table 16.2 (continued)

Authors (year)	Sample number (n)	Medication	Arm types and number of arms	Anode/cathode/current density (A/cm²)	Protocol	Results
Loo et al. (2018)	130	With and without antidepressant medication, stable dose >4 weeks, benzodiazepines and mood stabilizers for bipolar patients	Unipolar tDCS, unipolar sham, bipolar tDCS, bipolar sham (4)	F3/F8/0.07	30 min; 20 sessions in 4 weeks	Negative
Valiengo et al. (2017)	48	Only anticonvulsants were allowed when prescribed for previous stroke-related seizures	tDCS and sham (2)	F3/F4/0.08	30 min; 12 sessions in 6 weeks	Positive
Sampaio-Junior et al. (2018)	59	1st, 2nd, and third line pharmacotherapies per CANMAT guidelines and benzodiazepines	tDCS and Sham (2)	F3/F4/0.08	30 min; 12 sessions in 6 weeks	Positive

tDCS transcranial direct current stimulation, *F3* left dorsolateral prefrontal cortex, *F4* right dorsolateral prefrontal cortex, *F8* lateral right frontal area, *RSO* right supraorbital area, *CCT* cognitive control training

the group that received both interventions (tDCS and CCT, and not in each individually), while Brunoni et al. (2014) observed similar rates of response both in patients that received tDCS + CCT and sham tDCS + CCT [13]. Both RCTs recruited small samples. A larger trial (n = 192), investigating whether the clinical effects of cognitive-behavioral group therapy can be augmented by tDCS is still ongoing, with pending results [30].

In contrast to single-center trials, tDCS multicenter trials have tried to improve the generalizability of findings by evaluating the efficacy of the intervention in diverse populations. To date, the results of one multicenter trial by Loo et al., which randomized unipolar (n = 91) and bipolar (n = 39) patients to active or sham tDCS (with concurrent mood stabilizers and antidepressants) failed to show a significant between-group difference, as both groups improved over time [31]. Interestingly, this study used higher stimulation parameters than those used in previous trials (2.5 mA, applied for 30 min over 20 consecutive weekdays) [31]. The results of another multicenter trial involving active versus sham tDCS, the *DepressionDC* (5 sites, n = 152) are still pending publication [32]. In the *DepressionDC* trial, only unipolar patients are being randomized to active or sham tDCS as an add-on strategy to a stable antidepressant regimen and will undergo advanced tDCS technology, with recording of technical parameters (current, impedance, voltage) in every tDCS session [32]. The authors believe that this will allow for better control of stimulation, and further analysis of the interaction between technical parameters and relevant clinical outcomes.

The RCTs mentioned so far have dealt with primary depression. However, depression can also be associated with general medical conditions (i.e., neurologic, cardiologic, and endocrinologic). In this scenario, tDCS can be an interesting alternative, due to the possible contraindications of pharmacotherapy and its lower side effect tolerability in such patients. Of note, in an RCT to evaluate the efficacy of tDCS in post-stroke depression, Valiengo et al. (2017) randomized 48 patients to either active or sham tDCS, and observed that active tDCS was superior to sham in all endpoints [33]. Nevertheless, a recent meta-analysis (2018) concluded that a general statement about the efficacy of tDCS in post-stroke depression cannot be yet reached, due to the small sample sizes, heterogeneous methodologies, lack of uniform diagnostic criteria, and divergent data of available studies [34].

Although many of the cited studies recruited mixed samples of unipolar and bipolar patients, Sampaio Junior et al. (2018) randomized 59 patients uniquely with bipolar depression for either sham or active tDCS, under a stable pharmacological regimen with mood stabilizers [35]. The authors observed that tDCS showed superior improvement compared to sham [35]. Corroborating these findings, a recent meta-analysis (2017) concluded that bipolar depression responds well to tDCS, especially within 1 week of treatment [36]. However, since there is little data available to assess active tDCS versus other treatment modalities in bipolar depression, tDCS could only be evaluated in terms of response, rather than comparative efficacy [36]. Additional studies are still needed to clarify the effectiveness of tDCS in bipolar depression.

16.6   tDCS in the Maintenance Phase of the Depressive Episode: Results from Follow-Up Studies

The efficacy of tDCS as a continuation therapy for the maintenance phase of the depressive episode, and its role in relapse prevention, has been insufficiently investigated in the literature [37]. However, results from three follow-up studies, in which participants were pooled to receive tDCS as a continuation treatment for up to 6 months after an acute phase trial, showed promising results.

Aparicio et al. (2018) recruited 24 patients (16 with unipolar and 8 with bipolar depression) [38]. Sessions were performed twice a week over 6 months, with a mean survival duration of 17.5 weeks, a survival rate at the end of follow-up of 73.5%, and a trend for lower relapse rates in nontreatment resistant patients [38].

Martin et al. (2013) recruited 26 participants from two different studies, and offered sessions on a weekly basis for 3 months, and then, once per fortnight for the final 3 months [39]. The cumulative probability of surviving without relapse was 83.7% at 3 months, and 51.1% at 6 months, with medication-resistance being a predictor of poor response [39].

Finally, Valiengo et al. (2013) recruited 42 patients who responded to tDCS in the acute depressive phase (SELECT-trial) to receive a maximum of 9 tDCS sessions (every other week for 3 months, and then monthly for the remaining 3 months) [40]. The mean response duration was 11.7 weeks at a survival rate of 47%. Patients with treatment-resistant depression presented a lower 24-week survival rate as compared to nonrefractory patients (10% vs. 77%, OR = 5.52, $p < 0.01$) [40]. Perhaps the lower survival rate of the last trial, comparing with the other two, is associated with a less intensive course of tDCS sessions.

Future tDCS follow-up trials for depression should focus on optimization of maintenance phase parameters, such as frequency of sessions for longer periods than 6 months, in order to better understand the role of tDCS in depression relapse prevention.

16.7   tDCS in Depression: Recent Meta-Analyses

Three recent meta-analyses corroborate tDCS as an effective treatment in depression.

Brunoni et al. (2016), in a meta-analysis of individual patient data, observed that tDCS was significantly superior to sham for response (34% vs. 19% respectively, odds ratio (OR) = 2.44, 95% CI 1.38–4.32, number needed to treat (NNT) = 7), remission (23.1% vs. 12.7% respectively, OR = 2.38, 95% CI 1.22–4.64, NNT = 9) and depression improvement (B coefficient 0.35, 95% CI 0.12–0.57) [41]. The authors observed that treatment-resistant depression and higher tDCS doses (2 mA) were, respectively, negatively and positively associated with tDCS efficacy [41].

Subsequently, Mutz et al. (2019), in a systematic review and network meta-analysis about the comparative efficacy and acceptability of nonsurgical brain stimulation for the acute treatment of MDD in adults, observed tDCS to be efficacious across outcomes in both pairwise and network comparisons (response OR = 2.65,

95% CI 1.55–4.55) [42]. The authors considered that since tDCS is less expensive than transcranial magnetic stimulation (TMS), electroconvulsive therapy (ECT), and psychotherapy, the positive response finding can be relevant for policymakers who might consider tDCS as a clinical therapy outside the research setting [42].

Finally, Yuan (2019) reported an obviously significant difference between tDCS and control groups in both the Montgomery-Asberg Depression Rating Scale (MADRS) ($p < 0.00001$, mean difference = -5.18, 95% CI -7.13 to -3.23) and the Hamilton Depression Rating Scale (HDRS-17) ($p < 0.00001$, mean difference = -3.95, 95% CI -5.58 to -2.32) [43]. Furthermore, the author highlighted tDCS as a safe method, with few adverse events [43].

16.8   tDCS Safety and Tolerability

tDCS is widely considered a safe and well-tolerated technique, especially since the traditional current intensities are far below the thresholds which could cause brain injury [19]. Furthermore, since no action potentials are elicited, the seizure risk associated with tDCS remains negligible [19].

Common tDCS adverse events include local itching, tingling, burning sensation, and discomfort at the application site [8]. These effects occur in approximately 30% of patients, with erythema reaching an incidence of 80%, albeit low patient perception in clinical practice [8]. The risk of skin burns due to the electrical currents can be greatly diminished with a proper soaking of sponges with saline solution [19].

Very rare side effects include headaches, blurred vision, ringing in the ears, brighter or illuminated vision, fatigue, nausea, mild euphoria, reduced concentration, disorientation, insomnia, and anxiety (all with minimal difference between active and sham tDCS) [37]. Finally, meta-analyses have suggested that there is no increased risk of tDCS-induced mania/hypomania [44].

Despite its side effect profile, active tDCS has been considered as acceptable and safe as sham tDCS.

16.9   tDCS in Psychiatric Practice

Even though tDCS is not yet approved by the US Food and Drug Administration (FDA) for the treatment of depression, it bears a CE mark and, according to recent clinical guidelines, is possibly/probably effective for depression [37, 45].

The CANMAT 2016 Clinical Guidelines for the Management of Adults with MDD (Sect. 4. Neurostimulation Treatments) consider tDCS as a third-line treatment for the acute depressive phase [37]. These guidelines recommend that a minimum stimulation with 2 mA for at least 30 min per day for 2 weeks is necessary to observe an antidepressant effect, but had at that time no recommendations for maintenance treatment [37].

The guidelines by Lefaucheur et al. (2017), on the other hand, distinguished recommendations according to the specific tDCS montage: although the target electrode is placed over the left DLPFC (F3) in all cases, the cathode can be placed either over the orbitofrontal area (OFC) or the right DLPFC (F4) [45]. Regarding the OFC montage, there is a B level of evidence with 2 mA for 10 daily, 20–30 min sessions, in medicated or drug-free patients with MDD, and no drug-treatment resistance [45]. Concerning the right DLPFC (F4) montage, no recommendation could be made at that time [45], although larger studies that were published after these guidelines showed the F3/F4 montage to be efficacious (see Brunoni et al. 2017) [28].

At present, tDCS is still considered inferior in antidepressant efficacy in relation to TMS [37], but it is less expensive and more portable than the latter. These are the advantages that could make tDCS suitable for future home-use.

16.10 tDCS: Future Directions

The question of how to improve tDCS efficacy in MDD, in comparison with its first-line treatments (antidepressants and cognitive-behavioral psychotherapy) and TMS, remains open.

It is now understood that increasing current strength is not always a better alternative. In fact, one study showed that increasing current intensities (to 2.5 mA, as opposed to the recommended 2 mA) did not increment the efficacy of active tDCS [31]. On the other hand, recent research strategies have dealt with the combination of active tDCS with different modes of cognitive interventions aiming at synergistic, and not only additive, mechanisms. The rationale behind this dual strategy relies on the knowledge that the effects of NIBS techniques are known to be "state-dependent", that is, the "state" of the targeted cortical region influences their net effect [46]. In this sense, psychological methods such as cognitive-control therapy, which activate the same NIBS-stimulated regions, may improve clinical outcomes [46]. The dual strategy also offers patients the possibility to be engaged in meaningful cognitive activities during the period of electrical stimulation (usually half an hour), instead of letting depressive ruminations and negative effects dominate the mind at random.

Nowadays, in clinical practice, fixed current intensities and montages are used, without taking into consideration individual differences in brain function. Future RCTs involving tDCS should take into account these individual differences, which could affect the current distribution and clinical effect [14]. In this sense, individual modeling through brain scans and specific software can be used in two complementary strategies: (1) fixed current intensity and subsequent analysis of clinical effect (2), and diverse current intensities aiming at the same current dose at the neuronal level [14].

Future tDCS studies should also explore the effect of different biomarkers (i.e., genetic, epigenetic, biochemical, neuroimaging, neurocognitive) related to different subgroup responses. For instance, recent clinical findings suggest that baseline levels of the nerve growth factor (NGF) predict early depression improvement for tDCS versus escitalopram [47], and pre-treatment letter fluency, an ability associated with the left prefrontal cortex, was also observed to be a predictor of tDCS response [48].

Since tDCS is portable and relatively easy to apply, its home-use is also a topic for further exploration. Studies that have so far dealt with this issue involve small samples, are single-blinded, and focus on feasibility and safety [49]. Current recommendations for future home-use tDCS research include proper training of research staff, assessments of user participation capability, simple electrode preparation techniques and tDCS headgear, and strict dose control for each session, among others [50]. Home-use tDCS also avoids transportation costs and logistical problems regarding recruited patient samples in tDCS related research.

The self-use of tDCS is becoming more and more widespread (for instance, the "Do-It-Yourself" internet movement), with an increasing interest in its use for cognitive enhancement in otherwise healthy individuals. However, this behavior bears considerable risks, and its long-term clinical and side effects are still not properly understood [49]. Therefore, the scientific community and health regulatory agencies should prioritize the definition of objective and evidence-based clinical guidelines for home- and self-use tDCS, taking into account their multiple ethical considerations.

16.11 Conclusions

Depression is a global and incapacitating illness, whose first-line treatments are far from being completely efficient in the majority of cases, and bear with them a multitude of side effects. Psychotherapy, albeit free of medication side effects, is costly and time-consuming, and is not readily available in remote areas. NIBS techniques (like TMS and tDCS) are becoming increasingly recognized as efficient, safe, and tolerable interventions in the treatment of depression.

Early clinical trials comparing tDCS to placebo achieved mixed results (notably, with different protocols and montages), but more recent RCTs, involving larger patient samples and fixed montages, have shown tDCS to be more effective than placebo in the treatment of acute depression, with preliminary and promising results in maintenance open-label phases. Ensuing meta-analyses have confirmed these findings.

Even though tDCS is currently considered inferior to TMS in the treatment of the acute depressive episode, it has some advantages over TMS, like lower cost, portability and the possibility of self-use at home. These practical advantages offer a fair rationale for the continuation of tDCS-related research. tDCS augmentation with cognitive interventions, individual patterns of current distribution, and biomarkers associated with clinical response are considered relevant and interesting lines of research.

References

1. Kupfer DJ, Frank E, Phillips ML. Major depressive disorder: new clinical, neurobiological, and treatment perspectives. Lancet. 2012;379:1045–55.
2. DALYs GBD, Collaborators H. Global, regional, and national disability-adjusted life-years (DALYs) for 315 diseases and injuries and healthy life expectancy (HALE), 1990–2015: a systematic analysis for the Global Burden of Disease Study 2015. Lancet. 2016;388:1603–58.
3. Chachamovich E, Stefanello S, Botega N, Turecki G. Which are the recent clinical findings regarding the association between depression and suicide? Braz J Psychiatry. 2009;31(Suppl 1):S18–25.
4. American Psychiatric Association. Diagnostic and statistical manual of mental disorders. 5th ed. Washington, DC: American Psychiatric Association; 2013.
5. Rush AJ, Trivedi MH, Wisniewski SR, et al. Acute and longer-term outcomes in depressed outpatients requiring one or several treatment steps: a STAR*D report. Am J Psychiatry. 2006;163:1905–17.
6. Bikson M, Inoue M, Akiyama H, et al. Effects of uniform extracellular DC electric fields on excitability in rat hippocampal slices in vitro. J Physiol. 2004;557:175–90.
7. Woods AJ, Antal A, Bikson M, et al. A technical guide to tDCS, and related non-invasive brain stimulation tools. Clin Neurophysiol. 2016;127:1031–48.
8. Brunoni AR, Sampaio-Junior B, Moffa AH, et al. Noninvasive brain stimulation in psychiatric disorders: a primer. Braz J Psychiatry. 2019;41:70–81.
9. Hunter MA, Coffman BA, Gasparovic C, Calhoun VD, Trumbo MC, Clark VP. Baseline effects of transcranial direct current stimulation on glutamatergic neurotransmission and large-scale network connectivity. Brain Res. 2015;1594:92–107.
10. Grimm S, Beck J, Schuepbach D, et al. Imbalance between left and right dorsolateral prefrontal cortex in major depression is linked to negative emotional judgment: an fMRI study in severe major depressive disorder. Biol Psychiatry. 2008;63:369–76.
11. Kaiser RH, Andrews-Hanna JR, Wager TD, Pizzagalli DA. Large-scale network dysfunction in major depressive disorder: a meta-analysis of resting-state functional connectivity. JAMA Psychiat. 2015;72:603–11.
12. Greicius MD, Krasnow B, Reiss AL, Menon V. Functional connectivity in the resting brain: a network analysis of the default mode hypothesis. Proc Natl Acad Sci U S A. 2003;100:253–8.
13. Brunoni AR, Boggio PS, De Raedt R, et al. Cognitive control therapy and transcranial direct current stimulation for depression: a randomized, double-blinded, controlled trial. J Affect Disord. 2014;162:43–9.
14. Borrione L, Moffa AH, Martin D, Loo CK, Brunoni AR. Transcranial direct current stimulation in the acute depressive episode: a systematic review of current knowledge. J ECT. 2018;34:153–63.
15. Stagg CJ, Nitsche MA. Physiological basis of transcranial direct current stimulation. Neuroscientist. 2011;17:37–53.
16. Bulubas L, Mezger E, Keeser D, Padberg F, Brunoni A. Novel neuromodulatory approaches for depression: neurobiological mechanisms. In: Quevedo J, Carvalho AF, Zarate CA, editors. Neurobiology of depression. London: Academic Press; 2019. p. 347–60.
17. Ferrucci R, Bortolomasi M, Vergari M, et al. Transcranial direct current stimulation in severe, drug-resistant major depression. J Affect Disord. 2009;118:215–9.
18. Ferrucci R, Bortolomasi M, Brunoni A, et al. Comparative benefits of transcranial direct current stimulation (tDCS) treatment in patients with mild/moderate vs. severe depression. Clin Neuropsychiatry. 2009;6:246–51.
19. Palm U, Hasan A, Strube W, Padberg F. tDCS for the treatment of depression: a comprehensive review. Eur Arch Psychiatry Clin Neurosci. 2016;266:681–94.
20. Brunoni AR, Ferrucci R, Bortolomasi M, et al. Interactions between transcranial direct current stimulation (tDCS) and pharmacological interventions in the major depressive episode: findings from a naturalistic study. Eur Psychiatry. 2013;28:356–61.

21. Fregni F, Boggio PS, Nitsche MA, Marcolin MA, Rigonatti SP, Pascual-Leone A. Treatment of major depression with transcranial direct current stimulation. Bipolar Disord. 2006;8:203–4.
22. Fregni F, Boggio PS, Nitsche MA, Rigonatti SP, Pascual-Leone A. Cognitive effects of repeated sessions of transcranial direct current stimulation in patients with depression. Depress Anxiety. 2006;23:482–4.
23. Boggio PS, Rigonatti SP, Ribeiro RB, et al. A randomized, double-blind clinical trial on the efficacy of cortical direct current stimulation for the treatment of major depression. Int J Neuropsychopharmacol. 2008;11:249–54.
24. Palm U, Schiller C, Fintescu Z, et al. Transcranial direct current stimulation in treatment resistant depression: a randomized double-blind, placebo-controlled study. Brain Stimul. 2012;5:242–51.
25. Blumberger DM, Mulsant BH, Fitzgerald PB, et al. A randomized double-blind sham-controlled comparison of unilateral and bilateral repetitive transcranial magnetic stimulation for treatment-resistant major depression. World J Biol Psychiatry. 2012;13:423–35.
26. Blumberger DM, Tran LC, Fitzgerald PB, Hoy KE, Daskalakis ZJ. A randomized double-blind sham-controlled study of transcranial direct current stimulation for treatment-resistant major depression. Front Psych. 2012;3:74.
27. Brunoni AR, Valiengo L, Baccaro A, et al. The sertraline vs. electrical current therapy for treating depression clinical study: results from a factorial, randomized, controlled trial. JAMA Psychiat. 2013;70:383–91.
28. Brunoni AR, Moffa AH, Sampaio-Junior B, et al. Trial of electrical direct-current therapy versus escitalopram for depression. N Engl J Med. 2017;376:2523–33.
29. Segrave RA, Arnold S, Hoy K, Fitzgerald PB. Concurrent cognitive control training augments the antidepressant efficacy of tDCS: a pilot study. Brain Stimul. 2014;7:325–31.
30. Bajbouj M, Aust S, Spies J, et al. PsychotherapyPlus: augmentation of cognitive-behavioral therapy (CBT) with prefrontal transcranial direct current stimulation (tDCS) in major depressive disorder-study design and methodology of a multicenter double-blind randomized placebo-controlled trial. Eur Arch Psychiatry Clin Neurosci. 2018;268:797–808.
31. Loo CK, Husain MM, McDonald WM, et al. International randomized-controlled trial of transcranial direct current stimulation in depression. Brain Stimul. 2018;11:125–33.
32. Padberg F, Kumpf U, Mansmann U, et al. Prefrontal transcranial direct current stimulation (tDCS) as treatment for major depression: study design and methodology of a multicenter triple blind randomized placebo controlled trial (Depression DC). Eur Arch Psychiatry Clin Neurosci. 2017;267:751–66.
33. Valiengo LC, Goulart AC, de Oliveira JF, Bensenor IM, Lotufo PA, Brunoni AR. Transcranial direct current stimulation for the treatment of post-stroke depression: results from a randomised, sham-controlled, double-blinded trial. J Neurol Neurosurg Psychiatry. 2017;88:170–5.
34. Bucur M, Papagno C. A systematic review of noninvasive brain stimulation for post-stroke depression. J Affect Disord. 2018;238:69–78.
35. Sampaio-Junior B, Tortella G, Borrione L, et al. Efficacy and safety of transcranial direct current stimulation as an add-on treatment for bipolar depression: a randomized clinical trial. JAMA Psychiat. 2018;75:158–66.
36. Donde C, Amad A, Nieto I, et al. Transcranial direct-current stimulation (tDCS) for bipolar depression: a systematic review and meta-analysis. Prog Neuropsychopharmacol Biol Psychiatry. 2017;78:123–31.
37. Milev RV, Giacobbe P, Kennedy SH, et al. Canadian network for mood and anxiety treatments (CANMAT) 2016 clinical guidelines for the management of adults with major depressive disorder: section 4. Neurostimulation treatments. Can J Psychiatry. 2016;61:561–75.
38. Aparicio LVM, Rosa V, Razza LM, et al. Transcranial direct current stimulation (tDCS) for preventing major depressive disorder relapse: results of a 6-month follow-up. Depress Anxiety. 2019;36:262–8.
39. Martin DM, Alonzo A, Ho KA, et al. Continuation transcranial direct current stimulation for the prevention of relapse in major depression. J Affect Disord. 2013;144:274–8.

40. Valiengo L, Bensenor IM, Goulart AC, et al. The sertraline versus electrical current therapy for treating depression clinical study (select-TDCS): results of the crossover and follow-up phases. Depress Anxiety. 2013;30:646–53.
41. Brunoni AR, Moffa AH, Fregni F, et al. Transcranial direct current stimulation for acute major depressive episodes: meta-analysis of individual patient data. Br J Psychiatry. 2016;208:522–31.
42. Mutz J, Vipulananthan V, Carter B, Hurlemann R, Fu CHY, Young AH. Comparative efficacy and acceptability of non-surgical brain stimulation for the acute treatment of major depressive episodes in adults: systematic review and network meta-analysis. BMJ. 2019;364:l1079.
43. Wang Y. Transcranial direct current stimulation for the treatment of major depressive disorder: a meta-analysis of randomized controlled trials. Psychiatry Res. 2019;276:186–90.
44. Brunoni AR, Moffa AH, Sampaio-Junior B, Galvez V, Loo CK. Treatment-emergent mania/hypomania during antidepressant treatment with transcranial direct current stimulation (tDCS): a systematic review and meta-analysis. Brain Stimul. 2017;10:260–2.
45. Lefaucheur JP, Antal A, Ayache SS, et al. Evidence-based guidelines on the therapeutic use of transcranial direct current stimulation (tDCS). Clin Neurophysiol. 2017;128:56–92.
46. Sathappan AV, Luber BM, Lisanby SH. The dynamic duo: combining noninvasive brain stimulation with cognitive interventions. Prog Neuropsychopharmacol Biol Psychiatry. 2019;89:347–60.
47. Brunoni AR, Padberg F, Vieira ELM, et al. Plasma biomarkers in a placebo-controlled trial comparing tDCS and escitalopram efficacy in major depression. Prog Neuropsychopharmacol Biol Psychiatry. 2018;86:211–7.
48. Martin DM, Yeung K, Loo CK. Pre-treatment letter fluency performance predicts antidepressant response to transcranial direct current stimulation. J Affect Disord. 2016;203:130–5.
49. Palm U, Kumpf U, Behler N, et al. Home use, remotely supervised, and remotely controlled transcranial direct current stimulation: a systematic review of the available evidence. Neuromodulation. 2018;21:323–33.
50. Charvet LE, Kasschau M, Datta A, et al. Remotely-supervised transcranial direct current stimulation (tDCS) for clinical trials: guidelines for technology and protocols. Front Syst Neurosci. 2015;9:26.

Transcranial Direct Current Stimulation for the Treatment of Hallucinations in Patients with Schizophrenia

17

Jérôme Brunelin and Emmanuel Poulet

17.1 Introduction

Schizophrenia is a disabling disease affecting approximately 0.7% of the worldwide population [1]. Among the clinical dimensions of schizophrenia, one of the most debilitating symptoms is the presence of auditory verbal hallucinations (AVH). AVH affect 75% of patients with schizophrenia [2], have generally a negative content, and increase suicide risk [3]. Neuroimaging studies have repeatedly shown that AVH are associated with abnormal activity and connectivity of several cortical regions including Wernicke's and Broca's areas, the auditory cortex, the medial temporal lobe, the insula, and paracingulate region of the medial prefrontal cortex [4].

Currently, the first line of treatment for AVH consists of antipsychotics, with second-generation antipsychotics being more effective than classic neuroleptics. Clozapine remains the drug of choice for patients resistant to antipsychotic agents, while long-acting medications are advised to increase treatment adherence [5]. In adjunction to antipsychotic treatment, cognitive-behavioral therapy, including coping strategies [6] and electroconvulsive therapy [5], can also be proposed. However, despite this therapeutic armamentarium, AVH treatment-resistance remains high, and approximately 25–30% of patients report AVH even during adequate treatment. In such cases, the development of well-tolerated, non-pharmacological, noninvasive brain stimulation treatments targeting the brain region involved in the pathogenesis of AVH have been explored as treatments for these symptoms [7].

J. Brunelin (✉) · E. Poulet
INSEINSERM, U1028, CNRS, UMR5292, Lyon Neuroscience Research Center, PSYR2 Team, Lyon, France

University Lyon 1, Villeurbanne, France

Centre Hospitalier Le Vinatier, Bron, France
e-mail: jerome.brunelin@ch-le-vinatier.fr; emmanuel.poulet@chu-lyon.fr

© Springer Nature Switzerland AG 2020
B. Dell'Osso, G. Di Lorenzo (eds.), *Non Invasive Brain Stimulation in Psychiatry and Clinical Neurosciences*,
https://doi.org/10.1007/978-3-030-43356-7_17

Thus, within the last 10 years, transcranial direct current stimulation (tDCS) has been proposed as a therapeutic solution to decrease AVH in patients with schizophrenia [8, 9]. Here, we aim to provide an update of the literature examining the clinical effects of tDCS on AVH in patients with schizophrenia by conducting a review of randomized, sham-controlled studies on this topic.

17.2 Methods

17.2.1 Literature Search Strategy

We searched for articles published up until June 2019 in the PubMed and Web of Science databases using the following search terms: ("hallucinate" OR "hallucinated" OR "hallucinating" OR "hallucination" OR "hallucinations" OR "hallucinatory" OR "hallucinators" OR "hallucinatory") AND "schizophrenia" AND ("transcranial direct current stimulation" OR ("transcranial" AND "direct" AND "current" AND "stimulation") OR "transcranial direct current stimulation" OR "tdcs"). We also searched for articles in tDCS review articles and in the reference lists of retrieved articles.

17.2.2 Selection Criteria

The selection criteria were as follows: (1) original articles written in the English language, (2) sham-controlled trials, and (3) studies that included patients with schizophrenia. We excluded (1) case reports, (2) review articles, (3) meeting and conference abstracts, (4) open-label trials, (5) articles addressing the effects of other brain stimulation techniques (e.g., transcranial random-noise stimulation), and (6) studies that did not provide a clinical measure of hallucinations.

17.2.3 Data Extraction

For each study, the following data were extracted: (1) demographic and clinical characteristics of the patients including total sample size, diagnosis, age (in years), sex (male/female), handedness (right/left-handed), and antipsychotic medication dose; (2) tDCS parameters such as the type of device used, anode and cathode placement (according to the 10/20 international EEG system), electrode size (cm^2), intensity (mA), duration (min), and number and frequency of sessions (number of session per day); and (3) outcomes (the scale used to measure hallucinations) and main results (changes in hallucinations after tDCS).

17.3   Results

The primary search yielded 73 results on the PubMed database. After excluding studies according to our selection criteria, 11 randomized sham-controlled studies, investigating the effects of tDCS on hallucinations in patients with schizophrenia, were selected. Table 17.1 summarizes the methodologies and results of the selected studies.

Among the 11 retrieved studies, six found a significant decrease in AVH after active tDCS compared to sham, one reported a trend toward a significant decrease in AVH ([10], $p = 0.1$) and 4 reported no superiority of active tDCS over sham to decrease AVH [11–14].

These studies came from independent groups of researchers from different countries around the world (Australia, France, India, the Netherlands, Taiwan, and three groups in the United States). In total, nearly 400 patients were included in these studies and among them, more than half received active tDCS. Regarding the demographic and clinical characteristics of the patients, almost all studies included those diagnosed with schizophrenia according to DSM-IV or DSM-5 criteria. Some studies included patients with schizophrenia, patients with schizoaffective disorder, patients with psychosis NOS, patients with affective disorder, and patients with borderline personality disorder. Patients of both sexes were included. The mean age of included patients varied from 35.1 to 46.8. The large majority of studies included only right-handed patients, but some of them also included several left-handed patients. Patients were on antipsychotic medication in the large majority of studies, and the dose of medication varied from 493 to 1209 mg/day of chlorpromazine equivalents.

Regarding tDCS devices, all selected studies, except four, used the Eldith/Neuroconn DC stimulator device (NeuroConn GmbH, Ilmenau, Germany). The large majority of studies delivered tDCS for 20 minutes with a current intensity set at 2 mA, with 2 electrodes of 35 cm^2, the anode placed midway between FP1 and F3 (dorsolateral prefrontal cortex) and the cathode placed midway between T3 and P3 (temporoparietal junction). tDCS regimen usually consisted of 10 (up to 40) sessions, delivered twice a day over 5 consecutive days, with 3–5 hours between the two stimulation periods.

The main standardized psychometric scales used to measure AVH were: the Auditory Hallucination Rating Scale (AHRS), using its total score or its 'frequency' single item; and the Positive and Negative Syndrome Scale (PANSS), using the 'hallucinations' single item (P3).

Table 17.1 Description of randomized controlled studies investigating the clinical interest of transcranial Direct Current Stimulation (tDCS) for auditory hallucinations in patients with schizophrenia

Author (year)	Type	Diag	Device	Anode	Cathode	Size cm²	I mA	Duration min	n session	Group	n: Sex	Age	Laterality	Anti-psychotic dose	Scale	Main results	p
Kantrowitz et al. [23]	RCT	89 DSM IV (Active 12 Szaff)	BrainStim SYS Brainvision LLC	F3FP1	T3P3	38.8	2	20	10 (2/d)	Active	47: 32 M/15F	38.2 ± 9.9	47R	807 ± 768	AHRS	From 24.8 ± 5.7 to 19.5 ± 10.6	p = 0.03
//		(Sham 5 szaff)								Sham	42: 35 M/7F	40.1 ± 8.6	42R	628 ± 466	AHRS	From 25.2 ± 5.7 to 20.7 ± 10.1	
Lindenmayer et al. [24]	RCT	28 SZ DSM 5	Chattanooga Ionto system stimulator	F3FP1	T3P3	35	2	20	40 (2/d)	Active	15: 13 M/2F				AHRS	From 25.8 ± 3.1 to 20.2 ± 7.1	p ≤ 0.05
//		Age 40.2 ± 10.7 Anti-psychotic 891.81								Sham	13: 11 M/2F				AHRS	From 23.1 ± 4.4 to 20.2 ± 7.3	
Koops et al. [13]	RCT	54 (44 DSM IV SZ/ 12 NOS/ 2 Sz Aff/ 3 Aff disorder/ 3 borerline)	Neuroconn/ Eldith DC stimulator	F3FP1	T3P3	35	2	20	10 (2/d)	Active	28: 14 M/14F	44 ± 11	25R/3 L		AHRS	From 28 ± 6	p = 0.27
//										Sham	26: 11 M/15F	44 ± 12	24R/2 L		AHRS	From 30 ± 5	
Chang et al. [10]	RCT	60 SZ or Szaff DSM IV	Neuroconn/ Eldith DC stimulator	F3FP1	T3P3	35	2	20	10 (2/d)	Active	30: 14 M/16F	46.4 ± 10.3		493.8 ± 306.7	AHRS	From 29.1 ± 5.3; − 7.8 ± 1.8%	p = 0.1
//										Sham	30: 13 M/17F	42.2 ± 10.3		493.2 ± 284.9	AHRS	From 29.1 ± 4.8; −3.94 ± 1.8%	
Bose et al. [25]	RCT	25 SZ DSM IV	Neuroconn/ Eldith DC stimulator	F3FP1	T3P3	35	2	20	10 (2/d)	Active	12: 9 M/3F	31.3 ± 8.3	12R	621.5 ± 377.7 eq cpz	AHRS	From 31.0 ± 4.7 to 21.4 ± 4.9	p < 0.001
//										Sham	13: 5 M/8F	31.4 ± 7.6	13R	782.9 ± 336.6 eq cpz	AHRS	From 29.9 ± 2.9 to 27.9 ± 3.3	

Study	Design	Diagnosis	Device							Group	M:F	Age					p
Frohlich et al. [12]	RCT	19 SZ / 7 Szaff DSM IV	2 Neurocomm/Eldith DC stimulator + external trigger	F3FP1	Cz	35	2	20	5 (1/d)	Active	13: 9 M/4F	43.4 ± 12.6	10R/3 L	ND	AHRS	From 27.0 ± 6.9 to 20.6 ± 8.1	p = 0.52
//				Cz	T3/P3	35	2	20		Sham	13:11 M/2F	40.0 ± 10.7	11R/2 L	ND	AHRS	From 26.7 ± 6.3 to 18.2 ± 10.8	
Mondino et al. [26]	RCT	23 SZ DSM IV	Neurocomm/Eldith DC stimulator	F3FP1	T3P3	35	2	20	10 (2/d)	Active	11:8 M/3F	36.7 ± 9.7	10R/1 L	23.0 ± 11.4 olz eq	AHRS	From 27.2 ± 4.1 to 19.1 ± 7.1	p < 0.001
//										Sham	12:7 M/5F	37.3 ± 9.7	10R/2 L	25.4 ± 12.3 olz eq	AHRS	From 27.8 ± 8.0 to 24.9 ± 10.5	
Smith et al. [14]	RCT	19SZ/ 14Szaff DSM IV	Chattanooga Ionto system stimulator	F3	Fp2	5.08	2	20	5 (1/d)	Active	17: 14 M/3F	46.8 ± 11.1	ND	ND	PANSS P3	In the whole sample. From 2.6 ± 1.8 to 2.5 ± 1.8 in active; in sham from 2.7 ± 1.6 to 2.0 ± 1.4	p = 0.1
//										Sham	16: 10 M/6F	44.9 ± 9.2			PANSS P3	In patients with AVH at baseline P3 > 3 (N = 14). Diff pre-post sham −1.42 and in active −0.44	p = 0.07
Mondino et al. [27]	RCT	29 SZ DSM IV	Neurocomm/Eldith DC stimulator	F3FP1	T3P3	35	2	20	10 (2/d)	Active	15: 6 M/9	36.5 ± 9.5	13R/2 L	27.3 ± 20.0 olz eq	AHRS Freq item	−46%	p < 0.05
//										Sham	13:6 M/7F	39.2 ± 9.0	10R/3 L	34.0 ± 2.1 olz eq	AHRS Freq item	+7.5%	

(continued)

Table 17.1 (continued)

Author (year)	Type	Diag	Device	Anode	Cathode	Size cm²	I mA	Duration min	n session	Group	n: Sex	Age	Laterality	Antipsychotic dose	Scale	Main results	p
Fitzgerald et al. [11]	RCT	17 SZ/7 Szaff DSM IV	Neurocom/Eldith DC stimulator	F3	T3P3	35	2	20	15 (1/d)	Unilat	13	ND	ND	ND	PANSS P3	Active from 3.6 ± 2.3 to 3.0 ± 2.1; Sham from 3.2 ± 1.8 to 3.0 ± 2.0	p = 0.9
	Cross Over	Age 39.3 ± 11.7 Sex 15 M/9F		F3 + F4	T3P3 + T4P4	35	2	20	15 (1/d)	Bilat	11	ND	ND	ND	PANSS P3	Active from 3.8 ± 1.6 to 3.3 ± 2.1; sham from 3.5 ± 1.8 to 3.4 ± 7.7	p = 0.3
Brunelin et al. [28]	RCT	30 SZ DSM IV	Neurocom/Eldith DC stimulator	F3FP1	T3P3	35	2	20	10 (2/d)	Active	22 M/8F	40.4 ± 9.9	15R	994 ± 714 eq cpz	AHRS	From 28.3 ± 4.1 to 19.9 ± 5.8	p < 0.001
	//									Sham		35.1 ± 7.0	15R	1209 ± 998 eq cpz		From 27.2 ± 6.9 to 25.1 ± 7.7	

ND not done, *RCT* randomized controlled trial, *//* parallel 2-arm, *I* intensity (mA), *n* number, *Size* electrode size, *Diag* diagnostic according to DSM (Diagnostic and Statistical Manual of Mental Disorders), *SZ* patients with schizophrenia, *Szaff* patients with schizoaffective disorder
Antipsychotic dose: eq cpz: chlorpromazine equivalent (mg/day); olz eq: olanzapine equivalent (mg/day)
Scale: AHRS: Auditory Hallucination rating scale; PANSS: Positive and Negative syndrome scale

17.4   Discussion

The aim of this chapter was to provide an overview of the literature regarding the current use of tDCS to alleviate hallucinations in patients with schizophrenia. Our search of the PubMed and Web of Science databases yielded 11 RCT. Among them, six studies reported the superiority of active tDCS over sham stimulation to reduce hallucinations following repeated sessions of tDCS, whereas one reported only a trend toward significant difference (in favour of sham) and 4 did not report the superiority of active over sham stimulation.

Even if a relative homogeneity was observed between studies regarding the intensity of stimulation (2 mA) and the duration (20 minutes) of the tDCS sessions, some methodological, clinical, and demographic differences might explain the conflicting results observed between the studies. First, only the cross over study [11] failed to report any difference between active and sham, whereas all the positive studies were 2-arms parallel controlled studies. Since the duration of tDCS after-effects is still under debate, the crossover design seems not to be an appropriate way to investigate tDCS clinical effects. The parameters of stimulation also varied between positive and negative studies. While positive studies delivered at least 10 twice-daily sessions over 5 consecutive days with a 3–5 hours interval between sessions, three negative studies delivered once-daily sessions for either 5 days [12, 14] or 15 days [11]. The total and daily numbers of tDCS sessions are crucial parameters that can influence tDCS after-effects. This influence has been repeatedly reported by studies investigating the effects of tDCS applied over the motor cortex [15, 16]. In light of these studies, it can be hypothesized that 10 twice-daily sessions over 5 days would be more effective than 5 or 15 daily sessions to reduce AVH. Regarding the electrode montage, a large majority of the included studies used a frontotemporal electrode montage with the anode placed over the left dorsolateral prefrontal cortex (F3 or midway between F3 and Fp1) coupled with the cathode placed over the left temporoparietal junction (midway between T3 and P3). Smith et al. [14] used a different electrode montage with the anode over F3 and the cathode over Fp2 (supraorbital region), another study used a 3-electrode montage. One can hypothesize that not targeting the left temporoparietal junction, one of the main brain regions involved in the pathophysiology of AVH [17], may partly explain the negative results observed in this study.

Second, with regard to clinical characteristics, AVH features in terms of frequency, severity, emotional content, and level of pharmacoresistance may have an influence on the ability of tDCS to alleviate AVH. For instance, the AVH frequency varied between studies (from 3 or 5 AVH per week to continuous daily AVH). Interestingly, Hoffman et al. [18] observed differences in brain activity during AVH between continuous and intermittent hallucinators, especially in language-related areas that are the brain targets of non-invasive brain stimulation. In addition, it is important to note that the methods used to evaluate AVH severity (including AHRS) might not have been optimal and did not permit a full exploration of all the complexities of AVH phenomenon. Moreover, the four studies that did not report tDCS efficacy were those including mixed samples with patients suffering from either schizoaffective or affective disorder, NOS or schizophrenia. Conversely, all studies showing an effect of tDCS on AVH included patients with DSM schizophrenia exclusively. One may hypothesize then that tDCS is more effective on AVH in schizophrenia than in schizoaffective disorder.

Discrepancies between studies may also be explained by concomitant medication therapy (antipsychotic, benzodiazepine, and antidepressant). Indeed, a large body of studies in healthy volunteers has reported that medications (dopaminergic, serotonergic, and GABAergic drugs) might interact with the tDCS after-effects on neural plasticity. For instance, sulpiride, a blocker of the dopamine-D2 receptor, is known to nearly completely abolish the induction of tDCS after-effects in healthy volunteers [19]. Consistent with this, Agarwal et al. [20] reported that patients receiving antipsychotics with a high affinity for the dopamine D2 receptor showed significantly less improvement of AVH after tDCS compared to patients receiving low-affinity antipsychotics or a combination of both. Furthmore, Chhabra et al. [21] reported that patients with Val/Val polymorphism of Catechol-O-methyltransferase (COMT), an enzyme that degrades dopamine in the frontal regions, showed a greater improvement of AVH after tDCS than patients with a Met allele (Val/Met or Met/Met polymorphisms). These findings suggest that depending on their functional polymorphism, patients with schizophrenia could be less responsive to tDCS if they have a lower active dopamine degradation enzyme. Thus, medication, and especially antipsychotic dopaminergic medication, as well as dopamine metabolism have an influence on tDCS after-effects.

Another confounding factor might be the presence of comorbidities of patients with schizophrenia such as tobacco use disorder or borderline personality disorder [13, 14], which was not systematically reported in the included studies. In line with this, in an open study, Brunelin et al. [22] reported that tobacco smokers were nonresponders to tDCS (−6% of AVH score after tDCS), whereas nonsmokers showed a significant 46% decrease of AVH following the same tDCS regimen. It is important to note that in the Smith et al.'s study [14], reporting negative results, all patients were regular smokers. Further studies are needed to evaluate the optimal combination between tDCS, smoking status and medication.

In sum, current evidence suggests that active tDCS could reduce AVH by approximately 25%. The most commonly used parameters consisted of delivering 10 twice-daily sessions over 5 consecutive days (20 min, 2 mA) with the anode placed over the left dorsolateral prefrontal cortex and the cathode over the left temporoparietal junction. However, these findings primarily came from preliminary studies with small sample sizes, and some studies reported conflicting results. Further, large, randomized controlled trials evaluating the clinical effects of tDCS on AVH in patients with schizophrenia are needed in order to reach a firm conclusion on its efficacy.

References

1. McGrath J, Saha S, Chant D, Welham J. Schizophrenia: a concise overview of incidence, prevalence, and mortality. Epidemiol Rev. 2008;30(1):67–76.
2. Waters F, Fernyhough C. Hallucinations: a systematic review of points of similarity and difference across diagnostic classes. Schizophr Bull. 2017;43(1):32–43.

3. McCarthy-Jones S, Trauer T, Mackinnon A, Sims E, Thomas N, Copolov DL. A new phenomenological survey of auditory hallucinations: evidence for subtypes and implications for theory and practice. Schizophr Bull. 2014;40(1):231–5.
4. Zmigrod L, Garrison JR, Carr J, Simons JS. The neural mechanisms of hallucinations: a quantitative meta-analysis of neuroimaging studies. Neurosci Biobehav Rev. 2016;69:113–23.
5. Sommer IEC, Slotema CW, Daskalakis ZJ, Derks EM, Blom JD, van der Gaag M. The treatment of hallucinations in schizophrenia spectrum disorders. Schizophr Bull. 2012;38(4):704–14.
6. Kennedy L, Xyrichis A. Cognitive behavioral therapy compared with non-specialized therapy for alleviating the effect of auditory hallucinations in people with reoccurring schizophrenia: a systematic review and meta-analysis. Community Ment Health J. 2017;53(2):127–33.
7. Moseley P, Alderson-Day B, Ellison A, Jardri R, Fernyhough C. Non-invasive brain stimulation and auditory verbal hallucinations: new techniques and future directions. Front Neurosci. 2016;9:515.
8. Lefaucheur J-P, Antal A, Ayache SS, et al. Evidence-based guidelines on the therapeutic use of transcranial direct current stimulation (tDCS). Clin Neurophysiol. 2017;128(1):56–92.
9. Mondino M, Sauvanaud F, Brunelin J. A review of the effects of transcranial direct current stimulation for the treatment of hallucinations in patients with schizophrenia. J ECT. 2018;34(3):164–71.
10. Chang CC, Tzeng NS, Chao CY, Yeh CB, Chang HA. The effects of add-on fronto-temporal transcranial direct current stimulation (tDCS) on auditory verbal hallucinations, other psychopathological symptoms, and insight in schizophrenia: a randomized, double-blind, sham-controlled trial. Int J Neuropsychopharmacol. 2018;21(11):979–87.
11. Fitzgerald PB, McQueen S, Daskalakis ZJ, Hoy KE. A negative pilot study of daily bimodal transcranial direct current stimulation in schizophrenia. Brain Stimul. 2014;7(6):813–6.
12. Fröhlich F, Burrello TN, Mellin JM, et al. Exploratory study of once-daily transcranial direct current stimulation (tDCS) as a treatment for auditory hallucinations in schizophrenia. Eur Psychiatry. 2016;33:54–60.
13. Koops S, Blom JD, Bouachmir O, Slot MI, Neggers B, Sommer IE. Treating auditory hallucinations with transcranial direct current stimulation in a double-blind, randomized trial. Schizophr Res. 2018;201:329–36.
14. Smith RC, Boules S, Mattiuz S, et al. Effects of transcranial direct current stimulation (tDCS) on cognition, symptoms, and smoking in schizophrenia: a randomized controlled study. Schizophr Res. 2015;168(1–2):260–6.
15. Alonzo A, Brassil J, Taylor JL, Martin D, Loo CK. Daily transcranial direct current stimulation (tDCS) leads to greater increases in cortical excitability than second daily transcranial direct current stimulation. Brain Stimul. 2012;5(3):208–13.
16. Monte-Silva K, Kuo MF, Liebetanz D, Paulus W, Nitsche MA. Shaping the optimal repetition interval for cathodal transcranial direct current stimulation (tDCS). J Neurophysiol. 2010;103(4):1735–40.
17. Jardri R, Pouchet A, Pins D, Thomas P. Cortical activations during auditory verbal hallucinations in schizophrenia: a coordinate-based meta-analysis. Am J Psychiatry. 2011;168(1):73–81.
18. Hoffman RE, Hampson M, Wu K, et al. Probing the pathophysiology of auditory/verbal hallucinations by combining functional magnetic resonance imaging and transcranial magnetic stimulation. Cereb Cortex. 2007;17(11):2733–43.
19. Nitsche MA, Lampe C, Antal A, et al. Dopaminergic modulation of long-lasting direct current-induced cortical excitability changes in the human motor cortex. Eur J Neurosci. 2006;23(6):1651–7.
20. Agarwal SM, Bose A, Shivakumar V, et al. Impact of antipsychotic medication on transcranial direct current stimulation (tDCS) effects in schizophrenia patients. Psychiatry Res. 2016;235:97–103.
21. Chhabra H, Shivakumar V, Subbanna M, Kalmady SV, Bose A, Agarwal SM, Sreeraj VS, Dinakaran D, Narayanaswamy JC, Debnath M, Venkatasubramanian G. Gene polymorphisms and response to transcranial direct current stimulation for auditory verbal hallucinations in schizophrenia. Acta Neuropsychiatr. 2018;30(4):218–25.

22. Brunelin J, Hasan A, Haesebaert F, Nitsche MA, Poulet E. Nicotine smoking prevents the effects of frontotemporal transcranial direct current stimulation (tDCS) in hallucinating patients with schizophrenia. Brain Stimul. 2015;8(6):1225–7.
23. Kantrowitz JT, Sehatpour P, Avissar M, Horga G, Gwak A, Hoptman MJ, Beggel O, Girgis RR, Vail B, Silipo G, Carlson M, Javitt DC. Significant improvement in treatment resistant auditory verbal hallucinations after 5 days of double-blind, randomized, sham controlled, fronto-temporal, transcranial direct current stimulation (tDCS): a replication/extension study. Brain Stimul. 2019;12(4):981–91. pii: S1935-861X(19)30082–8.
24. Lindenmayer JP, Kulsa MKC, Sultana T, Kaur A, Yang R, Ljuri I, Parker B, Khan A. Transcranial direct-current stimulation in ultra-treatment-resistant schizophrenia. Brain Stimul. 2019;12(1):54–61.
25. Bose A, Shivakumar V, Agarwal SM, et al. Efficacy of fronto-temporal transcranial direct current stimulation for refractory auditory verbal hallucinations in schizophrenia: a randomized, double-blind, sham-controlled study. Schizophr Res. 2018;195:475–80.
26. Mondino M, Jardri R, Suaud-Chagny M-F, Saoud M, Poulet E, Brunelin J. Effects of fronto-temporal transcranial direct current stimulation on auditory verbal hallucinations and resting-state functional connectivity of the left temporo-parietal junction in patients with schizophrenia. Schizophr Bull. 2016;42(2):318–26.
27. Mondino M, Haesebaert F, Poulet E, Suaud-Chagny M-F, Brunelin J. Fronto-temporal transcranial direct current stimulation (tDCS) reduces source-monitoring deficits and auditory hallucinations in patients with schizophrenia. Schizophr Res. 2015;161(2–3):515–6.
28. Brunelin J, Mondino M, Gassab L, et al. Examining transcranial direct-current stimulation (tDCS) as a treatment for hallucinations in schizophrenia. Am J Psychiatry. 2012;169(7):719–24.

Transcranial Direct Current Stimulation for Obsessive–Compulsive Disorder

18

Shayanth Manche Gowda, Venkataram Shivakumar, Janardhanan C. Narayanaswamy, and Ganesan Venkatasubramanian

18.1 Introduction

Obsessive–compulsive disorder (OCD) is characterized by obsessions and/or compulsions. Obsessions are repetitive, intrusive, irrational, anxiety-provoking, ego dystonic thoughts, urges, or images that are generally not pleasurable. Compulsions are repetitive behaviours or mental acts that the individual feels driven to perform in response to an obsession [1, 2]. OCD is often considered as a chronic and disabling mental disorder with an estimated lifetime prevalence of 1.0–3% [3, 4]. It accounts for 2.5% of the total global years lost to disability and is among the top 20 causes of illness-related disability in people aged 15–44 years [5]. OCD is a heterogeneous condition characterized by a wide range of symptoms, which are grouped into a smaller number of unique symptom dimensions, such as the need for symmetry, forbidden thoughts, cleaning, and hoarding [6]. These symptom dimensions of OCD have unique patterns of comorbidity [7], heritability [8], neuropsychological profile [9], neuroanatomical correlates [10], possibly a differential course [11] and treatment response [12, 13].

A significant proportion, i.e. 40–60% of the patients with OCD, do not respond satisfactorily to the first-line pharmacological treatment, including SRIs [14], and approximately 30% of patients with OCD fail to respond to any empirically based intervention, including cognitive behavioural therapy [15].

Treatment methods like deep brain stimulation (DBS) and stereotactic surgeries are considered in treatment refractory OCD. These options require a neurosurgical intervention in a specialized setting and they are sometimes associated with adverse effects. Moreover, the acceptance of invasive treatment modalities as a treatment option by patients is also a concern. In this context, non-invasive brain stimulation

S. M. Gowda · V. Shivakumar · J. C. Narayanaswamy (✉) · G. Venkatasubramanian
OCD Clinic and WISER Neuromodulation Program, Department of Psychiatry, National
Institute of Mental Health and Neurosciences (NIMHANS), Bengaluru, Karnataka, India
e-mail: jcn.nimhans@gmail.com; venkat.nimhans@gmail.com

© Springer Nature Switzerland AG 2020
B. Dell'Osso, G. Di Lorenzo (eds.), *Non Invasive Brain Stimulation in Psychiatry and Clinical Neurosciences*,
https://doi.org/10.1007/978-3-030-43356-7_18

249

(NIBS) techniques could bridge this gap and could potentially emerge as treatment options as augmenting strategies to address partial responders, residual symptoms with conventional treatment, and treatment-resistant/refractory OCD. Repetitive transcranial magnetic stimulation (rTMS) has been evaluated with a moderate success rate across studies in treatment-resistant OCD [16, 17]. Transcranial direct current stimulation (tDCS) is a novel and a re-emerging non-invasive neuromodulatory treatment option of interest with promising preliminary evidence in the last decade for OCD. The application of tDCS therapeutically modulates brain network activity and, hence, an overview of neural circuitry abnormality of OCD might be beneficial.

18.2   Neurobiology of OCD and the Potential Target Regions for tDCS

Many studies involving neuropsychological functioning, structural and functional neuroimaging as well as treatment studies in OCD have implicated the potential role of neural circuitry dysfunction. Cortico–striato–thalamo–cortical (CSTC) circuit abnormalities remain one of the prominent pathophysiological abnormalities in OCD [18, 19]. CSTC circuit has direct and indirect pathways. In the direct pathway, an excitatory glutamatergic signal projects from cortex on to the striatum, which further sends an inhibitory GABA-ergic signal to the internal part of the globus pallidus and sub-thalamic nucleus. This results in disinhibition of the thalamus and an increased excitatory effect on the cortex. In the indirect pathway, an excitatory glutamatergic signal projects from cortex to striatum, which further projects an inhibitory GABA-ergic signal on to the external part of the globus pallidus and the subthalamic nucleus, sending an excitatory signal to the internal part of the globus pallidus, which further sends inhibitory signals to the thalamus. The net result of the indirect pathway is increased inhibition of the thalamus and decreased excitation on the cortex. In this way, the direct pathway functions as a self-reinforcing positive feedback loop and contributes to the initiation and continuation of behaviours, whereas the indirect pathway provides a mechanism of negative feedback, which is essential for the inhibition of behaviours and switching between behaviours. In patients with OCD, an imbalance between the direct and indirect pathways results in excessive activity in the direct pathway over the indirect pathway, leading to hyperactivation of the orbitofrontal–subcortical pathway.

The CSTC circuits are parallel, partially non-overlapping circuits with origin from different cortical regions. These are as described subsequently.

18.2.1 Motor Circuit/Sensorimotor Circuit

This connects the sensorimotor and motor cortices, consisting of the pre-supplementary motor area (pre-SMA)/supplementary motor area (SMA) with the putamen, which further projects on to the globus pallidus interna and externa and caudal substantia nigra. The internal pallidal segment, in turn, projects to the ventrolateral thalamic nucleus and finally back to the sensorimotor cortex [20].

Table 18.1 Summary of functions of the brain structures implicated in OCD

Regions of brain	Functions	Functional status in OCD	Suggested montage placement
OFC and associated networks	Reversal learning Emotional and motivation behaviour Motor and response inhibition Monitors reward values	Hyperactive	Cathodal stimulation for inhibiting the hyperactive OFC
dlPFC and associated networks	Set shifting Executive functions (planning and working memory, attention, spatial information and integration of emotional and cognitive processing)	Preliminary evidences to suggest hyperactive left dlPFC and hypoactive right dlPFC	Cathodal stimulation of left dlPFC and anodal stimulation of right dlPFC might hold promise towards co-occurring anxiety and depressive symptoms but to suggest any ideal montage to address OC symptoms at this of time is difficult
Pre-SMA	Response inhibition Behavioural switching (from unwanted action to the desired action) Conflict monitoring	Unclear about the activity level— conflicting findings Considering Compensatory hyperactivity during response inhibition task	Anodal stimulation to activate the hypoactive pre-SMA
Cerebellum	Motor coordination Visuo-spatial information Cognitive and affective functions	Hypoactive	Anodal simulation to activate the hypoactive cerebellum

OFC orbito-frontal cortex, *dlPFC* dorsolateral prefrontal cortex, *Pre-SMA* pre-supplementary motor area

Functional neuroimaging studies in healthy individuals have consistently reported that better response inhibition control, i.e. shorter stop signal reaction time is associated with greater activation of pre-SMA [21, 22], which further strengthens the role of pre-SMA in response inhibition [23]; for details refer to Table 18.1. Lesions of the superior medial parts of the frontal lobes involving pre-SMA [24] and transcranial magnetic stimulation of pre-SMA have shown to worsen the response inhibition [25]. A few tDCS studies in healthy individuals with anodal stimulation of pre-SMA have shown improvement in response inhibition [26, 27]. Response inhibition has been implicated as endophenotype in OCD: poorer response inhibition performance in patients with OCD has shown to be associated with hyperactivity in the pre-SMA [28]. Many researchers have interpreted this finding in a contrasting manner regarding the causal versus consequential (compensatory) hyperactivity of pre-SMA, which is crucial to choose an electrode montage in tDCS (anodal-stimulating versus cathodal-inhibiting). Brain network activity is not static, rather it undergoes changes continuously as per the internal and external demands; hence, the functional activity of pre-SMA during resting state in comparison to

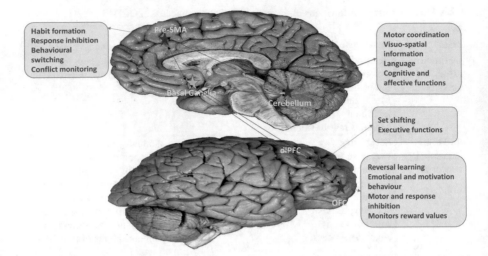

Fig. 18.1 Functions of the brain regions evaluated in tDCS studies. *Pre-SMA* (pre-supplementary motor area), *dlPFC* (dorsolateral prefrontal cortex), *OFC* (orbito-frontal cortex)

demanding task differs [29–31]. Schematic representation of functions of the brain regions and its neural circuits implicated in OCD, which are studied as targets for tDCS stimulation, is given in Fig. 18.1.

18.2.2 Dorsal Cognitive Circuit

This circuit includes projections from the dorsal prefrontal regions, including the dorsolateral prefrontal cortex (dlPFC) and dorsal anterior cingulate cortex (ACC) on to the dorsolateral caudate nucleus, which is further connected to dorsomedial parts of the globus pallidus and rostral substantia nigra [18]. Disrupted cortico-cortical interactions between dlPFC and OFC are known to reduce the top-down cognitive control under negative emotional distraction, resulting in dysfunctions of cognitive and emotional processing in OCD patients [32], as shown in Table 18.1. Functional neuroimaging in patients with OCD has implicated interhemispheric imbalance, while correction of the interhemispheric imbalance is supplemented with clinical improvement in OCD symptoms [33]. Similarly, interhemispheric imbalance is thought to exist between left and right anterior neural circuits involving dlPFC, i.e. hyperactivation of left dlPFC and hypoactivation of the right anterior neural circuits with attempts to improve this imbalance through neuromodulation [34]. Furthermore, dlPFC circuitry abnormalities appear to be associated with executive function deficits (working memory) in OCD.

18.2.3 Ventral Cognitive Circuit

This circuit is formed by neural projections from the anterolateral orbitofrontal cortex (OFC) to the ventromedial caudate nucleus, which in turn innervates the dorsomedial part of the internal pallidum and rostromedial substantia nigra. OFC has extensive neural interconnections between dlPFC and amygdala and modulates the cognitive and emotional regulation. It is crucial for the motor and response inhibition; impaired function in this loop results in set shifting difficult and ritualized behavioural responses [18] as shown in Table 18.1. Hyperactivity of the OFC–ACC loop in patients with OCD is well established [35, 36]. Both medial orbitofrontal cortex (mOFC) and lateral orbitofrontal cortex (lOFC) have separate neural connections and sub-serve different functions. Furthermore, both these structures are differentially affected in OCD, with lOFC loop circuits showing signs of hyperactivity, and mOFC circuits showing signs of hypoactivity [37].

In patients with OCD, functional connectivity between the ventral striatum and other prefrontal regions is increased [38] and the overall illness severity correlates with the alteration in the functional connectivity between ventral caudate regions and OFC [39]. Treatment with deep brain stimulation (DBS) and repetitive transcranial direct current stimulation (rTMS) appears to reduce the functional hyperconnectivity between prefrontal cortical regions and the ventral striatum/head of the caudate nucleus and improvement in the clinical symptoms of OCD [40, 41].

18.2.4 Cerebellum

The CSTC circuit/orbitofronto-striato-pallido-thalamic loop has also interconnections with other regions of the brain such as the cerebellum, which is essential for the visuo-spatial information [42]. Apart from the motor coordination, cerebellum also serves the function of language, cognitive and affective behavioural functions [43, 44]. Structural abnormality in the cerebellum has been reported in patients with OCD [45, 46]. At resting state, hypoactivity in the bilateral cerebellum correlates with symptom severity in patients with OCD [36]. Improvement in cerebellar hypoactivity with pharmacological (selective serotonin reuptake inhibitors, SSRIs) treatment has been studied [47]. rTMS stimulation of cerebellum in schizophrenia patients is well tolerated and resulted in improvement of psychotic, depressive and cognitive symptoms, providing preliminary evidence to target hypoactive cerebellum in OCD for neurostimulation [48].

18.3 Summary of tDCS Studies in OCD

It is important to point out that, until today, the number of tDCS studies conducted in OCD is very limited. Most of the studies have used an open-label design or are case-level observations. There is only one blinded sham-controlled RCT.

A total of three studies have primarily stimulated dlPFC [34, 49, 50] as shown in Table 18.2 and the sample sizes of these studies are too small to comment on the efficacy. However, all these three studies are unique to use different stimulation parameters such as anodal and cathodal stimulation of left dlPFC as well as bilateral stimulation of dlPFC, which have not yielded significant improvement in OC symptoms. Similar to rTMS studies, the role of tDCS targeting dlPFC is limited only to address the co-occurring anxiety and depressive symptoms.

Table 18.2 tDCS studies with dlPFC as the primary target

Type of study and sample size (N)	Electrodes	tDCS parameters Current Electrode size Duration of session No of sessions	Findings
Volpato et al. (2013) [34]	Sham-controlled study N = 1	Cathode: left dlPFC Anode: posterior neck-base	2 mA 35 cm² 20 min 10 sessions (1/day)	No improvement in OC symptoms Improvement in depressive (−34% HAM-D) and anxiety (−17.8% HMA-A) symptoms with verum tDCS
Palm et al. (2017) [49]	Case study N = 1	Anode: left dlPFC Cathode: right dlPFC	2 mA 35 cm² 30 min 20 sessions (2/day, 3 h apart)	Improvement in OC symptoms (−22% YBOCS), depressive (−10% HAM-D) and anxiety symptoms (−21% HAM-A) decreased
Dinn et al. (2016) [50]	Open-label study N = 5	Anode: left dlPFC Cathode: right OFC	2 mA 35 cm² 20 min 15 sessions (1/day)	Post tDCS improvement in OC symptoms (−23% OCI), but the improvement did not persist till 1-month follow up Improvement in depression (−30% BDI)

tDCS transcranial direct current stimulation, *dlPFC* dorsolateral prefrontal cortex, *HAM-D* Hamilton depression rating scale, *HAM-A* Hamilton anxiety rating scale. *OCI* Obsessive–Compulsive Inventory, *BDI* Beck Depression Inventory, *YOCS* Yale-brown obsessive–compulsive scale

There have been four studies, which have primarily targeted OFC, as shown in Table 18.3. Out of these, three studies have also studied anodal stimulation of possible hypoactive cerebellum in patients with OCD with some promising results [51–53]. However, these findings have not been replicated in larger, sham-controlled designs yet. Among these studies, only one study [54] has a relatively higher sample size (n = 42). However, since this study has used a different kind of leads with wide range of electrical doses (2–3 mA), generalizing this finding with the other tDCS studies is difficult. Other studies targeting same area have not yielded such higher and sustained improvement in OC symptoms. In view of promising findings from the rTMS studies, which have targeted OFC, it would be interesting to examine the effect of tDCS on OFC of patients with OCD in well-designed studies.

Recently, there have been attempts to stimulate SMA/pre-SMA through tDCS, as shown in Table 18.4. A randomized controlled partial crossover study of 10 patients with OCD has shown worsening of OCD symptoms with anodal stimulation and

Table 18.3 tDCS studies with OFC as the primary target

Study	Type of study and sample size (*N*)	Electrodes	tDCS parameters Current Electrode size Duration of session No. of sessions	Findings
Mondino et al. (2015) [51]	Case study *N* = 1	Cathode: left OFC Anode: right cerebello-occipital region	2 mA 35 cm² 20 min 10 sessions (2/ day; 2 h apart)	Improvement in OC symptoms (−26% YBOCS)
Bation et al. (2015) [52]	Open-label study *N* = 8	Anode: right cerebellum Cathode: left OFC	2 mA 35 cm² 20 min 10 sessions (2/ day; 3 h apart)	Improvement in OC symptoms (−26.4% YBOCS) Effects lasted up to 3 months
Alizadeh Goradel et al. (2016) [53]	Case study *N* = 1	Anode: right occipital Cathode: left OFC	2 mA 25 cm² 20 min 10 sessions (1/ day)	Improvement in OC symptoms (−64% YBOCS), depression (−87% BDI); and anxicty (−100% HAM-A)
Najafi et al. (2017) [54]	Open-label study *N* = 42	Anode: parieto-temporo-occipital areas Cathode: right OFC	2–3 mA Three leads each in cathode and anode 5.5 cm² 30 min 15 sessions (1/ day)	Improvement in OC symptoms (−63.4% YBOCS) Maintenance of the effect at 3 months' follow up (−77.6% YBOCS)

tDCS transcranial direct current stimulation, *OFC* orbito-frontal cortex, *YOCS* Yale-brown obsessive–compulsive scale, *HAM-A* Hamilton anxiety rating scale

improvement with cathodal stimulation of pre-SMA [58]. However, the only published parallel-arm RCT with sham-controlled, blinded design ($n = 25$) with anodal stimulation of left pre-SMA has shown significant improvement in OCD with active tDCS compared to sham stimulation [60]. This finding is in tune with earlier two case reports from the same group [55, 56]. However, an open-label study targeting SMA with cathodal tDCS reported clinically significant improvement in 15% of the participants [61]. The effect of cathodal tDCS on pre-SMA needs to be examined using RCT design.

In summary, anodal stimulation of SMA/pre-SMA to improve the OCD symptoms has emerging evidence. Promising results of cathodal stimulation of left OFC along with anodal stimulation of cerebellum deserve further evaluation using controlled studies.

Table 18.4 tDCS studies with SMA/pre-SMA as the primary target

Study	Type of study and sample size (N)	Electrodes	tDCS parameters Current Electrode size Duration of session No of sessions	Findings
Narayanaswamy et al. (2015) [55]	Case series N = 2	Anode: left pre-SMA Cathode: right OFC	2 mA 35 cm² 20 min 20 sessions (2/day, at least 3 h between 2 sessions)	Improvement in OC symptom (− >40% YBOCS) in both the subjects Improvement in depressive as well as anxiety symptoms
Hazari et al. (2016) [56]	Case study N = 1	Anode: left pre-SMA Cathode: right OFC	2 mA 35 cm² 20 min 20 sessions (2/day, at least 3 h between 2 sessions)	Improvement in OC symptom (−80% YBOCS) during 7 months Similar improvement with booster session on relapse
D'Urso et al. (2016) [57]	Case study N = 1	Anode: pre-SMA Cathode: right deltoid And then, reverse montage	2 mA 25 cm² 20 min 10 sessions (1/day)	Worsening of OC symptoms after anodal tDCS Improvement in OC symptoms (−30% YBOCS) after cathodal tDCS
D'Urso et al. (2016) [58]	Randomized controlled partial crossover study N = 12 (10 subjects completed the RCT)	Active electrode- midline pre-SMA Reference electrode: right deltoid (cathode or anode based on the cross-over design)	2 mA 25 cm² 20 min 10 sessions (1/day)	Cathodal tDCS was significantly more effective than anodal tDCS In the active cathodal arm, improvement in OC symptoms (−17.5% YBOCS) with 10 sessions, (−20.1% YBOCS) with 20 sessions
Silva et al. (2016) [59]	Case study N = 2	Cathode: bilateral SMA Anode: right deltoid	2 mA 25 cm² 30 min 10 sessions (1/day)	Subject 1: no improvement at week 4, YBOCS score dropped by 18% at week 12 Patient 2: YBOCS score reduced by 17% at week 4; reduction of 55% at week 12

Table 18.4 (continued)

Gowda et al. (2019) [60]	Randomized, double-blinded, sham-controlled trial $N = 25$	Anode: left pre-SMA Cathode: right OFC	2 mA 35 cm^2 20 min 20 sessions (2/day, at least 3 h between 2 sessions)	The improvement in OC symptom was significantly greater in the verum tDCS (4 out of 12) compared to sham tDCS (0 out of 13) Subjects who responded with verum tDCS all of them have shown >35% improvement in YBOCS
Kumar et al. (2019) [61]	Open-label study $N = 20$	Cathode: supplementary motor area (SMA) Anode: right occipital area	2 mA 25 cm^2 20 min 20 sessions (2/day, at least 3 h between 2 sessions)	There was 35% YBOCS reduction in 15% of the participants

tDCS transcranial direct current stimulation, *pre-SMA* pre-supplementary motor area, *YOCS* Yale-brown obsessive–compulsive scale

18.4 What May be the Future of tDCS for OCD?

In view of its easy application, tolerability and relatively lower cost involved, tDCS is a non-invasive neuromodulation strategy, which merits further evaluation in OCD. Considering the challenge posed by treatment resistance to SSRIs in OCD, tDCS might evolve as one of the treatment options. At present, field studies are numerically limited and characterized by methodological inconsistencies and small sample sizes. Therefore, more controlled studies are required to confirm some of the preliminary observations.

Conventional tDCS is associated with diffuse stimulation over the required target area and it may be less specific. Novel advancements, such as high-definition tDCS (HD-tDCS), might be a potential strategy to overcome this limitation. In addition, neuronavigation-based approaches would be a step forward to enhance treatment precision. Furthermore, there is a need to examine the mechanism of symptom improvement with tDCS. Use of computational modelling of electrical current appears to be a significant advancement in tDCS research [62]. Neuroimaging, mainly using functional MRI, as well as neurocognitive assessment may be important tools in this regard. Finally, in oder to examine the effect of tDCS in OCD, we also propose that well-designed studies may be conducted in larger samples, using uniform methodology and multi-site collaborative efforts.

Acknowledgments This work is partly supported by the Wellcome trust DBT India Alliance intermediate fellowship grant to Dr. Janardhanan C. Narayanaswamy (IA/CPHI/16/1/502662) and the Swarnajayanti Fellowship Grant of the Department of Science and Technology (Government of India) to Ganesan Venkatasubramanian (DST/SJF/LSA-02/2014-15).

References

1. Rasmussen SA, Eisen JL. Clinical features and phenomenology of obsessive compulsive disorder. Psychiatr Ann. 1989;19(2):67–73.
2. American Psychiatric Association. DSM 5. Washington, DC: American Psychiatric Association; 2013.
3. Adam Y, Meinlschmidt G, Gloster AT, Lieb R. Obsessive–compulsive disorder in the community: 12-month prevalence, comorbidity and impairment. Soc Psychiatry Psychiatr Epidemiol. 2012;47(3):339–49.
4. Ruscio AM, Stein DJ, Chiu WT, Kessler RC. The epidemiology of obsessive-compulsive disorder in the National Comorbidity Survey Replication. Mol Psychiatry. 2010;15(1):53–63.
5. Ayuso-Mateos JL. Global burden of obsessive-compulsive disorder in the year 2000. Geneva: World Health Organization; 2006.
6. Mataix-Cols D, do Rosario-Campos MC, Leckman JF. A multidimensional model of obsessive-compulsive disorder. Am J Psychiatry. 2005;162(2):228–38.
7. Prabhu L, Cherian AV, Viswanath B, Kandavel T, Math SB, Reddy YJ. Symptom dimensions in OCD and their association with clinical characteristics and comorbid disorders. J Obsess-Compuls Relat Disord. 2013;2(1):14–21.
8. Katerberg H, Delucchi KL, Stewart SE, Lochner C, Denys DA, Stack DE, et al. Symptom dimensions in OCD: item-level factor analysis and heritability estimates. Behav Genet. 2010;40(4):505–17.
9. Hashimoto N, Nakaaki S, Omori IM, Fujioi J, Noguchi Y, Murata Y, et al. Distinct neuropsychological profiles of three major symptom dimensions in obsessive–compulsive disorder. Psychiatry Res. 2011;187(1):166–73.
10. Mataix-Cols D, Wooderson S, Lawrence N, Brammer MJ, Speckens A, Phillips ML. Distinct neural correlates of washing, checking, and hoarding symptom dimensions in obsessive-compulsive disorder. Arch Gen Psychiatry. 2004;61(6):564–76.
11. Eisen JL, Sibrava NJ, Boisseau CL, Mancebo MC, Stout RL, Pinto A, et al. Five-year course of obsessive-compulsive disorder: predictors of remission and relapse [CME]. J Clin Psychiatry. 2013;74(3):233–9.
12. Mataix-Cols D, Rauch SL, Manzo PA, Jenike MA, Baer L. Use of factor-analyzed symptom dimensions to predict outcome with serotonin reuptake inhibitors and placebo in the treatment of obsessive-compulsive disorder. Am J Psychiatry. 1999;156(9):1409–16.
13. Mataix-Cols D, Rauch SL, Baer L, Eisen JL, Shera DM, Goodman WK, et al. Symptom stability in adult obsessive-compulsive disorder: data from a naturalistic two-year follow-up study. Am J Psychiatry. 2002;159(2):263–8.
14. Pallanti S, Hollander E, Bienstock C, Koran L, Leckman J, Marazziti D, et al. Treatment non-response in OCD: methodological issues and operational definitions. Int J Neuropsychopharmacol. 2002;5(2):181–91.
15. Schruers K, Koning K, Luermans J, Haack MJ, Griez E. Obsessive-compulsive disorder: a critical review of therapeutic perspectives. Acta Psychiatr Scand. 2005;111(4):261–71.
16. Berlim MT, Neufeld NH, Van den Eynde F. Repetitive transcranial magnetic stimulation (rTMS) for obsessive–compulsive disorder (OCD): an exploratory meta-analysis of randomized and sham-controlled trials. J Psychiatr Res. 2013;47(8):999–1006.
17. Rehn S, Eslick GD, Brakoulias V. A meta-analysis of the effectiveness of different cortical targets used in repetitive transcranial magnetic stimulation (rTMS) for the treatment of obsessive-compulsive disorder (OCD). Psychiatry Q. 2018;89(3):645–65.
18. Milad MR, Rauch SL. Obsessive-compulsive disorder: beyond segregated cortico-striatal pathways. Trends Cogn Sci. 2012;16(1):43–51.
19. Saxena S, Rauch SL. Functional neuroimaging and the neuroanatomy of obsessive-compulsive disorder. Psychiatr Clin N Am. 2000;23(3):563–86.
20. Russo M, Naro A, Mastroeni C, Morgante F, Terranova C, Muscatello MR, et al. Obsessive-compulsive disorder: a "sensory-motor" problem? Int J Psychophysiol. 2014;92(2):74–8.

21. Chao HH, Luo X, Chang JL, Li CS. Activation of the pre-supplementary motor area but not inferior prefrontal cortex in association with short stop signal reaction time—an intra-subject analysis. BMC Neurosci. 2009;10:75.

22. Congdon E, Mumford JA, Cohen JR, Galvan A, Aron AR, Xue G, et al. Engagement of large-scale networks is related to individual differences in inhibitory control. Neuroimage. 2010;53(2):653–63.

23. Aron AR. From reactive to proactive and selective control: developing a richer model for stopping inappropriate responses. Biol Psychiatry. 2011;69(12):e55–68.

24. Picton TW, Stuss DT, Alexander MP, Shallice T, Binns MA, Gillingham S. Effects of focal frontal lesions on response inhibition. Cereb Cortex. 2007;17(4):826–38.

25. Chen C-Y, Muggleton NG, Tzeng OJ, Hung DL, Juan C-H. Control of prepotent responses by the superior medial frontal cortex. Neuroimage. 2009;44(2):537–45.

26. Hsu T-Y, Tseng L-Y, Yu J-X, Kuo W-J, Hung DL, Tzeng OJ, et al. Modulating inhibitory control with direct current stimulation of the superior medial frontal cortex. Neuroimage. 2011;56(4):2249–57.

27. Kwon YH, Kwon JW. Response inhibition induced in the stop-signal task by transcranial direct current stimulation of the pre-supplementary motor area and primary sensoriomotor cortex. J Phys Ther Sci. 2013;25(9):1083–6.

28. de Wit SJ, de Vries FE, van der Werf YD, Cath DC, Heslenfeld DJ, Veltman EM, et al. Presupplementary motor area hyperactivity during response inhibition: a candidate endophenotype of obsessive-compulsive disorder. Am J Psychiatry. 2012;169(10):1100–8.

29. Cocchi L, Zalesky A, Nott Z, Whybird G, Fitzgerald PB, Breakspear M. Transcranial magnetic stimulation in obsessive-compulsive disorder: a focus on network mechanisms and state dependence. Neuroimage Clin. 2018;19:661–74.

30. Cocchi L, Zalesky A, Fornito A, Mattingley JB. Dynamic cooperation and competition between brain systems during cognitive control. Trends Cogn Sci. 2013;17(10):493–501.

31. de Vries FE, de Wit SJ, Cath DC, van der Werf YD, van der Borden V, van Rossum TB, et al. Compensatory frontoparietal activity during working memory: an endophenotype of obsessive-compulsive disorder. Biol Psychiatry. 2014;76(11):878–87.

32. Han HJ, Jung WH, Yun JY, Park JW, Cho KK, Hur JW, et al. Disruption of effective connectivity from the dorsolateral prefrontal cortex to the orbitofrontal cortex by negative emotional distraction in obsessive-compulsive disorder. Psychol Med. 2016;46(5):921–32.

33. Goncalves OF, Carvalho S, Leite J, Pocinho F, Relvas J, Fregni F. Obsessive compulsive disorder as a functional interhemispheric imbalance at the thalamic level. Med Hypotheses. 2011;77(3):445–7.

34. Volpato C, Piccione F, Cavinato M, Duzzi D, Schiff S, Foscolo L, et al. Modulation of affective symptoms and resting state activity by brain stimulation in a treatment-resistant case of obsessive–compulsive disorder. Neurocase. 2013;19(4):360–70.

35. Maia TV, Cooney RE, Peterson BS. The neural bases of obsessive-compulsive disorder in children and adults. Dev Psychopathol. 2008;20(4):1251–83.

36. Hou J, Wu W, Lin Y, Wang J, Zhou D, Guo J, et al. Localization of cerebral functional deficits in patients with obsessive-compulsive disorder: a resting-state fMRI study. J Affect Disord. 2012;138(3):313–21.

37. Fettes P, Schulze L, Downar J. Cortico-striatal-thalamic loop circuits of the orbitofrontal cortex: promising therapeutic targets in psychiatric illness. Front Syst Neurosci. 2017;11:25.

38. Sakai Y, Narumoto J, Nishida S, Nakamae T, Yamada K, Nishimura T, et al. Corticostriatal functional connectivity in non-medicated patients with obsessive-compulsive disorder. Eur Psychiatry. 2011;26(7):463–9.

39. Harrison BJ, Pujol J, Cardoner N, Deus J, Alonso P, López-Solà M, et al. Brain corticostriatal systems and the major clinical symptom dimensions of obsessive-compulsive disorder. Biol Psychiatry. 2013;73(4):321–8.

40. Figee M, Luigjes J, Smolders R, Valencia-Alfonso C-E, Van Wingen G, De Kwaasteniet B, et al. Deep brain stimulation restores frontostriatal network activity in obsessive-compulsive disorder. Nat Neurosci. 2013;16(4):386.

41. Dunlop K, Woodside B, Olmsted M, Colton P, Giacobbe P, Downar J. Reductions in cortico-striatal hyperconnectivity accompany successful treatment of obsessive-compulsive disorder with dorsomedial prefrontal rTMS. Neuropsychopharmacology. 2016;41(5):1395.
42. Nakao T, Okada K, Kanba S. Neurobiological model of obsessive–compulsive disorder: evidence from recent neuropsychological and neuroimaging findings. Psychiatry Clin Neurosci. 2014;68(8):587–605.
43. De Smet HJ, Paquier P, Verhoeven J, Marien P. The cerebellum: its role in language and related cognitive and affective functions. Brain Lang. 2013;127(3):334–42.
44. Koziol LF, Budding D, Andreasen N, D'Arrigo S, Bulgheroni S, Imamizu H, et al. Consensus paper: the cerebellum's role in movement and cognition. Cerebellum. 2014;13(1):151–77.
45. de Wit SJ, Alonso P, Schweren L, Mataix-Cols D, Lochner C, Menchon JM, et al. Multicenter voxel-based morphometry mega-analysis of structural brain scans in obsessive-compulsive disorder. Am J Psychiatry. 2014;171(3):340–9.
46. Narayanaswamy JC, Jose D, Kalmady SV, Agarwal SM, Venkatasubramanian G, Reddy YJ. Cerebellar volume deficits in medication-naïve obsessive compulsive disorder. Psychiatry Res Neuroimaging. 2016;254:164–8.
47. Sanematsu H, Nakao T, Yoshiura T, Nabeyama M, Togao O, Tomita M, et al. Predictors of treatment response to fluvoxamine in obsessive-compulsive disorder: an fMRI study. J Psychiatr Res. 2010;44(4):193–200.
48. Demirtas-Tatlidede A, Freitas C, Cromer JR, Safar L, Ongur D, Stone WS, et al. Safety and proof of principle study of cerebellar vermal theta burst stimulation in refractory schizophrenia. Schizophr Res. 2010;124(1–3):91–100.
49. Palm U, Leitner B, Kirsch B, Behler N, Kumpf U, Wulf L, et al. Prefrontal tDCS and sertraline in obsessive compulsive disorder: a case report and review of the literature. Neurocase. 2017;23(2):173–7.
50. Dinn WM, Aycicegi-Dinn A, Göral F, Karamursel S, Yildirim EA, Hacioglu-Yildirim M, et al. Treatment-resistant obsessive-compulsive disorder: insights from an open trial of transcranial direct current stimulation (tDCS) to design a RCT. Neurol Psychiatry Brain Res. 2016;22(3–4):146–54.
51. Mondino M, Haesebaert F, Poulet E, Saoud M, Brunelin J. Efficacy of cathodal transcranial direct current stimulation over the left orbitofrontal cortex in a patient with treatment-resistant obsessive-compulsive disorder. J ECT. 2015;31(4):271–2.
52. Bation R, Poulet E, Haesebaert F, Saoud M, Brunelin J. Transcranial direct current stimulation in treatment-resistant obsessive–compulsive disorder: an open-label pilot study. Prog Neuropsychopharmacol Biol Psychiatry. 2016;65:153–7.
53. Alizadeh Goradel J, Pouresmali A, Mowlaie M, Sadeghi MF. The effects of transcranial direct current stimulation on obsession-compulsion, anxiety, and depression of a patient suffering from obsessive-compulsive disorder. Pract Clin Psychol. 2016;4(2):75–80.
54. Najafi K, Fakour Y, Zarrabi H, Heidarzadeh A, Khalkhali M, Yeganeh T, et al. Efficacy of transcranial direct current stimulation in the treatment resistant patients who suffer from severe obsessive-compulsive disorder. Indian J Psychol Med. 2017;39(5):573–8.
55. Narayanaswamy JC, Jose D, Chhabra H, Agarwal SM, Shrinivasa B, Hegde A, et al. Successful application of add-on transcranial direct current stimulation (tDCS) for treatment of SSRI resistant OCD. Brain Stimul. 2015;8(3):655–7.
56. Hazari N, Narayanaswamy JC, Chhabra H, Bose A, Venkatasubramanian G, Reddy YJ. Response to transcranial direct current stimulation in a case of episodic obsessive compulsive disorder. J ECT. 2016;32(2):144–6.
57. D'Urso G, Brunoni AR, Anastasia A, Micillo M, de Bartolomeis A, Mantovani A. Polarity-dependent effects of transcranial direct current stimulation in obsessive-compulsive disorder. Neurocase. 2016;22(1):60–4.
58. D'Urso G, Brunoni AR, Mazzaferro MP, Anastasia A, de Bartolomeis A, Mantovani A. Transcranial direct current stimulation for obsessive-compulsive disorder: a randomized, controlled, partial crossover trial. Depress Anxiety. 2016;33(12):1132–40.

59. Silva RM, Brunoni AR, Miguel EC, Shavitt RG. Transcranial direct current stimulation for treatment-resistant obsessive-compulsive disorder: report on two cases and proposal for a randomized, sham-controlled trial. Sao Paulo Med J. 2016;134(5):446–50.
60. Gowda SM, Narayanaswamy JC, Hazari N, Bose A, Chhabra H, Balachander S, et al. Efficacy of pre-supplementary motor area transcranial direct current stimulation for treatment resistant obsessive compulsive disorder: a randomized, double blinded, sham controlled trial. Brain Stimul. 2019;12(4):922–9.
61. Kumar S, Kumar N, Verma R. Safety and efficacy of adjunctive transcranial direct current stimulation in treatment-resistant obsessive-compulsive disorder: an open-label trial. Indian J Psychiatry. 2019;61(4):327–34.
62. da Silva RMF, Batistuzzo MC, Shavitt RG, Miguel EC, Stern E, Mezger E, et al. Transcranial direct current stimulation in obsessive-compulsive disorder: an update in electric field modeling and investigations for optimal electrode montage. Expert Rev Neurother. 2019;19(10):1025–35.

Transcranial Direct Current Stimulation in Addiction

19

Giovanni Martinotti, Andrea Miuli, Mauro Pettorruso,
Hamed Ekhtiari, Colleen A. Hanlon,
Primavera A. Spagnolo, and Massimo Di Giannantonio

19.1 tDCS: The Rationale of Use in Addiction

Although medications currently used for psychiatric disorders have shown efficacy, the nonspecific receptor selectivity and the inability to intervene in certain
brain target regions for homeostatic mechanisms still represent a huge obstacle in
pharmacotherapy of psychiatric disorders [1]. In the field of drug addiction, one
of the most prevalent psychiatric disorders, despite the enormous efforts to find
effective medications, there are only a handful of approved pharmacological treatments with limited efficacy, as demonstrated by the high long-term relapse rates
[2, 3]. Many different molecules have been tested. Unfortunately, the results of
these trials have not been completely successful in meeting expectations [4–7].
These pitfalls in new drug development for addiction treatment, together with a

G. Martinotti (✉)
Department of Neuroscience, Imaging and Clinical Sciences, 'G. D'Annunzio' University,
Chieti, Italy

Department of Pharmacy, Pharmacology and Clinical Sciences, University of Hertfordshire,
Hatfield, UK

SRP 'Villa Maria Pia', Rome, Italy
e-mail: giovanni.martinotti@gmail.com

A. Miuli · M. Pettorruso · M. Di Giannantonio
Department of Neuroscience, Imaging and Clinical Sciences, 'G. D'Annunzio' University,
Chieti, Italy

H. Ekhtiari
Laureate Institute for Brain Research, Tulsa, OK, USA

C. A. Hanlon
Medical University of South Carolina (MUSC), Charleston, SC, USA

P. A. Spagnolo
National Institute on Neurological Disorders and Stroke, National Institute of Health,
Bethesda, MD, USA

© Springer Nature Switzerland AG 2020
B. Dell'Osso, G. Di Lorenzo (eds.), *Non Invasive Brain Stimulation
in Psychiatry and Clinical Neurosciences*,
https://doi.org/10.1007/978-3-030-43356-7_19

better understanding of their neurobiology, have paved the ground for new treatment approaches and developments, as the case of non-invasive brain stimulation (NIBS).

Prolonged exposure to addictive agents results in multiple circuit dysfunctions through neuronal adaptation and toxicity mechanisms [8]. Significant alterations in neural circuits can result in deficits in reward processing, salience attribution, motivation, inhibitory control, learning and memory consolidation. This allows the birth of a complex phenotype, characterized by different symptomatic dimensions, each related to specific circuits. Transcranial neuromodulation techniques, such as transcranial direct current stimulation (tDCS), could mitigate these deficits targeting different neural circuits [9]. Among these, the Dorso-Lateral-Prefrontal-Cortex (DLPFC), as the main node in the executive control network, certainly represents one of the main targets.

A large body of literature implicates the DLPFC in the cognitive deficits observed in many psychiatric disorders, including lack of inhibitory control, impulsivity, altered decision making, which are also observed in individuals with addiction [10, 11]. Moreover, neuroimaging studies have revealed that the activity in this area is significantly reduced in association with craving for substances like alcohol [12], cocaine [13], nicotine [14] and heroin [15]. An increased activity of the DLPFC is associated with reduction of craving as showed in an fMRI study in subjects abstaining from the use of nicotine even for only 4 hours [16]. This means that intervention targeting this region may result in reduced drug-seeking and -taking behaviours. Craving is frequently correlated with impulsivity [17], and the stimulation of the DLPFC could also exert positive effects on impulse control and attention regulation [1]. Therefore, the stimulation of the DLPFC can modulate activity in this area as well as in interconnected areas within the ECN, thus increasing inhibitory control over craving and restoring executive functioning.

Stimulation of the DLPFC or other potential targets can be achieved by using non-invasive brain stimulation interventions such as tDCS. This device, with the transmission of positive or negative charges, acts on the resting membrane potential of neurons causing depolarization (anodic-positive stimulation) or hyperpolarization (cathodic-negative stimulation), respectively [18–20]. The flow is conventionally considered as directed from the anode to the cathode, creating a closed circuit [21]. Several neurobiological mechanisms explain the neuromodulation and neuroplasticity induced by tDCS: (1) the increase of the intracellular concentration of Ca^{++} (in particular using anodal tDCS) [22]; (2) the modulation of the excitability of glutamatergic synaptic receptors in pyramidal neurons and the inhibition of the release of GABA [23–25]; (3) probable modulation of brain-derived neurotrophic factor (BDNF) levels [26].

The cognitive modulation associated with tDCS is probably related to all these neurobiological aspects, but may also be determined by the activation of the ventromedial prefrontal cortex (vmPFC), modulated by alterations established at the level of DLPFC following repeated anodic stimulation. The indirect effects on vmPFC could therefore be the means by which tDCS act on self-control and decision making, strongly altered cognitive processes in people with drug-use disorders, also reducing the risk of relapse [27]. It is believed that tDCS is a reasonable alternative to existing addiction therapies.

19.2 tDCS as a Therapeutic Tool in Addiction Medicine

Recently, several studies have been evaluating the efficacy of tDCS for addictive disorders. In particular, a systematic review conducted in 2017 summarized results from 18 different studies using tDCS. Several substances were considered in the review (caffeine, alcohol, cannabis, cocaine, heroin, nicotine, methamphetamines and novel psychoactive substances) and 16 articles studied the efficacy of tDCS applied to the DLPFC, whereas two articles evaluated the efficacy of tDCS to the frontal-parietal-temporal area (FPT), indicating how DLPFC stimulation has received considerable scientific evidence. With regard to the clinical efficacy, while all DLPFC studies showed a reduction in craving, in studies with the placement of electrodes on FPT, only one showed significant data. Electrodes were placed with the anode on the right and the cathode on the left in six studies, with the anode on the left and the cathode on the right in six studies and with anode right/left—cathode right/left in four studies [28]. Lapenta and colleagues examined 29 articles on the use of tDCS in the treatment of addictions reviewing not only the clinical efficacy but also the related neurophysiological and cognitive implications of this technique. This work considered food, nicotine, alcohol, cocaine, crack, methamphetamine and cannabis supporting the role of tDCS in the treatment of addictions both in terms of craving and quantity of substances taken, and in terms of improvement of executive and cognitive functions [9]. Finally, Ekhtiari and colleagues published in 2019 a consensus paper describing the current knowledge of tDCS and TMS in the field of addiction. This review highlights how the most used amperage is 2 mA and that most studies (71%) did not include any follow-up (there were only two studies with 1-year follow-up). An interesting aspect is when tDCS stimulation should be applied, with the definition of four different groups: (1) before the participant sought standard treatment (2) while the subject was treatment seeking but before undergoing standard treatment, (3) within the first month of standard treatment (mainly detoxification and stabilization) and (4) after the initial recovery period (more than 1 month). Another interesting issue is how craving, the main outcome of treatment effectiveness, has been rated in the different studies: the use of VAS scale or the amount of intake of substance should probably be associated with cue-reactivity behavioural paradigms or biological metrics [29].

19.2.1 tDCS in Nicotine-Use Disorder

Tobacco-use disorder, as well as causing countless organic damage with a high impact on public health costs, has recently been strongly linked to the onset of depressive episodes [30]. Thus, given that NIBS has been shown to be effective in treating depressive disorders, these interventions can be used as a treatment for comorbid tobacco-use disorders and depression.

One of the first studies investigating the efficacy of tDCS in cigarette addiction was the one of Fregni and coll. in 2008. They tested 24 subjects randomized to receive three different tDCS modalities in a single session: (1) sham tDCS; (2) anodal tDCS over the right DLPFC (R-DLPFC); (3) anodal tDCS over the left DLPFC (L-DLPFC). All the active tDCS protocols were set with 2 mA for 20 minutes of stimulation. A significant reduction on craving was observed only in the active tDCS protocols [31]. In another study, Boggio and colleagues assessed the effects of five consecutive sessions of tDCS on the DLPFC. Twenty-six patients were randomized to two separate groups: L-DLPFC anodal stimulation (2 mA/20 min) and sham stimulation. Results showed a small but significant reduction in cigarette consumption and craving in the treated group compared to the placebo group [32]. Xu and colleagues used the same protocol (L-DLPFC 2 mA/20-minute anodal vs. sham stimulation), applying the cathode above the right supraorbital area. They tested also the attention level of the participant during the stimulation with a computer task to assess the efficacy of tDCS not only on the craving level but also on cognition and mood in dependent smokers after overnight abstinence. Results showed a reduction of negative effect in these subjects that was strictly related with craving level, but no efficacy on attention and cognition was observed [33]. In another study, Falcone and colleagues investigated, in a sample of 25 subjects, not only the reduction of the intensity of craving or the number of cigarettes smoked, but also the ability to resist smoking. Using anodal stimulation of LDLPFC and cathodal stimulation of right supraorbital area (compared with sham), the research team applied a single 20-minute session with an intensity of 1.0 mA. Every participant underwent tDCS seeing smoking-related cues: patients had the option to smoke at any time or receive $1 for every 5 min they abstained. At the end of the study, an increase in latency was observed between the consumption of cigarettes with a significant reduction in the amount of tobacco consumed only in the group of patients who underwent an active stimulation [34]. A very recent study performed by Ghorbani Behnam *and colleagues* examined not only the efficacy of the 'anodal LDLPFC/cathodal RDLPFC' stimulation versus sham, but also versus bupropione, the gold standard in the pharmacological treatment of tobacco addiction. In fact, subjects were divided ramdomly into five groups: (1) treatment with 300-mg bupropion (8 weeks); (2) active tDCS (20 sessions for 4 weeks); (3) sham stimulation like group 2; (4) active tDCS (20 sessions for 12 weeks), and (5) sham stimulation like group 4. The main finding of the study was that the longer-period tDCS group had a better percentage of 6-month abstinence rate (25.7%) compared with the short-period tDCS group (7%), showing no significant differences with respect to the bupropion group (6-month abstinence rate of 20%). Both the two active tDCS protocols were also better than the sham stimulation groups [35]. More information about the functional connectivity after the stimulation of tDCS in these treatments is given by a recent study of Yang *and colleagues*. Placing the anode over the F3 and the cathode over the F4 (10–20 EEG system), 32 smokers were stimulated for 30 minutes, in an MRI scanner, at 1-mA intensity. During this period of

treatment, after the acquisition of an anatomical scan, they also completed a go/
no-go task, a monetary incentive delay task, a cue-reactivity task and an emotion
task. This study revealed considerable information on the neuromodulation of different areas: the neural activity of left superior frontal gyrus and the left middle
frontal gyrus were reduced only in the active stimulation group and a significant
functional connection was shown between the L-DLPFC and the right parahippocampal gyrus during the resting-state analysis [36]. Finally, Fectau et al., in a study
of 2014, analysed the effect on tobacco consumption using a different position of
the electrodes: 'right anodal/left cathodal' in a crossover, blind at four levels (group
allocator, subjects, tDCS provider, outcome assessor), randomized, sham-controlled
trial. They stimulated 12 adults with two periods of 5 consecutive days (2-mA intensity for 30 minutes) separated by 3 months' free of stimulation in which every participant had written a diary of tobacco consumption. This study provided a significant
result of efficacy in reducing the number of cigarettes smoked and the desire to
smoke in the active stimulation with respect to the sham tDCS [37].

19.2.2 tDCS in Alcohol-Use Disorder

One of the first studies was conducted on 13 patients who received an active 'anodal/
L-DLPFC and cathodal/R-DLPFC' stimulation (2 mA for 20 minutes), an active
'anodal/R-DLPFC and cathodal/L-DLPFC' stimulation (2 mA for 20 minutes), and
a sham stimulation bilaterally over DLPFC, in three separate sessions, while watch-
ing alcohol consumption videos. The study showed a reduction in alcohol craving
in both active groups, with no effect in the placebo group [38]. Another study, using
a similar setting (2 mA/20 minutes), focused on an anodal stimulation over the
L-DLPFC (cathode was on right supradeltoid area) to prevent alcohol-use relapses,
investigating also cognitive and frontal executive processes, craving, depressive and
anxiety symptoms during 5 consecutive weeks of treatment and after 4 weeks of
follow-up in 13 alcoholics. Active tDCS group ($n = 6$) showed a reduction of depressive symptoms and craving for alcohol. This study also provided event-related
potentials (ERPs) investigation, finding how active tDCS was able to block the
increase in neural activation triggered by alcohol-related cues in prefrontal cortex
(PFC) [39]. Consistently, in another study, Klauss and colleagues treated 35 subjects with bilateral active stimulation for 5 consecutive days (2 mA/13 minutes,
twice per day, with an interval of 20 minutes) versus sham stimulation. In this case,
the research group used a 'cathodal/L-DLPFC and anodal/R-DLPFC' configuration, showing a reduction in relapse and an improvement in quality of life perception [40]. Also in another study of 2018, Klauss and coll. stimulated with the same
electrode configuration (2 mA/20 minutes) a group of Alcohol-Use Disorder (AUD)
patients to prevent relapses for alcohol use. Active or sham-tDCS were applied daily
for a total of ten sessions and alcohol craving was monitored weekly for 5 weeks.
Even if craving scores progressively decreased in both groups, the reduction of
alcohol craving was significant only in the active stimulation group [41, 42]. After
these studies on a sample of AUD patients, Wietschorke and collaborators

stimulated 30 detoxified patients ('cathodal/L-DLPFC and anodal/R-DLPFC' stimulation, 1 mA/20 minutes per session, vs. sham stimulation over DLPFC) also with the presentation of emotional and alcohol-related pictures to detect any change in alcohol cue reactivity. The results of this study showed a reduction of craving intensity for alcohol in the real tDCS group but also a negative emotional internal process linked to alcohol desire [43]. Although the evidence in supporting the use of tDCS in AUD appears to be relevant, there are some studies with negative results. In particular, there are two recent studies made by den Uyl's research group that compared the efficacy of tDCS and cognitive bias modification (CBM) in AUD patients. CBM is a psychological therapy, which assumes that changes in cognitive biases lead to changes in anxiety and depression symptoms [44]. Hazardous drinkers were randomized in four groups: real CBM/active tDCS, real CBM/sham tDCS, control CBM/active tDCS, or control CBM/sham tDCS. In both these studies, a nonsignificant effect of tDCS was shown [45, 46].

19.2.3 tDCS in Cocaine- and Stimulant-Use Disorder

With regards to the treatment of Cocaine-Use Disorder (CUD), there has been increasing attention to tDCS.

One of the first studies aimed to assess the efficacy of tDCS on risk-taking behaviours in CUD was conducted by Gorini and colleagues using either left DLPFC anodal/right DLPFC cathodal stimulation, right DLPFC anodal/left DLPFC cathodal stimulation, or sham stimulation. Thirty-six subjects (18 CUD and 18 controls) underwent a 20-minute stimulation at 1.5 mA and tested with Balloon Analogue Risk Task (BART) and game-of-dice task (GDT). In the first task, a significant effect of tDCS in comparison with sham stimulation was shown, whereas with GDT similar results could not be observed [47]. The placement of cathode over F3 and anode over F4 (10–20 International EEG system) was also made in another study investigating the efficacy of tDCS on craving level for crack-cocaine. Seventeen patients underwent tDCS stimulation for 20 minutes at 2 mA for 5 consecutive days, while 19 patients received sham-tDCS. The results of this study showed the efficacy of active tDCS for reduction in crack-cocaine craving [48]. In contrast with these positive findings, the study of Klauss et al. in 2018 did not appear to support the therapeutic role of tDCS as regards to crack-cocaine craving. Thirty-five patients with crack-cocaine-use disorder, after receiving a standard treatment with psychosocial intervention combined with pharmacotherapy, underwent 4 weeks of tDCS treatment (2 mA/20 minutes per session), with the cathode placed over the left DLPFC and the anode over the right DLPFC. Crack-cocaine craving scores progressively decreased in both sham ($n = 16$) and real tDCS ($n = 19$) groups during the treatment period, showing no significant difference between two groups at 1-month and 2-month follow-up on crack-cocaine-use relapse rate [41, 42].

The neuromodulating effect of tDCS using EEG procedures has been investigated as well. In 2014, the N2 component (200–350 ms) of EEG in anterior cingulate cortex (AAC) (which seems to be involved in drug-related attention bias [49]) was examined during the tDCS stimulation and visual presentation of a picture of drug-related cues. Thirteen subjects with crack-cocaine addiction underwent 20-minute stimulation at 2 mA with left cathodal/right anodal tDCS over the DLPFC. The main finding of this study was that left cathodal but not the right anodal tDCS seemed to reduce activity in the ACC during crack-related image visualization [50].

Another study of ERPs under drug-related cues, more specifically in its P3 segment (300–500 ms), showed that, in a sample of AUD and CUD patients, the activity in the ventral medial prefrontal cortex (vmPFC) changed in terms of activity after 5 consecutive daily sessions of tDCS treatment (2 mA, cathodal left and anodal right DLPFC) [51]. In an additional study, the same group described an increased connection between the vmPFC and the nucleus accumbens (NAcc) always during some cocaine cues. The authors concluded that these results may explain the efficacy of tDCS in CUD [52].

For what concerns the treatment of another stimulant drug such as methamphetamine (METH), Shahbabaie et al. [53] investigated, in 32 abstinent male METH abusers, the efficacy of 20-minute right DLPFC anodal tDCS (2 mA) in a sham-controlled trial. During the stimulation, subjects were exposed to METH cues. Results demonstrated a significant reduction of craving in active tDCS versus sham condition and increased craving levels during METH-related cue exposure in the active tDCS group [53].

19.2.4 tDCS in Opiate-Use Disorder

The application of tDCS for the treatment of Opiate-Use Disorder is still in its infancy.

Wang et al. [54] in a sham-controlled study in heroin-addicted subjects treated with a single stimulation at 1-mA tDCS over the frontal-parietal-temporal (FPT) area reported positive findings, emphasizing a possible role of FPT in the 'circuits of the addiction' and a possible role of tDCS at this level [54].

Differently, Sharifi-Fardshad et al. [55] used the classical paradigm of right cathodal/left anodal and right anodal/left cathodal tDCS over DLPFC. In a sample of 40 opiate addicts divided into two groups of active stimulation (2 mA/20 minutes) and 1 sham, they showed a significant craving reduction in the anodal stimulation of DLPFC in line with the scientific evidence for other addictions [55].

19.2.5 tDCS in Other Substance-Use Disorders

In cannabis-use disorders, Boggio et al. [56] tested 25 patients divided into three groups: left anodal/right cathodal tDCS of the DLPFC ($n = 8$), right anodal/left cathodal tDCS of the DLPFC ($n = 9$), or sham stimulation ($n = 8$). The paradigm of stimulation was set at 1 mA for 10 min in a single stimulation session. In this study, right anodal/left cathodal tDCS of DLPFC was significantly associated with a diminished craving for marijuana. These preliminary results, although promising, need to be replicated.

19.2.5.1 tDCS in Gambling Disorder

Recently, tDCS has also been evaluated for the treatment of behavioural addictions, particularly gambling disorder (GD).

Considering the 'anodal right DLPFC/cathodal left DLPFC' configuration, Soyata et al. [57] in an RCT with 20 GD patients showed that 20 sessions with 20-minute stimulation (2 mA of intensity) drastically improved Iowa Gambling Task (IGT) and Wisconsin Card Sorting Test (WCST) scores in the whole sample. Using magnetic resonance spectroscopy (MRS), Dickler et al. [58] demonstrated that anodic stimulation of the right DLPFC in 16 subjects affected by GD increased right prefrontal GABA metabolite signal levels. Moreover, positive correlations between right prefrontal GABA level and impulsivity, risk-taking behaviour and gambling craving in the active tDCS session were also found and may explain some of the effects of tDCS in GD [58]. A recent study by Martinotti et al. [59] used the same 'Anodal right DLPFC/Cathodal left DLPFC' configuration and was consistent with what previously observed. With an amperage of 1.5 mA/20 minutes for 5 consecutive days and with a weekly follow-up of 3 months in a small sample of gamblers, the authors showed a long-lasting effect of tDCS [59]. Four articles on healthy controls [60–63] compared the previous electrode setting with a configuration 'Anodal right DLPFC/Cathodal left DLPFC'. Minati and colleagues, in a sham-controlled study, with a set-up of 2 mA displayed during the performance of Games-Howell test, found significant results only in the 'anodal right sample' [60]. Boggio and colleagues, using 2 mA/15 minutes only one session [56], and Ye and colleagues, evaluating weighted risk aversion using 2 mA/18 minutes per one single session [64], found a significant improvement of symptoms and risk performance with 'Anodal right DLPFC/Cathodal left DLPFC' compared with 'Cathodal Right DLPFC/Anodal Left DLPFC'. Fecteau et al. compared these two configurations and the monolateral anodal stimulation of right DLPFC or left DLPFC (the cathode was placed over the contralateral supraorbital area) in a sham-controlled randomized study applying a single session using 2 mA during the performance of Balloon Analogue Risk Task (BART). There were no differences between the two bilateral configurations, but both were better than sham and unilateral placement [62]. Another approach consists of the consecutive stimulation: first stimulation anodal left DLPFC/cathodal right DLPFC, second stimulation anodal right DLPFC/cathodal left DLFPC. Martinotti et al., in a case report, used this procedure setting at 1.5 mA for 20 minutes during 2 weeks of active stimulation and 24 weeks of follow-up and showed an improvement in an urge to gamble as well as in depression, anxiety and impulsivity symptoms [65]. Besides, the monocephalic right DLPFC anodal stimulation has also shown positive results. Ye et al. [63] studied in healthy volunteers five different monocephalic tDCS protocols on a risk preference task: right anodal, right cathodal, left anodal, left cathodal and sham stimulation always on DLPFC during a single session at 2 mA/18 minutes. Only the anodal right DLPFC stimulation showed an improvement in decision making, in particular, patients chose more often safe option [63].

But DLPFC is not the only target identified for tDCS stimulation in the treatment of GD. Van't Wout et al. [66] used, in healthy volunteers, an 'Anodal PO8/cathodal Fp1' configuration and tried to explain the 'emotional' response obtained after a 20-minute single session of stimulation at 2 mA intensity. The research group revealed a significantly less intense 'emotive response' at the Gambling Task after the tDCS stimulation. Ouellet et al. stimulated the OFC in healthy volunteers with three methodologies: anodal left/cathodal right, anodal right/cathodal left, or sham stimulation for a single session in a random order. Active stimulation duration was 30 minutes at 1.5-mA intensity. Electrodes were placed at Fp1 and Fp2 sites, over to the frontal poles, which include the OFC. In this study, respect to sham stimulation, active tDCS, regardless of left anodal or right anodal stimulation, showed a significantly greater increase in performances at computerized neurocognitive tasks, measuring the decision making (IGT) and the impulse control (Stroop Colour-Word Test, SCWT) [67].

19.2.5.2   HD-tDCS in Gambling Disorder

High-definition-tDCS (HD-tDCS) is a neuromodulation method, which, using the same technical and rational principle as tDCS, also reaches deeper areas of the brain in reason of a specific focal stimulation obtained with multichannel electrical stimulations through smaller electrodes placed in an EEG helmet, rather than larger electrodes used in conventional tDCS montage. This configuration guarantees a greater precision in stimulation, allowing a more correct identification of the current flow between electrodes. Using this paradigm, He et al. [68] showed that 'Anodal right/ Cathodal left' stimulation had some benefit into the IGT performance and not the 'Anodal left/Cathodal right' configuration. All the experiments were conducted for one session and 1.5 mA/20 minutes [68]. HD-tDCS is also useful for 'monolateral' protocols. Guo et al., in a single blind, randomized controlled trial SB-RCT, used two protocols: anodal left and cathodal left both at 1.5 mA/20 minutes for a single session evaluating the performance of BART test. The same group found that focalized unilateral cathodal HD-tDCS on L-DLPFC could improve risk decision making [69]. Moving away from a canonical one-sided or two-sided setting, Wang et al. used HD-tDCS placing nine electrodes in a complex configuration, mainly in accordance with the international EEG system. In the first protocol, the seven anodes were placed over Cz, Ex10, C2, FT10, Ex5, FC2 and FCz and the two cathodes over Fpz and Afz; in the second, the seven anodes were placed over Fz, TP7, O2, P8, FC6, FC5 and O9 and the two cathodes over Pz and CPz. In this way, they used an anodal stimulation activating the rostral anterior cingulate cortex/ventral medial prefrontal cortex (rACC/vmPFC) and the posterior cingulate cortex (PCC). In one single session at the intensity of 2 mA, they showed that electric brain stimulation over these regions lowered the performance in the IGT (Ying [70]).

19.2.6 tDCS in Food Addiction

Obesity is still one of the major public health concerns and there is a growing need for new treatment options. tDCS is a neuromodulation technique that has been shown to reduce food craving and consumption, particularly when used on the DLPFC with the anode on the right and the cathode on the left hemisphere.

In a study in healthy subjects, active stimulation session tDCS (2 mA for 20 minutes) was applied under three different conditions: (1) anodal/left and cathodal/right on DLPFC, (2) cathodal/right and anodal/left on DLPFC and (3) placebo. A reduction in food craving was observed, comparing DLPFC right anodal/left cathodal stimulation with other groups and a lower caloric intake in both active groups compared to placebo [71]. Another study applied one tDCS session (2 mA for 20 minutes with anode on right DLPFC) in healthy subjects finding a significant reduction of craving [72]. In a recent study, 18 (10 women and 8 men) adults with obesity completed the Dutch eating behaviour questionnaire-restraint and the Barratt Impulsiveness Scale, and received 20 minutes of tDCS active (2 mA) and a tDCS sham session [73]. The craving and food consumption were evaluated in both sessions using a test with a photo of the desired food and a test that considers the total kilocalories, preferred and less preferred, present in three very tasty foods. No significant effect of tDCS was found with respect to controls, but significant differences were found in favour of the active stimulation analysing particular sub-populations: women with a lower level of impulsivity; men planning to decrease the calorie intake; men with a higher level of impulsivity. This is the first study reporting significant reductions in craving and food consumption in a sample of obese patients using the most popular tDCS assembly in appetite studies. The results also highlight the cognitive heterogeneity of individuals with obesity and the importance of considering these differences in the assessment of the efficacy of DLPFC-targeted tDCS in future obesity-related studies. These data need to be confirmed in larger trials.

19.3   Safety of tDCS in SUDs

Serious side effects have rarely been observed with tDCS [74]. Nitsche [75] performed tDCS on approximately 500 healthy subjects between 2000 and 2003. No serious side effects such as seizures or psychiatric symptoms occurred, but only a slight tingling sensation at the electrode during the first seconds of stimulation, or the perception of a brief flash of light if the pulse was suddenly triggered or interrupted [18, 20]. One of the most common side effects is the presence of erythema below the skin surface touched by the electrodes [76]. In some rare cases, this lesion could evolve in a persistent skin lesion similar to burns, and contact dermatitis appeared after stimulation, even in healthy subjects. This lesion seems to be linked with the dose of a single tDCS session, which is defined by the electrode montage [77]. The tDCS seems to be safe from the cutaneous point of view also in patients with impaired skin [78]. It has also been shown that patients with uni/bipolar depression may develop post-treatment mania or hypomania: causal relationships between tDCS and psychological changes, however, remain uncertain and are currently being studied [79]. Although a few cases of seizure have been reported, the causal reaction is unclear. In fact, Liebetanz et al. [80] demonstrated that anodal tDCS did not reduce the epileptogenic threshold in a dedicated study in rats. In the same study, the cathodal stimulation generated a long-lasting increase of epileptogenic threshold, suggesting cathodal tDCS as a possible tool to treat drug-refractory partial epilepsy [80]. The same group, in 2009, established that a stimulus of 52 mA is required to produce brain lesions with tDCS, 400 C/m², much higher than the density of electric charge to which a human is exposed during stimulation (e.g. 343–960 C/m² in standard protocols: 1–2 mA 20 minutes, with surface electrodes between 25 and 35 cm², coated with sponges soaked in saline solution) [81]. In humans, tDCS has shown a very good level of safety in the field of epilepsy [82, 83]. Other common side effects are temporary headache and dizziness, in most of the cases not very intense [84]. In addition, several studies support the safety of tDCS by monitoring parameters such as neuron-specific enolase (NSE: neuronal damage marker), with the evaluation with MRI (M A [85]), electroencephalography (EEG) and neuropsychological tests [86].

A relevant point is represented by the development of epileptic seizures during stimulation in subjects with addiction. The use of many excitatory substances (such as cocaine and methamphetamine) as well as alcohol withdrawal seem to determine a lower epileptogenic threshold [87]. To avoid the risk of epileptic seizure in these populations, it is very important to ensure an accurate evaluation of patients' status in terms of intoxication and/or withdrawal. Although there is no report of epileptic seizures in these patients in association with the use of tDCS, a conservative approach needs to be proposed, avoiding the stimulation procedures in these specific conditions.

19.4 Current Limitations and Future Perspectives

Although in the last decade there has been increasing interest in investigating the efficacy of tDCS for the treatment of addictive disorders, there are still a number of technical challenges and limitations.

First, the configuration of the device limits focality: the large sponge electrodes commonly used (25 and 35 cm²) do not allow to precisely target a brain area or node. One practical aspect of this problem is that the common process to apply electrodes is the international 10–20 EEG system, but future work will benefit from the use of subject-specific computational models based on anatomical MRI and neuronavigation processes for targeting tDCS. Another technical aspect, well considered in rTMS protocols, is the possibility to record the brain activity during the simulation using EEG [1].

In terms of efficacy in addiction, different protocols have been proposed. A meta-analysis [88] assessed the effects of 17 studies revealing a significant medium effect size (Hedge's $g = 0.476$) favouring non-invasive DLPFC neurostimulation over sham stimulation in the reduction of substance or food craving with no significant differences between rTMS and tDCS or between left and right DLPFC stimulation. The cumulative effect of repetitive sessions of tDCS should also be taken into account. This is because, as reported for the treatment of depression [89] and also in SUDs, it has been noted that the improvement is gradual and probably dependent on the number of stimulations over time.

Concerning the issue of choosing and selecting subjects to be studied, the need to recruit 'real patients' is quite evident, as the majority of patients with SUD have a polyabuse of substances (the presence of addiction to a single drug is rather rare) and, for the same reason, there is growing interest in subjects with psychiatric comorbidity (7.9 million individuals in 2015 had co-occurring SUDs and mental illness in the U.S.) [90]. One of the aspects that well describe how the presence of comorbidity is useful in the design of these protocols is that, for example, nicotine use has been associated with a reduction in the clinical efficacy of tDCS treatment in schizophrenic subjects [91]. Moreover, studies able to understand the potential benefits of concurrent therapies (pharmacological, behavioural) used in combination with brain stimulation may increase a participant's chances of becoming abstinent [90]. Another aspect of the sample selection is the distinction and selection of ethnic strain. As the genetic differences between populations could influence different enzymes or the development of different pathologies, there is a growing need to create protocols of NIBS taking into account the differences between ethnic groups [92].

Moreover, pre-registration of study protocols with primary and secondary outcomes is encouraged to promote transparency. Shared protocols will enable higher methodological standards and reproducibility. Protocols should ideally contain (1) a detailed description of materials and equipment, (2) step-by-step administration instructions with accompanying video examples, where appropriate, (3) information on troubleshooting strategies, and (4) guides for data processing, analysis and interpretation. These protocols could then be used to establish multicentre trials. Finally, the use of an online data and registration platform will facilitate comparative and integrative analysis. The establishment of shared research questions, protocols and data repository does not come without its challenges. Both within and across cultures, there exist different norms and ideas about what constitutes a clinically significant change. For instance, not all the cultures emphasize 'abstinence only' as a goal in addiction treatment, necessitating the ongoing awareness and open discussion of these types of assumptions. Further, a risk in prioritizing well-established procedures and findings is the reduction in acknowledgment of innovative approaches and newly formed theories [29].

All this is reflected, therefore, in the need for well-controlled trials evaluating tDCS efficacy, given the broad scope for heterogeneity in results, as a consequence of task dependence [93] and variations in current density, resulting from interindividual anatomical differences [23, 24] and intraindividual state differences [94].

In conclusion, the current limitations and future perspectives in the field of tDCS should take better account of: (1) the increasing need for online pre-recorded clinical trials and protocol sharing via interconnected platforms [29]; (2) a good selection of the population of the study (taking into account ethnic differences, comorbidities, current therapies and the selection of a 'real patient') [90]; (3) a need of double-blind randomized clinical trials (DB-RCTs) with a long period of follow-up; (4) EEG and/or MEG techniques to determine specific brain oscillations; (5) brain imaging, for observing long-term structural and functional effects of tDCS on addictive patients; (6) tDCS dose, electrode montage and placement with optimal current density [9].

19.5   Conclusions

The interest of the clinical and scientific world around the tDCS, in recent years, is consistently growing. Although it has already been demonstrated that tDCS might be a promising therapeutic tool for a large number of psychiatric disorders [95], it is still premature to conclude that tDCS is an efficient technique in reducing substance abuse craving. However, a recent review reported that tDCS stimulation was effective in craving reduction in 8 of 16 clinical trials over DLPFC and in 1 of 2 clinical trials over FPT [28], showing some level of evidence and, certainly, high potentiality. As regards to the region of stimulation, even if previous studies indicated the left DLPFC as the 'golden target' for tDCS therapy in the treating of SUDs [96], the positive results on craving were substantially equivalent both with 'anodal right DLPFC/cathodal left DLPFC' than with 'anodal LDLPFC/cathodal RDLPFC' [28]. An interesting fact concerns the safety of this neuromodulation technique: no major side effects have been reported (in most cases only mild erythema or itching sensation under the electrodes) [97] with low risk of developing epileptic seizures, always related to individual predisposition or concurrent abstinence from benzodiazepines or alcohol [87, 98].

Other areas of development could involve the evaluation of comorbid psychiatric symptoms, with specific attention on the dimension of anhedonia, frequently impaired in addicted subjects [99]. Moreover, the effect of tDCS in other new types of addictions could be explored, given the rise of novel psychoactive substances in the addiction scenario [100, 101], as well as its use in combination with pharmacotherapies able to enhance its effects, such as the increase of the intracellular concentration of Calcium [102] and the modulation of the excitability of glutamatergic synaptic receptors in pyramidal neurons and the inhibition of the release of GABA [103].

Strong limitations concerning the study design, the small sample size, the high level of heterogeneity of protocols, the lack of studies with long follow-up periods highlight the need for further studies.

Through larger, sham-controlled studies with more uniform reporting standards in tDCS research, we will be better prepared to deliver something meaningful to our patients. Finally, we acknowledge that SUD is a very complex disease that probably cannot be approached by a single methodology, like a brain stimulation intervention. By performing rigorous studies with tDCS, however, we will be able to confidently approach the next frontier of experimental medicine in SUD—combining targeted brain stimulation with pharmacotherapy and behavioural management in order to optimize treatment efficacy for different patients [29].

Conflict of Interest None

References

1. Bashir S, Yoo W-K. Neuromodulation for addiction by transcranial direct current stimulation: opportunities and challenges. Ann Neurosci. 2016;23(4):241–5. https://doi.org/10.1159/000449485.
2. O'Brien CP. Review. Evidence-based treatments of addiction. Philosophical Transactions of the Royal Society of London. Series B. Bio Sci. 2008;363(1507):3277–86. https://doi.org/10.1098/rstb.2008.0105.
3. Chiamulera C, Padovani L, Corsi M. Drug discovery for the treatment of substance use disorders: novel targets, repurposing, and the need for new paradigms. Current Opinion in Pharmacol. 2017;35:120–4. https://doi.org/10.1016/j.coph.2017.08.009.
4. Achab S, Khazaal Y. Psychopharmacological treatment in pathological gambling: a critical review. Current Pharmaceutical Design. 2011;17(14):1389–95. https://doi.org/10.2174/138161211796150774.
5. Muller CP, Schumann, G. Drugs as instruments: a new framework for non-addictive psychoactive drug use. Behav Brain Sci. 2011;34(6): 293–310. https://doi.org/10.1017/S0140525X11000057.
6. Bolt DM, Piper ME, Theobald WE, Baker TB. Why two smoking cessation agents work better than one: role of craving suppression. J Cons Clini Psychol. 2012;80(1):54–65. https://doi.org/10.1037/a0026366.
7. Mariani JJ, Levin FR. Psychostimulant treatment of cocaine dependence. Psych Clin North Am. 2012;35(2);425–39. https://doi.org/10.1016/j.psc.2012.03.012.
8. Koob GF, Volkow ND. Neurobiology of addiction: a neurocircuitry analysis. The Lancet. Psychiatry. 2016;3(8):760–73. https://doi.org/10.1016/S2215-0366(16)00104-8.
9. Lapenta OM, Marques LM, Rego GG, Comfort WE, Boggio PS. tDCS in addiction and impulse control disorders. J ECT. 2018;34(3):182–92. https://doi.org/10.1097/YCT.0000000000000541.
10. Lipton DM, Gonzales BJ, Citri A. Dorsal striatal circuits for habits, compulsions and addictions. Front Syst Neurosci. 2019;13:28. https://doi.org/10.3389/fnsys.2019.00028.
11. Jasinska AJ, Stein EA, Kaiser J, Naumer MJ, Yalachkov Y. Factors modulating neural reactivity to drug cues in addiction: a survey of human neuroimaging studies. Neurosci Biobehav Rev. 2014;38:1–16. https://doi.org/10.1016/j.neubiorev.2013.10.013.
12. Olbrich HM, Valerius G, Paris C, Hagenbuch F, Ebert D, Juengling FD. Brain activation during craving for alcohol measured by positron emission tomography. Aust N Z J Psychiatry. 2006;40(2):171–8. https://doi.org/10.1080/j.1440-1614.2006.01765.x.
13. Bonson KR, Grant SJ, Contoreggi CS, Links JM, Metcalfe J, Weyl HL, et al. Neural systems and cue-induced cocaine craving. Neuropsychopharmacology. 2002;26(3):376–86. https://doi.org/10.1016/S0893-133X(01)00371-2.
14. Wang Z, Faith M, Patterson F, Tang K, Kerrin K, Wileyto EP, et al. Neural substrates of abstinence-induced cigarette cravings in chronic smokers. J Neurosci. 2007;27(51):14035–40. https://doi.org/10.1523/JNEUROSCI.2966-07.2007.
15. Zijlstra F, Booij J, van den Brink W, Franken IHA. Striatal dopamine D2 receptor binding and dopamine release during cue-elicited craving in recently abstinent opiate-dependent males. Eur Neuropsychopharmacol. 2008;18(4):262–70. https://doi.org/10.1016/j.euroneuro.2007.11.002.
16. McBride D, Barrett SP, Kelly JT, Aw A, Dagher A. Effects of expectancy and abstinence on the neural response to smoking cues in cigarette smokers: an fMRI study. Neuropsychopharmacology. 2006;31(12):2728–38. https://doi.org/10.1038/sj.npp.1301075.
17. Dezfouli A, Piray P, Keramati MM, Ekhtiari H, Lucas C, Mokri A. A neurocomputational model for cocaine addiction. Neural Comput. 2009;21(10):2869–93. https://doi.org/10.1162/neco.2009.10-08-882.

18. Nitsche MA, Fricke K, Henschke U, Schlitterlau A, Liebetanz D, Lang N, et al. Pharmacological modulation of cortical excitability shifts induced by transcranial direct current stimulation in humans. J Physiol. 2003;553(Pt 1):293–301. https://doi.org/10.1113/jphysiol.2003.049916.
19. Nitsche MA, Paulus W. Excitability changes induced in the human motor cortex by weak transcranial direct current stimulation. J Physiol. 2000;527(Pt 3):633–9. https://doi.org/10.1111/j.1469-7793.2000.t01-1-00633.x.
20. Nitsche MA, Liebetanz D, Lang N, Antal A, Tergau F, Paulus W. Safety criteria for transcranial direct current stimulation (tDCS) in humans. Clin Neurophysiol. 2003;114(11):2220–2.
21. Priori A. Brain polarization in humans: a reappraisal of an old tool for prolonged non-invasive modulation of brain excitability. Clin Neurophysiol. 2003;114(4):589–95.
22. Roche N, Geiger M, Bussel B. Mechanisms underlying transcranial direct current stimulation in rehabilitation. Ann Phys Rehabil Med. 2015;58(4):214–9. https://doi.org/10.1016/j.rehab.2015.04.009.
23. Kim J-H, Kim D-W, Chang WH, Kim Y-H, Kim K, Im C-H. Inconsistent outcomes of transcranial direct current stimulation may originate from anatomical differences among individuals: electric field simulation using individual MRI data. Neurosci Lett. 2014;564:6–10. https://doi.org/10.1016/j.neulet.2014.01.054.
24. Kim YJ, Ku J, Cho S, Kim HJ, Cho YK, Lim T, Kang YJ. Facilitation of corticospinal excitability by virtual reality exercise following anodal transcranial direct current stimulation in healthy volunteers and subacute stroke subjects. J Neuroeng Rehabil. 2014;11:124. https://doi.org/10.1186/1743-0003-11-124.
25. Stagg CJ, Best JG, Stephenson MC, O'Shea J, Wylezinska M, Kincses ZT, et al. Polarity-sensitive modulation of cortical neurotransmitters by transcranial stimulation. J Neurosci. 2009;29(16):5202–6. https://doi.org/10.1523/JNEUROSCI.4432-08.2009.
26. Stagg CJ, Nitsche MA. Physiological basis of transcranial direct current stimulation. Neuroscientist. 2011;17(1):37–53. https://doi.org/10.1177/1073858410386614.
27. Zhao H, Qiao L, Fan D, Zhang S, Turel O, Li Y, et al. Modulation of brain activity with noninvasive Transcranial Direct Current Stimulation (tDCS): clinical applications and safety concerns. Front Psychol. 2017;8:685. https://doi.org/10.3389/fpsyg.2017.00685.
28. Lupi M, Martinotti G, Santacroce R, Cinosi E, Carlucci M, Marini S, et al. Transcranial direct current stimulation in substance use disorders: a systematic review of scientific literature. J ECT. 2017;33(3):203–9. https://doi.org/10.1097/YCT.0000000000000401.
29. Ekhtiari H, Tavakoli H, Addolorato G, Baeken C, Bonci A, Campanella S, et al. Transcranial electrical and magnetic stimulation (tES and TMS) for addiction medicine: a consensus paper on the present state of the science and the road ahead. Neurosci Biobehav Rev. 2019;104:118–40. https://doi.org/10.1016/j.neubiorev.2019.06.007.
30. Cheslack-Postava K, Wall MM, Weinberger AH, Goodwin RD. Increasing depression and substance use among former smokers in the United States, 2002-2016. Am J Prev Med. 2019;57(4):429–37. https://doi.org/10.1016/j.amepre.2019.05.014.
31. Fregni F, Liguori P, Fecteau S, Nitsche MA, Pascual-Leone A, Boggio PS. Cortical stimulation of the prefrontal cortex with transcranial direct current stimulation reduces cue-provoked smoking craving: a randomized, sham-controlled study. J Clin Psychiatry. 2008;69(1):32–40.
32. Boggio PS, Liguori P, Sultani N, Rezende L, Fecteau S, Fregni F. Cumulative priming effects of cortical stimulation on smoking cue-induced craving. Neurosci Lett. 2009;463(1):82–6. https://doi.org/10.1016/j.neulet.2009.07.041.
33. Xu J, Fregni F, Brody AL, Rahman AS. Transcranial direct current stimulation reduces negative affect but not cigarette craving in overnight abstinent smokers. Front Psych. 2013;4:112. https://doi.org/10.3389/fpsyt.2013.00112.
34. Falcone M, Bernardo L, Ashare RL, Hamilton R, Faseyitan O, McKee SA, et al. Transcranial direct current brain stimulation increases ability to resist smoking. Brain Stimul. 2016;9(2):191–6. https://doi.org/10.1016/j.brs.2015.10.004.
35. Ghorbani Behnam S, Mousavi SA, Emamian MH. The effects of transcranial direct current stimulation compared to standard bupropion for the treatment of tobacco dependence:

a randomized sham-controlled trial. Eur Psychiatr. 2019;60:41–8. https://doi.org/10.1016/j.eurpsy.2019.04.010.

36. Yang L-Z, Shi B, Li H, Zhang W, Liu Y, Wang H, et al. Electrical stimulation reduces smokers' craving by modulating the coupling between dorsal lateral prefrontal cortex and parahippocampal gyrus. Soc Cogn Affect Neurosci. 2017;12(8):1296–302. https://doi.org/10.1093/scan/nsx055.

37. Fecteau S, Agosta S, Hone-Blanchet A, Fregni F, Boggio P, Ciraulo D, Pascual-Leone A. Modulation of smoking and decision-making behaviors with transcranial direct current stimulation in tobacco smokers: a preliminary study. Drug Alcohol Depend. 2014;140:78–84. https://doi.org/10.1016/j.drugalcdep.2014.03.036.

38. Boggio PS, Sultani N, Fecteau S, Merabet L, Mecca T, Pascual-Leone A, et al. Prefrontal cortex modulation using transcranial DC stimulation reduces alcohol craving: a double-blind, sham-controlled study. Drug Alcohol Depend. 2008;92(1–3):55–60. https://doi.org/10.1016/j.drugalcdep.2007.06.011.

39. da Silva MC, Conti CL, Klauss J, Alves LG, do Nascimento Cavalcante HM, et al. Behavioral effects of transcranial direct current stimulation (tDCS) induced dorsolateral prefrontal cortex plasticity in alcohol dependence. J Physiol Paris. 2013;107(6):493–502. https://doi.org/10.1016/j.jphysparis.2013.07.003.

40. Klauss J, Penido Pinheiro LC, Silva Merlo BL, de Almeida Correia Santos G, Fregni F, Nitsche MA, Miyuki Nakamura-Palacios E. A randomized controlled trial of targeted prefrontal cortex modulation with tDCS in patients with alcohol dependence. Int J Neuropsychopharmacol. 2014;17(11):1793–803. https://doi.org/10.1017/S1461145714000984.

41. Klauss J, Anders QS, Felippe LV, Ferreira LVB, Cruz MA, Nitsche MA, Nakamura-Palacios EM. Lack of effects of extended sessions of Transcranial Direct Current Stimulation (tDCS) over dorsolateral prefrontal cortex on craving and relapses in crack-cocaine users. Front Pharmacol. 2018;9:1198. https://doi.org/10.3389/fphar.2018.01198.

42. Klauss J, Anders QS, Felippe LV, Nitsche MA. Multiple sessions of Transcranial Direct Current Stimulation (tDCS) reduced craving and relapses for alcohol use : a randomized placebo-controlled trial in alcohol use disorder. Front Pharmacol. 2018;9:716. https://doi.org/10.3389/fphar.2018.00716.

43. Wietschorke K, Lippold J, Jacob C, Polak T, Herrmann MJ. Transcranial direct current stimulation of the prefrontal cortex reduces cue-reactivity in alcohol-dependent patients. J Neural Transm. 2016;123(10):1173–8. https://doi.org/10.1007/s00702-016-1541-6.

44. Hallion LS, Ruscio AM. A meta-analysis of the effect of cognitive bias modification on anxiety and depression. Psychol Bull. 2011;137(6):940–58. https://doi.org/10.1037/a0024355.

45. den Uyl TE, Gladwin TE, Lindenmeyer J, Wiers RW. A clinical trial with combined transcranial direct current stimulation and attentional bias modification in alcohol-dependent patients. Alcohol Clin Exp Res. 2018;42(10):1961–9. https://doi.org/10.1111/acer.13841.

46. den Uyl TE, Gladwin TE, Wiers RW. Electrophysiological and behavioral effects of combined transcranial direct current stimulation and alcohol approach bias retraining in hazardous drinkers. Alcohol Clin Exp Res. 2016;40(10):2124–33. https://doi.org/10.1111/acer.13171.

47. Gorini A, Lucchiari C, Russell-Edu W, Pravettoni G. Modulation of risky choices in recently abstinent dependent cocaine users: a transcranial direct-current stimulation study. Front Hum Neurosci. 2014;8:661. https://doi.org/10.3389/fnhum.2014.00661.

48. Batista EK, Klauss J, Fregni F, Nitsche MA, Nakamura-Palacios EM. A randomized placebo-controlled trial of targeted prefrontal cortex modulation with bilateral tDCS in patients with crack-cocaine dependence. Int J Neuropsychopharmacol. 2015;18(12) https://doi.org/10.1093/ijnp/pyv066.

49. Goldstein RZ, Volkow ND. Dysfunction of the prefrontal cortex in addiction: neuroimaging findings and clinical implications. Nat Rev Neurosci. 2011;12(11):652–69. https://doi.org/10.1038/nrn3119.

50. Conti CL, Nakamura-Palacios EM. Bilateral transcranial direct current stimulation over dorsolateral prefrontal cortex changes the drug-cued reactivity in the anterior cingulate

cortex of crack-cocaine addicts. Brain Stimul. 2014;7(1):130–2. https://doi.org/10.1016/j.brs.2013.09.007.

51. Conti CL, Moscon JA, Fregni F, Nitsche MA, Nakamura-Palacios EM. Cognitive related electrophysiological changes induced by non-invasive cortical electrical stimulation in crack-cocaine addiction. Int J Neuropsychopharmacol. 2014;17(9):1465–75. https://doi.org/10.1017/S1461145714000522.

52. Nakamura-Palacios EM, Lopes IBC, Souza RA, Klauss J, Batista EK, Conti CL, et al. Ventral medial prefrontal cortex (vmPFC) as a target of the dorsolateral prefrontal modulation by transcranial direct current stimulation (tDCS) in drug addiction. J Neural Transm. 2016;123(10):1179–94. https://doi.org/10.1007/s00702-016-1559-9.

53. Shahbabaie A, Golesorkhi M, Zamanian B, Ebrahimpoor M, Keshvari F, Nejati V, et al. State dependent effect of transcranial direct current stimulation (tDCS) on methamphetamine craving. Int J Neuropsychopharmacol. 2014;17(10):1591–8. https://doi.org/10.1017/S1461145714000686.

54. Wang Y, Shen Y, Cao X, Shan C, Pan J, He H, et al. Transcranial direct current stimulation of the frontal-parietal-temporal area attenuates cue-induced craving for heroin. J Psychiatr Res. 2016;79:1–3. https://doi.org/10.1016/j.jpsychires.2016.04.001.

55. Sharifi-Fardshad M, Mehraban-Eshtehardi M, Shams-Esfandabad H, Shariatirad S, Molavi N, Hassani-Abharian P. Modulation of drug craving in crystalline-heroin users by transcranial direct current stimulation of dorsolateral prefrontal cortex. Addict Health. 2018;10(3):173–9. https://doi.org/10.22122/ahj.v10i3.613.

56. Boggio PS, Campanha C, Valasek CA, Fecteau S, Pascual-Leone A, Fregni F. Modulation of decision-making in a gambling task in older adults with transcranial direct current stimulation. Eur J Neurosci. 2010;31(3):593–7. https://doi.org/10.1111/j.1460-9568.2010.07080.x.

57. Soyata AZ, Aksu S, Woods AJ, İşçen P, Saçar KT, Karamürscl S. Effect of transcranial direct current stimulation on decision making and cognitive flexibility in gambling disorder. Eur Arch Psychiatry Clin Neurosci. 2019;269(3):275–84.

58. Dickler M, Lenglos C, Renauld E, Ferland F, Edden RA, Leblond J, Fecteau S. Online effects of transcranial direct current stimulation on prefrontal metabolites in gambling disorder. Neuropharmacology. 2018;131:51–7. https://doi.org/10.1016/j.neuropharm.2017.12.002.

59. Martinotti G, Lupi M, Montemitro C, Miuli A, Di Natale C, Spano MC, et al. Transcranial direct current stimulation reduces craving in substance use disorders. J ECT. 2019;35(3):207–11. https://doi.org/10.1097/YCT.0000000000000580.

60. Minati I, Campanha C, Critchley HD, Boggio PS. Effects of transcranial direct-current stimulation (tDCS) of the dorsolateral prefrontal cortex (DLPFC) during a mixed-gambling risky decision-making task. Cogn Neurosci. 2012;3(2):80–8. https://doi.org/10.1080/17588928.2011.628382.

61. Boggio PS, Zaghi S, Villani AB, Fecteau S, Pascual-Leone A, Fregni F. Modulation of risk-taking in marijuana users by transcranial direct current stimulation (tDCS) of the dorsolateral prefrontal cortex (DLPFC). Drug Alco Depend. 2010;112(3):220–5. https://doi.org/10.1016/j.drugalcdep.2010.06.019.

62. Fecteau S, Pascual-Leone A, Zald DH, Liguori P, Theoret H, Boggio PS, Fregni F. Activation of prefrontal cortex by transcranial direct current stimulation reduces appetite for risk during ambiguous decision making. J Neurosci: The Official Journal of the Society for Neuroscience. 2007;27(23):6212–18. https://doi.org/10.1523/JNEUROSCI.0314-07.2007.

63. Ye H, Huang D, Wang S, Zheng H, Luo J, Chen S. Activation of the prefrontal cortex by unilateral transcranial direct current stimulation leads to an asymmetrical effect on risk preference in frames of gain and loss. Brain Res. 2016;1648(Pt A):325–32. https://doi.org/10.1016/j.brainres.2016.08.007.

64. Ye H, Chen S, Huang D, Wang S, Luo J. Modulating activity in the prefrontal cortex changes decision-making for risky gains and losses: a transcranial direct current stimulation study. Behav Brain Res. 2015;286:17–21. https://doi.org/10.1016/j.bbr.2015.02.037.

65. Martinotti G, Chillemi E, Lupi M, De Risio L, Pettorruso M, Giannantonio MD. Gambling disorder and bilateral transcranial direct current stimulation: a case report. J Behav Addict. 2018;7(3):834–7. https://doi.org/10.1556/2006.7.2018.85.

66. van't Wout M, Silverman H. Modulating what is and what could have been: The effect of transcranial direct current stimulation on the evaluation of attained and unattained decision outcomes. Cogn Aff Behav Neurosci. 2017;17(6):1176–85. https://doi.org/10.3758/s13415-017-0541-9.

67. Ouellet J, McGirr A, Van den Eynde F, Jollant F, Lepage M, Berlim MT. Enhancing decision-making and cognitive impulse control with transcranial direct current stimulation (tDCS) applied over the orbitofrontal cortex (OFC): a randomized and sham-controlled exploratory study. J Psychiatr Res. 2015;69:27–34. https://doi.org/10.1016/j.jpsychires.2015.07.018.

68. He Q, Chen M, Chen C, Xue G, Feng T, Bechara A. Anodal stimulation of the left DLPFC increases IGT scores and decreases delay discounting rate in healthy males. Front Psychol. 2016;7:1421. https://doi.org/10.3389/fpsyg.2016.01421.

69. Guo H, Zhang Z, Da S, Sheng X, Zhang X. High-definition transcranial direct current stimulation (HD-tDCS) of left dorsolateral prefrontal cortex affects performance in Balloon Analogue Risk Task (BART). Brain Behav. 2018;8(2):e00884. https://doi.org/10.1002/brb3.884.

70. Wang Y, Ma N, He X, Li N, Wei Z, Yang L, et al. Neural substrates of updating the prediction through prediction error during decision making. Neuroimage. 2017;157:1–12. https://doi.org/10.1016/j.neuroimage.2017.05.041.

71. Fregni F, Orsati F, Pedrosa W, Fecteau S, Tome FAM, Nitsche MA, et al. Transcranial direct current stimulation of the prefrontal cortex modulates the desire for specific foods. Appetite. 2008;51(1):34–41. https://doi.org/10.1016/j.appet.2007.09.016.

72. Goldman RL, Borckardt JJ, Frohman HA, O'Neil PM, Madan A, Campbell LK, et al. Prefrontal cortex transcranial direct current stimulation (tDCS) temporarily reduces food cravings and increases the self-reported ability to resist food in adults with frequent food craving. Appetite. 2011;56(3):741–6. https://doi.org/10.1016/j.appet.2011.02.013.

73. Ray MK, Sylvester MD, Helton A, Pittman BR, Wagstaff LE, McRae TR, Turan B, Fontaine KR, Amthor FR, Boggiano MM. The effect of expectation on transcranial direct current stimulation (tDCS) to suppress food craving and eating in individuals with overweight and obesity. Appetite. 2019;136:1–7.

74. Bikson M, Grossman P, Thomas C, Zannou AL, Jiang J, Adnan T, et al. Safety of transcranial direct current stimulation: evidence based update 2016. Brain Stimul. 2016;9(5):641–61. https://doi.org/10.1016/j.brs.2016.06.004.

75. Nitsche MA, Fricke K, Henschke U, Schlitterlau A, Liebetanz D, Lang N, Paulus W. Pharmacological modulation of cortical excitability shifts induced by transcranial direct current stimulation in humans. J Physiol. 2003;553(Pt 1):293–301. https://doi.org/10.1113/jphysiol.2003.049916.

76. Poreisz C, Boros K, Antal A, Paulus W. Safety aspects of transcranial direct current stimulation concerning healthy subjects and patients. Brain Res Bull. 2007;72(4–6):208–14. https://doi.org/10.1016/j.brainresbull.2007.01.004.

77. Peterchev AV, Wagner TA, Miranda PC, Nitsche MA, Paulus W, Lisanby SH, et al. Fundamentals of transcranial electric and magnetic stimulation dose: definition, selection, and reporting practices. Brain Stimul. 2012;5(4):435–53. https://doi.org/10.1016/j.brs.2011.10.001.

78. Shiozawa P, da Silva ME, Raza R, Uchida RR, Cordeiro Q, Fregni F, Brunoni AR. Safety of repeated transcranial direct current stimulation in impaired skin: a case report. J ECT. 2013;29(2):147–8. https://doi.org/10.1097/YCT.0b013e318279c1a1.

79. Loo C, Katalinic N, Mitchell PB, Greenberg B. Physical treatments for bipolar disorder: a review of electroconvulsive therapy, stereotactic surgery and other brain stimulation techniques. J Affect Disord. 2011;132(1–2):1–13. https://doi.org/10.1016/j.jad.2010.08.017.

80. Liebetanz D, Klinker F, Hering D, Koch R, Nitsche MA, Potschka H, et al. Anticonvulsant effects of transcranial direct-current stimulation (tDCS) in the rat cortical ramp model of focal epilepsy. Epilepsia. 2006;47(7):1216–24. https://doi.org/10.1111/j.1528-1167.2006.00539.x.

81. Liebetanz D, Koch R, Mayenfels S, Konig F, Paulus W, Nitsche MA. Safety limits of cathodal transcranial direct current stimulation in rats. Clin Neurophysiol. 2009;120(6):1161–7. https://doi.org/10.1016/j.clinph.2009.01.022.

82. Galvez V, Ho K-A, Alonzo A, Martin D, George D, Loo CK. Neuromodulation therapies for geriatric depression. Curr Psychiatry Rep. 2015;17(7):59. https://doi.org/10.1007/s11920-015-0592-y.
83. Kirton A, Ciechanski P, Zewdie E, Andersen J, Nettel-Aguirre A, Carlson H, et al. Transcranial direct current stimulation for children with perinatal stroke and hemiparesis. Neurology. 2017;88(3):259–67. https://doi.org/10.1212/WNL.0000000000003518.
84. Khedr EM, El Gamal NF, El-Fetoh NA, Khalifa H, Ahmed EM, Ali AM, et al. A double-blind randomized clinical trial on the efficacy of cortical direct current stimulation for the treatment of Alzheimer's disease. Front Aging Neurosci. 2014;6:275. https://doi.org/10.3389/fnagi.2014.00275.
85. Nitsche MA, Niehaus L, Hoffmann KT, Hengst S, Liebetanz D, Paulus W, Meyer B-U. MRI study of human brain exposed to weak direct current stimulation of the frontal cortex. Clin Neurophysiol. 2004;115(10):2419–23. https://doi.org/10.1016/j.clinph.2004.05.001.
86. Tadini L, El-Nazer R, Brunoni AR, Williams J, Carvas M, Boggio P, et al. Cognitive, mood, and electroencephalographic effects of noninvasive cortical stimulation with weak electrical currents. J ECT. 2011;27(2):134–40. https://doi.org/10.1097/YCT.0b013e3181e631a8.
87. Leach JP, Mohanraj R, Borland W. Alcohol and drugs in epilepsy: pathophysiology, presentation, possibilities, and prevention. Epilepsia. 2012;53(Suppl 4):48–57. https://doi.org/10.1111/j.1528-1167.2012.03613.x.
88. Jansen JM, Daams JG, Koeter MWJ, Veltman DJ, van den Brink W, Goudriaan AE. Effects of non-invasive neurostimulation on craving: a meta-analysis. Neurosci Biobehav Rev. 2013;37(10 Pt 2):2472–80. https://doi.org/10.1016/j.neubiorev.2013.07.009.
89. Loo CK, Mitchell PB. A review of the efficacy of transcranial magnetic stimulation (TMS) treatment for depression, and current and future strategies to optimize efficacy. J Affect Disord. 2005;88(3):255–67. https://doi.org/10.1016/j.jad.2005.08.001.
90. Coles AS, Kozak K, George TP. A review of brain stimulation methods to treat substance use disorders. Am J Addict. 2018;27(2):71–91. https://doi.org/10.1111/ajad.12674.
91. Brunelin J, Hasan A, Haesebaert F, Nitsche MA, Poulet E. Nicotine smoking prevents the effects of frontotemporal Transcranial Direct Current Stimulation (tDCS) in hallucinating patients with schizophrenia. Brain Stimul. 2015;8(6):1225–7. https://doi.org/10.1016/j.brs.2015.08.002.
92. Yang L-Z, Yang Z, Zhang X. Non-invasive brain stimulation for the treatment of nicotine addiction: potential and challenges. Neurosci Bull. 2016;32(6):550–6. https://doi.org/10.1007/s12264-016-0056-3.
93. Hsu T-Y, Juan C-H, Tseng P. Individual differences and state-dependent responses in transcranial direct current stimulation. Front Hum Neurosci. 2016;10:643. https://doi.org/10.3389/fnhum.2016.00643.
94. Horvath JC, Vogrin SJ, Carter O, Cook MJ, Forte JD. Effects of a common transcranial direct current stimulation (tDCS) protocol on motor evoked potentials found to be highly variable within individuals over 9 testing sessions. Exp Brain Res. 2016;234(9):2629–42. https://doi.org/10.1007/s00221-016-4667-8.
95. Dubljevic V, Saigle V, Racine E. The rising tide of tDCS in the media and academic literature. Neuron. 2014;82(4):731–6. https://doi.org/10.1016/j.neuron.2014.05.003.
96. Hayashi T, Ko JH, Strafella AP, Dagher A. Dorsolateral prefrontal and orbitofrontal cortex interactions during self-control of cigarette craving. Proc Natl Acad Sci U S A. 2013;110(11):4422–7. https://doi.org/10.1073/pnas.1212185110.
97. Ekici B. Transcranial direct current stimulation-induced seizure: analysis of a case. Clin EEG Neurosci. 2015;46:169. https://doi.org/10.1177/1550059414540647.
98. Martinotti G, Di Nicola M, Romanelli R, Andreoli S, Pozzi G, Moroni N, Janiri L. High and low dosage oxcarbazepine versus naltrexone for the prevention of relapse in alcohol-dependent patients. Hum Psychopharmacol. 2007;22(3):149–56.
99. Spano MC, Lorusso M, Pettorruso M, Zoratto F, Di Giuda D, Martinotti G, di Giannantonio M. Anhedonia across borders: transdiagnostic relevance of reward dysfunction for noninvasive brain stimulation endophenotypes. CNS Neurosci Ther. 2019;25(11):1229–36.

100. Martinotti G, Lupi M, Acciavatti T, Cinosi E, Santacroce R, Signorelli MS, et al. Novel psychoactive substances in young adults with and without psychiatric comorbidities. Biomed Res Int. 2014;2014:815424. https://doi.org/10.1155/2014/815424.
101. Schifano F, Leoni M, Martinotti G, Rawaf S, Rovetto F. Importance of cyberspace for the assessment of the drug abuse market: preliminary results from the Psychonaut 2002 project. Cyberpsychol Behav. 2003;6(4):405–10.
102. Martinotti G, Di Nicola M, Tedeschi D, Mazza M, Janiri L, Bria P. Efficacy and safety of pregabalin in alcohol dependence. Adv Ther. 2008;25(6):608–18.
103. Martinotti G, Orsolini L, Fornaro M, Vecchiotti R, De Berardis D, Iasevoli F, Di Giannantonio, M. Aripiprazole for relapse prevention and craving in alcohol use disorder: current evidence and future perspectives. Exp Opi Inv Drug. 2016;25(6):719–728. https://doi.org/10.108 0/13543784.2016.1175431.

Transcranial Direct Current Stimulation in Neurodevelopmental Disorders

20

Giordano D'Urso, Elena Toscano, Gianpiero Gallo, and Andrea de Bartolomeis

20.1 Introduction

Neurodevelopmental disorders are a group of heterogeneous disorders of the Central Nervous System, emerging in the early childhood and entailing an abnormal brain function. These conditions may affect emotions, cognition, language, behavior, sensory, and motor functions. The prevalence of neurodevelopmental disorders has risen dramatically over the recent decades, especially as regards Autism Spectrum Disorder (ASD) and Attention-Deficit/Hyperactivity Disorder (ADHD). Unfortunately, the available treatments, i.e., medications, cognitive, behavioral, and rehabilitative interventions, have only limited effectiveness and their use is even controversial. Thus, considering the huge suffering of patients and their families as well as the economic burden of neurodevelopmental disorders, there is an urgent need to find and to assess efficacy, feasibility, and safety of new treatments. In this context, Non-Invasive Brain Stimulation (NIBS) techniques are attracting a growing interest, particularly for the possibility to tackle at circuits' level the pathophysiology of the different diseases. This new treatment approach is being increasingly used in clinical psychiatry—especially for treatment-resistant disorders—to such an extent that is leading to the establishment of facilities entirely dedicated to psychiatric neuromodulation [1].

In fact, in the last two decades, NIBS has yielded significant results in the treatment of adults with psychiatric disorders, allegedly through the induction of neuroplasticity. In particular, these techniques showed efficacy in adults suffering from psychiatric conditions that often emerge in childhood and adolescence, even if the full-blown manifestation occurs later in the adulthood. This is the case, for example, for obsessive–compulsive disorder (OCD) [2].

G. D'Urso (✉) · E. Toscano · G. Gallo · A. de Bartolomeis
Section of Psychiatry, Department of Neuroscience, Reproductive Sciences and Odontostomatology, University of Naples "Federico II", Naples, Italy
e-mail: giordano.durso@unina.it

© Springer Nature Switzerland AG 2020
B. Dell'Osso, G. Di Lorenzo (eds.), *Non Invasive Brain Stimulation in Psychiatry and Clinical Neurosciences*,
https://doi.org/10.1007/978-3-030-43356-7_20

Consequently, NIBS techniques have been recently proposed in pediatric populations affected by brain disorders as tools to explore and affect plasticity in a developing brain, as well as to treat the associated behavioral problems. In fact, through their effects on synaptic plasticity, NIBS techniques might affect the neurodevelopmental trajectories related to disease and therefore exert a therapeutic action. Transcranial direct current stimulation (tDCS) has the great advantage, over transcranial magnetic stimulation (TMS), of not requiring the immobilization of subjects, a condition very hard to achieve in patients with neurodevelopmental disorders, who are often hyperactive and noncompliant. In this chapter, we describe the available studies assessing the effect of tDCS in treating neurodevelopmental disorders.

20.2   tDCS in Autism Spectrum Disorder

ASD is a complex neurodevelopmental condition with an increasing prevalence, characterized by persistent deficits in social communication and interaction as well as by restricted and repetitive patterns of behaviors or interests. The onset is typically in the early developmental period and the symptoms cause significant impairment of functioning [3]. ASD is clinically and etiologically heterogeneous, encompassing a wide range of cognitive and verbal disabilities, sensory abnormalities, and behavioral symptoms. The causes and the pathophysiology of ASD are not yet clear. Rightward brain lateralization, inhibition/excitation unbalance, abnormal brain connectivity, altered synaptic maturation, and dysfunction of the mirror neurons system are some of the proposed mechanisms.

No specific treatments for ASD exist and those used hitherto (i.e., behavioral, educational, and medical interventions) mainly target comorbid/associated symptoms. In the last years, NIBS interventions have been increasingly considered in the treatment of ASD, especially tDCS for its ease of use. Nevertheless, despite the growing interest, to date, tDCS has been only marginally used in autistic patients. The published studies on tDCS in ASD patients are summarized below. They are grouped on the basis of their neurophysiological rationale and/or of the functions and symptoms targeted by the intervention.

20.2.1 Inhibition/Excitation (I/E) Unbalance

The very first tDCS trials involving autistic patients were conducted in young adults, with the aim of replicating the encouraging results obtained with low-frequency (inhibitory) TMS over the left dorsolateral prefrontal cortex (L-DLPFC) [4]. In a preliminary report from our group, cathodal (inhibitory) tDCS over L-DLPFC was used to treat the behavioral symptoms of a 26-year-old patient with ASD and severe mental retardation [5]. The rationale of this intervention was based on the theory of the inhibition/excitation unbalance, which holds that neurophysiological alterations, behavior abnormalities, and cognitive deficits of ASD patients are due to an impaired brain growth, leading to the disruption of basic cytoarchitectural structures, called the "cell minicolumns." In short, the minicolumns in healthy subjects consist of radially oriented arrays of pyramidal projection neurons (excitatory), surrounded by a combination of GABAergic interneurons (inhibitory) that serve to dynamically modulate pyramidal cell inputs and outputs. In the cerebral cortex of subjects with ASD, the peripheral compartment of the minicolumns is narrower than that of the age-matched controls, especially in the prefrontal cortical areas. This alteration entails a reduced inhibitory function by the GABAergic interneurons and a consequent prevailing excitatory action stemming from the pyramidal cells. Accordingly, the adjacent minicolumns tend to stimulate one another, causing an abnormal activation across the cerebral cortex even in response to low inputs. This mechanism can theoretically explain many cognitive, sensorial, and motor manifestations of ASD. Consistent with this theory, we hypothesized that using cathodal inhibitory tDCS over a cortical hub such as DLPFC could restore inhibition in it and in interconnected networks, thereby leading to a clinical improvement. Our first patient, who had not responded to different psychosocial and pharmacological interventions, underwent 10 consecutive week-day sessions of 1.5 mA/20 minutes tDCS, with the cathode over the L-DLPFC and the anode over the contralateral deltoid. Other treatments were kept unvaried during tDCS. Behavioral symptoms were assessed with the Aberrant Behavior Checklist (ABC), administered to the parents both before and after the tDCS course. At the end of the study, a clinically significant improvement of behavioral symptoms was observed, as evidenced by a 40.2% decrease in the total ABC score compared to the baseline. Furthermore, clinical improvement was still present at 3-month follow-up visit.

In a second study, we aimed to replicate the previous finding in a larger sample of young adult autistic patients with severe behavioral problems, and to assess the safety, feasibility, and efficacy of tDCS in these subjects, by means of an open-label phase II design [6]. Twelve autistic patients with intellectual disabilities and speech impairment were enrolled. All of them received ten daily sessions of cathodal tDCS over the L-DLPFC (1.5 mA, 20 minutes). tDCS treatments were carried out at the centers where patients were already attending an outpatient daily program of occupational rehabilitation. All participants underwent active treatment while concomitant therapies (rehabilitative and pharmacological) remained the same for 1 month before the trial and through the study. Behavioral symptoms were assessed with the ABC, which was administered before and after tDCS treatment. Two out of twelve enrolled subjects interrupted the treatment because they were unable to tolerate the treatment procedures. Eight out of ten study completers improved in their abnormal behaviors, reaching an average reduction of 26.7% of the total ABC score. More specifically, the most statistically significant change was seen in the "hyperactivity and lack of compliance" subscale of ABC. The remaining two patients were unresponsive to the treatment. Interestingly, these were the least severely ill patients at baseline (in terms of ABC total score), and scored the lowest ratio between the hyperactivity/noncompliance subscale and the total score at the baseline. These data may suggest a positive correlation between the effect size of tDCS on ASD patients and the clinical severity at baseline.

Starting from this early evidence, Gomez and colleagues aimed to replicate it on a sample of 10-year-old or younger autistic children [7]. The patients underwent twenty tDCS sessions (1 mA; 20 minutes) with the cathode over the L-DLPFC and the anode over the right arm. Clinical outcomes were measured in all participants before and after 1, 3, and 6 months from treatment completion, using the ABC, ATEC (Autism Treatment Evaluation Checklist), and ADI (Autism Diagnostic Interview). Moreover, a subset of participants also underwent an EEG recording to assess the effect of treatment on ERP and functional connectivity. A significant reduction in the total score on the three clinical scales was observed, which was maintained during the first 6 months after treatment, with only a slight and nonsignificant increase in the last evaluation. ERP (event-related potential) analysis during a passive oddball task showed a shortening of P300 latency after stimulation, without modulation of P300 amplitude. Since delayed latency and smaller amplitude of P300 have been linked to abnormal connectivity of the frontal lobes and to attention deficits of ASD patients, the authors interpreted the shortening of the P300 latency as indicating an increase of functional brain connectivity. This study has a certain merit of assessing the long-term effects of treatment with the longest follow-up among all tDCS trials involving autistic patients.

20.2.2 Right Lateralization

Starting from the evidence of a relative hypoactivity of the left hemisphere compared to the right in autistic patients, Amatachaya and colleagues conducted the only available tDCS trial using a randomized double-blind placebo-controlled design [8]. They applied anodal (excitatory) or sham tDCS over the L-DLPFC (with cathodal reference over the right shoulder) of 20 autistic children for 5 consecutive days (1 mA, 20 minutes for active stimulation; same electrode placement, but switching off the stimulation after 30 seconds for sham tDCS). After 4 weeks of washout, each participant underwent the other stimulation condition. During the treatment, no changes were made to the pharmacological therapies in progress. Three main outcomes were assessed before and after the treatment: the CARS (Childhood Autism Rating Scale)—which is a measure of autism severity, the ATEC—to assess the effectiveness of the treatment, and the CGAS (Children's Global Assessment Scale)—to estimate patients' psychosocial functioning. At the end of the study, the results outlined a significantly greater pre- to post-treatment decrease in all scores for the active tDCS compared to the sham, with the exception of the language domain of the ATEC.

In a follow-up study, the same authors started from the hypothesis that the behavioral improvements they observed with the stimulation of the left prefrontal cortex were mediated by an increase of alpha frequency and, consequently, of synaptic connectivity [9]. They randomized 20 male children to receive a single session of active and sham tDCS over the L-DLPFC. The outcomes of the study were peak alpha frequency (PAF), assessed before, immediately after, at 24, 48, and 72 hours after active and sham tDCS, and ATEC, administered to the patients' caregivers' pre- and post-tDCS session. According to the hypothesis, the results showed a significant pre- to post-session improvement in two domains of ATEC (social and health/behavior domains) and a significant increase in PAF at the stimulation site after active—but not sham—tDCS. Furthermore, the increase in PAF was significantly associated with improvements in psychosocial functioning, as measured with the ATEC.

20.2.3 Social Cognition

Impaired social cognition and social skills are among the hallmarks of ASD, with substantial challenges found in empathy and theory of mind, i.e., the ability to take the perspective of the others and infer their mental state. Social cognition refers to mental processes required to complete social tasks, while social skills refer to utilizing social cognition to perform tasks required to engage social interactions. The right temporoparietal junction (rTPJ) plays a role in social cognitive processes that are considered relevant for empathy and Theory of Mind (ToM) and is associated with ToM deficits in individuals with ASD. In healthy subjects, anodal tDCS applied over the rTPJ improves social functioning in tasks for perspective taking and evaluation of self against others, while cathodal tDCS applied over the same area reduces accuracy in ToM and cognitive empathy tasks.

Wilson and colleagues investigated for the first time the use of tDCS applied over the rTPJ to target social functioning in adults with ASD. In a first case report, eight consecutive tDCS sessions were administered to an 18-year-old high-functioning autistic patient [10]. The anode was placed over the rTPJ (CP6 according to the 10/10 EEG system) and the cathode on the ipsilateral deltoid (1.5 mA; 30 minutes). The ATEC was administered before tDCS, after the last session, and at 2-month follow-up to assess behavioral symptoms. Moreover, informal follow-up was made 1 year after tDCS. The ATEC results showed a substantial improvement in social functioning from baseline to post-tDCS, which remained unchanged up to 1-year follow-up, suggesting that tDCS could be a promising intervention modality to safely enhance treatments targeting social cognition and social skills.

In a second study, the same authors wanted to extend this preliminary observation by investigating the effect of anodal tDCS over the rTPJ combined with computer-based social skills treatment interventions [11]. Their hypothesis was that active anodal tDCS would result in greater improvements in verbal fluency (VF) and social skills (Test of Adolescent Social Skills-Modified, TASSK-M) performance compared to sham. Active (2 mA; 30 minutes) or sham (0–2.0 mA during 20 seconds, then decreased to 0 mA after 30 seconds; 30 minutes) tDCS, with the same positioning of the electrodes used in the previous study, was randomly assigned to six adults autistic patients with normal or higher cognitive functioning with a within-subjects, double-blind design. Tasks were performed before, during, and post-tDCS stimulation. The results suggested the effectiveness of tDCS paired with social skills treatments with significantly higher scores on the VF test after active tDCS compared to the sham, especially in the emotion-word section of the test.

20.2.4 Executive Functions

ASD patients often display deficits in executive functions (EFs), which in turn contribute to the core autistic features of impaired social skills and social cognition. In particular, affected subjects may have a Working Memory (WM) deficit, consisting of difficulties in maintaining, updating, and manipulating information held in temporary storage. tDCS was shown to enhance WM in both healthy adults and clinical populations when applied over the DLPFC. In the first study assessing the effect of tDCS on the WM of autistic patients, Steenburgh and colleagues hypothesized that WM performance of autistic patients would improve during frontal tDCS and that such enhancement would generalize to an untrained task [12]. The authors enrolled twelve high-functioning adult patients, who received 40 minutes of 1.5 mA bifrontal-tDCS (F3/F4 according to the EEG 10/20 system) while they were engaged in a battery of WM tasks. Using a single-blind crossover design, each participant underwent three consecutive sessions of tDCS in randomized counterbalanced order on three separate days (left anodal/right cathodal stimulation, right anodal/left cathodal stimulation, or sham stimulation). At the end of the treatment, participants engaged again in WM tasks before taking the Brief Test of Attention (BTA). The authors observed that both active conditions improved the overall WM performance and that tDCS benefits transferred to an untrained task completed shortly after right anodal stimulation. In a subsequent open trial, Rothärmel and colleagues administered ten consecutive 2 mA/15 minutes cathodal tDCS sessions over the L-DLPFC to eight high-functioning ASD patients [13]. EFs were assessed with the Stroop test, Trail-Making Test [TMT] A and B, Modified Wisconsin Card Sorting Test [mWCST], and Verbal Fluency Test, whereas behavioral dysexecutive syndrome was evaluated with the Behavioral Dysexecutive Syndrome Inventory and the Repetitive and Restricted Behavior scale. After tDCS, the authors observed an improvement in initiation (using the TMT-A) and flexibility (TMT-B; letter Verbal Fluency Test; mWCST), which are known to be the most impaired EFs in autism. Moreover, they reported a beneficial effect on such behavioral symptoms as repetitive behaviors, restricted interests, and hypoactivity. Taken together, the aforementioned results suggest that tDCS is a promising method to enhance EF in adults with high-functioning ASD.

20.2.5 Language

Language impairment is very common among ASD patients. The combination of tDCS with speech therapy might represent a new tool to improve language abilities in autism, considering the potential of tDCS to enhance learning through an action on synaptic plasticity. An open-label, noncontrolled study by Schneider and Hopp investigated the effect of tDCS on syntax acquisition in a sample of 10 children and adolescents with ASD and severe language impairment [14]. The authors applied one session of anodal tDCS (2 mA, 30 minutes) over the L-DLPFC with the cathode placed over the right supraorbital region. Using a modified version of the Bilingual

Aphasia Test (BAT), which assesses various linguistic skills such as comprehension, repetition, lexical access, reading, and writing for each level of language, authors investigated vocabulary and syntax comprehension both before and after tDCS. They performed first a vocabulary test, during which patients had to touch a stimulus upon verbal request. Thereafter, a session of syntax training was performed by exposure to scaffolding sentences approximating the syntax to be tested in the following syntax comprehension test, during which children had to select a picture corresponding to a sentence presented in its canonical subject–verb–object sequence. Results demonstrated an improvement in syntax acquisition and vocabulary scores after tDCS, suggesting that this treatment can be an effective tool to improve language abilities in children with ASD.

20.2.6 Catatonia

In a case report, Costanzo and colleagues described the effect of bilateral tDCS over the DLPFC in a 14-year-old girl with ASD and drug-resistant catatonia [15]. Recent evidence suggests that Catatonia-ASD is a frequent comorbidity, probably because these two conditions share abnormalities in neural circuitries, such as alterations in prefrontal and parietal activation as well as in functional connectivity between these two brain regions. The best treatment for catatonia is Electroconvulsive Therapy (ECT), which also turned out to be effective on comorbid conditions, even when these were not ECT typical indications [16]. However, this treatment is still stigmatized and underutilized in many countries [17]. For this reason, tDCS has been proposed in adolescents as a safer and less invasive alternative to ECT. The catatonic patient described by Costanzo and colleagues had not responded to many different pharmacological treatments (benzodiazepines, antipsychotics, antidepressants, anticonvulsants). She underwent 28 consecutive, daily tDCS sessions—while keeping her drug regimen unvaried—with the cathode over the R-DLPFC and the anode over the L-DLPFC (1 mA; 20 minutes). Catatonic symptoms, assessed with the Kanner Catatonia Rating Scale, showed a 30% decrease at the end of the treatment, and the effects were maintained at a 1-month follow-up evaluation.

To sum up, patients with ASD can benefit from tDCS, which is able to reduce not only associated and comorbid symptoms but also core autistic manifestations; being safe, inexpensive, and easy to administer, it could have a substantial role in the management of autistic symptoms for which no specific treatments currently exist.

20.3   tDCS in Attention-Deficit/Hyperactivity Disorder

ADHD is a neurodevelopmental disorder characterized by inattention and inappropriate levels of hyperactivity and/or impulsivity. In childhood, it has a prevalence of 7%, and is often associated with other disorders such as oppositional-defiant, tic, anxiety, and mood disorders [18].

Symptoms appear by the age of 12 and, in a great portion of patients, persist in the adulthood. In the long term, ADHD can lead to a wide range of adverse outcomes such as, for example, poor educational achievement, substance-related disorders, gambling, anticonservative conducts, thus causing high individual and social costs.

Many fMRI studies in ADHD patients have shown dysfunctions in fronto-cingulo-striato-thalamic and fronto-parieto-cerebellar networks that mediate cognitive control, attention, timing, and WM. Furthermore, there is emerging evidence of abnormalities in orbitofrontal, ventromedial prefrontal, and limbic areas that mediate motivation and emotion control. In addition, the poor deactivation of the default mode network (DMN) suggests abnormally hypoengaged task-positive and hyper-engaged task-negative networks, both dysfunctions being related to impaired cognition.

The pharmacological treatment of ADHD is represented mainly by stimulants (i.e., methylphenidate) and an inhibitor of norepinephrine reuptake (atomoxetine). Unfortunately, these treatments can worsen the comorbid conditions and/or cause intolerable side effects, such as decreased appetite, sleep problems, headache, nausea, and delayed growth. Alternative treatments, namely, neurofeedback, cognitive training, dietary interventions, and behavioral therapy, have been demonstrated to have small effect sizes, be time consuming, and require high motivation and compliance of patients and their families. Therefore, there is a considerable need for new treatment strategies in the management of ADHD. tDCS may be a valuable therapeutic option, also considering its recognized ability to improve cognitive functions such as attention and working memory.

The first study in this field assessed the effects of tDCS on declarative memory of children with ADHD [19]. In healthy people, the frontal brain areas originate slow oscillations during slow-wave sleep, which are thought to be beneficial for the declarative memory. Deficits in declarative memory of ADHD children have been associated with a malfunctioning of this mechanism. tDCS was used to induce slow oscillations during early slow-wave sleep in 12 ADHD male children and 12 healthy controls. Two anodes were placed bilaterally over the left and the right DLPFC (F3 and F4 according to the EEG system), while the cathodes were placed over the ipsilateral mastoids. Sinusoidal stimulation was started 4 minutes after patients had entered non-REM sleep stage 2 for the first time and it was applied in a series of five 5-min intervals separated by 1-min intervals without stimulation. The current strength of each anodal electrode ranged from 0 to 250 mA at a frequency of 0.75 Hz. Each participant received both active and sham stimulation, 1 week apart. Declarative memory was assessed through a computer memory task. Results showed an increase of slow oscillation during the slow-wave sleep and an improvement of declarative memory only for ADHD subjects. Furthermore, in ADHD children, memory consolidation improved to the level of healthy controls. Using the same stimulation protocol, Munz et al. replicated these early results and additionally demonstrated an improvement in behavioral inhibition in 14 children with ADHD [20].

In a subsequent study, Bandeira and colleagues extensively assessed the executive functions of nine children after five consecutive tDCS sessions [21]. The cathode was placed over the right supraorbital area and the anode over F3 (2 mA; 30 minutes). During tDCS sessions, subjects were engaged in activities entailing the activation of the DLPFC (i.e., card-matching game, during which they were asked to match pictures and to create associations between pictures). At the end of the treatment, an increase of visual attention and inhibitory control was observed, while no differences were detected in WM and attention.

In a randomized, double-blind, sham-controlled, crossover trial, Soff et al. treated fifteen adolescents with ADHD with either anodal (1 mA) or sham tDCS over the L-DLPFC for 5 days. Active treatment caused a reduction of inattention and impulsivity at the standardized working memory test (Quantified Behavior Test, QbTest) compared to sham, and this effect was stable 7 days after the last stimulation [22].

Another study from the same group used fMRI to assess the neurofunctional correlates of tDCS effects on WM. Sixteen adolescents with ADHD underwent either anodal tDCS or sham (1 mA; 20 minutes) over the L-DLPFC with simultaneous fMRI during n-back WM task [23]. Anodal stimulation and not sham improved WM performance and led to a greater activation of the DLPFC and of other interconnected regions, i.e., left premotor cortex, left supplementary motor cortex, and precuneus.

A different stimulation protocol was used by Cachoeira and colleagues in a randomized, double-blind, sham-controlled trial on seventeen patients with ADHD [24]. They applied the anode over the R-DLPFC and the cathode over the L-DLPFC (five sessions; 2 mA; 20 minutes), thereby inverting the generally used positions. The rationale of this different montage stands in the evidence of an R-DLPFC hypoactivation in ADHD patients during attention tasks and of a WM improvement after anodal stimulation of this area in healthy subjects. Behavioral and neuropsychological assessments were performed at four different time points. tDCS turned out to reduce ADHD behavioral symptoms and improve several aspects of attention. Interestingly, the improvement was stable 4 weeks after the last stimulation.

A different brain area, i.e., the right inferior frontal gyrus (rIFG), was targeted in another trial involving 21 male adolescents with ADHD and 21 healthy controls aged from 13 to 17 years [25]. Each participant received one session of anodal, cathodal, and sham stimulation (separated by at least 1 week) while completing the Flanker task, a test assessing the ability to control interferential stimuli. The results showed that anodal tDCS and not cathodal or sham reduced commission errors and reaction time. In particular, the rate of commission errors after tDCS was comparable to that of healthy controls.

The predominant role of R-DLPFC in inhibitory control was indirectly confirmed by the study of Solstaninejad and colleagues, who reported no effect of anodal tDCS over the L-DLPFC, while an improvement was observed after cathodal tDCS of the same area, probably via an interhemispheric communication mechanism [26].

Similar results were reported in another study by the same group, which in addition examined the effects of tDCS over the orbitofrontal cortex (OFC) [27]. Twenty-five children with ADHD underwent one session of four different tDCS conditions: left DLPFC anodal/right DLPFC cathodal, left DLPFC anodal/right OFC cathodal, left DLPFC cathodal/right OFC anodal, and sham. The current intensity was 1 mA and each stimulation was delivered for 15 minutes with a 72-hour interval between the different conditions. Participants underwent Go/No-Go task, N-back test, Wisconsin Card Sorting Test (WCST), and Stroop task after each tDCS session. The different conditions turned out to affect distinct cognitive functions. Anodal tDCS over the L-DLPFC improved executive control functions, while left DLPFC cathodal/right OFC anodal tDCS increased inhibitory control. Both anodal and cathodal stimulation of OFC benefited cognitive flexibility.

In conclusion, analyzed data indicate that tDCS may reduce symptoms and improve neuropsychological functioning in children and adolescents with ADHD, showing to a potential role of this technique as a treatment option for different aspects of this complex disorder.

20.4   tDCS in Tourette Syndrome

Tourette Syndrome (TS) is a neurodevelopmental disorder with the onset in the early childhood, characterized by motor and vocal tics and causing important distress and severe functional impairment.

Neurophysiological studies have shown an abnormal excitability of motor cortex (MC) in TS patients, while functional neuroimaging demonstrated a correlation between the activity of supplementary motor area (SMA) and tic severity [28].

Based on this evidence, Mrackic-Sposta et al. used cathodal tDCS over the left motor cortex of two adult TS patients [29]. Each patient received five sessions of active and five of sham tDCS (2 mA, 15 minutes) with a 2-week washout interval between the two conditions. The Yale Global Tic Severity Scale (YGTSS) was administered at baseline and at the end of each session. The results showed a reduction of tics in both patients only after active stimulation, suggesting that cathodal tDCS over left MC might induce an adaptive mechanism of widespread reduction of excitability in the motor system, which in turn prevents the release of unwanted movements.

In another report, a 16-year-old treatment-refractory TS patient underwent ten daily tDCS sessions (2 mA; 30 minutes) with the cathode placed over the pre-SMA and the anode over the right deltoid muscle [30]. Interestingly, the same electrode montage was shown to be effective in reducing the symptoms of OCD, a condition frequently found in combination with TS [31, 32]. An fMRI scan was performed before and immediately after the treatment. Tic severity was assessed at four time points, starting from baseline up to 6 months post-treatment and showed a progressive decrease of YGTSS scores. The post-treatment resting-state fMRI showed reduced activity in the left precentral region and in the left cerebellum of the sensorimotor resting-state network. This result is in line with previous evidence showing a correlation between motor symptom severity and an increased activity in the sensorimotor region and cerebellum.

In conclusion, although very little evidence is available, the preliminary results suggest a possible role for cathodal tDCS over MC/pre-SMA in the treatment of TS patients.

20.5   tDCS in Dyslexia

Developmental dyslexia is a specific learning disorder consisting of a persistent deficit in learning to read, occurring in 5–17% of children, which cannot be explained by a deficit in sensory or cognitive functions, or by a lack of motivations or of adequate reading instruction [33]. It has been associated with hypoactivation of the left parieto-temporal regions, left occipito-temporal regions—which is the most consistent finding—and with hyperactivation of the inferior frontal regions. Other evidence suggest hypofunctioning of the left superior temporal gyrus (STG) and reduction in gray matter volume in brain areas involved in speech and language processing.

Conventional remediation methods are based on cognitive training programs focused on the deficient aspects of reading skills. These programs have been shown to modify activation in critically involved brain areas and often improve reading, by inducing compensatory processes. Unfortunately, such improvements are rarely stable. Therefore, there is an urgent need for new and more effective treatment strategies in order to prevent the everyday-life severe functional impairment of patients with dyslexia.

A possible progress could be the integration of cognitive interventions with NIBS techniques, targeted to the brain areas putatively activated by the specific training, in order to obtain a synergic effect. This approach has already been used for the treatment of other psychiatric conditions, such as, for example, depression [34].

To our knowledge, only tDCS—among all brain stimulation techniques—has been used in patients with dyslexia. In a first study, Costanzo and colleagues hypothesized that stimulating the hypoactive parieto-temporal cortex could improve reading abilities in dyslexic subjects [35]. Nineteen children and adolescents with dyslexia were enrolled and performed different neuropsychological tests for reading abilities at baseline and after each session of stimulation. tDCS treatment design included four counterbalanced conditions: in two active conditions, 1-mA tDCS was administered for 20 minutes over bilateral parieto-temporal areas (in the midway between P7/8 and TP7/8) with left anodal/right cathodal (to enhance left lateralization of the target area) or left cathodal/right anodal (to enhance right lateralization) montages; two control conditions, sham stimulation with the left anodal/right cathodal montage, and a condition without tDCS stimulation, were included. In the text-reading accuracy, the results showed a significant improvement (error reduction) after left anodal/right cathodal parieto-temporal tDCS, with no significant effect in other reading-related measures and for other treatment conditions.

A second study from the same group investigated the effects of multiple tDCS sessions combined with a cognitive training and whether these effects were long lasting in a sample of eighteen children and adolescents with dyslexia, who were randomly assigned to active or sham left anodal/right cathodal parieto-temporal stimulation [36]. The patients received eighteen 20-minute sessions of 1 mA tDCS combined with cognitive reading tasks focused on the improvement of reading accuracy. The results demonstrated that reading errors were significantly reduced only in patients receiving active tDCS and the improvement was stable up to 1 month after the end of the treatment.

Finally, the same authors used the previously detailed 18-session protocol in 26 dyslexic patients, with the aim of assessing the duration of the effect. The results showed that only the active group received long-lasting benefits in reading abilities, and these persisted up to the last follow-up visit, 6 months after the end of the treatment [37].

Other authors investigated the effects of tDCS applied to the STG on auditory temporal resolution and speech long-latency auditory-evoked potentials [38]. Seventeen children and adolescents with dyslexia were randomized to receive four stimulation conditions: left anodal/right cathodal tDCS (to increase cortical excitability in left STG and inhibit it in right STG), left anodal tDCS with the cathode on contralateral shoulder (to increase cortical excitability only in left STG), sham tDCS, and baseline status without applying tDCS. All participants underwent the gap in noise (GIN) test and long-latency auditory-evoked potentials recording at baseline and after 20 minutes of tDCS. The results showed a significant increase in correct responses in the GIN test, as well as reduced latency and increased amplitude of the P1, N1, and P2 waves only in the active stimulation conditions.

Finally, Heth and colleagues investigated the effects of tDCS on text-reading fluency and accuracy when the visual extrastriate area V5—which modulates incoming visual information and has a role in word identification—is targeted by the stimulation [39]. Twenty-three 18-year and older dyslexic subjects were enrolled and randomly assigned to five 1.5 mA or sham sessions of 20-minute tDCS with the anode placed over the left V5 area and the cathode over the right orbitofrontal cortex. The results demonstrated a significant improvement of reading speed and fluency only after active tDCS, suggesting a therapeutic potential of tDCS applied to the visual network in dyslexic subjects.

20.6   tDCS in Stuttering

Stuttering, or childhood-onset fluency disorder, is a neurodevelopmental disorder affecting 5% of children, and persisting in 1% of adults, characterized by disfluent speech with involuntary repetitions, prolongations of speech sounds, and blocks at the levels of syllables and words [40]. Although its etiology is still unclear, converging evidence from neuroimaging studies shows that people who stutter (PWS) have significant abnormalities in critical brain regions supporting speech, such as a deficient structural connectivity in white matter of left-hemispheric speech areas (inferior frontal cortex, IFC) and a right-hemispheric compensatory hyperactivity. In fact, in healthy subjects the left and not the right IFC has a prominent role in motor planning as well as in integration of sensory signals during speech production. Furthermore, many previous studies consistently demonstrated a reduced activation in Wernicke's area (WA) and its right homologue region (RW). Fluency therapies use techniques for altering speech patterns to reduce overt stuttering, but the results may not persist without continued practice and can be difficult to fully integrate into everyday speech. There is a value, therefore, in developing novel interventions to improve therapy outcomes for PWS, including tDCS.

In a first study, Chesters and colleagues investigated whether a single session of tDCS could improve fluency in PWS [41]. The authors enrolled 16 subjects (mean age: 30 years) who received, in two separate sessions, either anodal (1 mA; 20 minutes) or sham stimulation with the anode over the L-IFC (FC5 according to 10–20 EEG system, which is centered on Broca's region) and the cathode over the right supraorbital ridge. Stuttering was significantly reduced at two outcome time points for the sentence-reading task, in both the tDCS and sham conditions, probably due to practice, but not during the paragraph-reading or conversation tasks.

In a subsequent study, the same authors applied anodal stimulation to the L-IFC during speech production with temporary fluency inducers [42]. Thirty adult participants were enrolled in a randomized, double-blind, controlled trial of five daily sessions of anodal tDCS over the L-IFC, covering also the ventral sensorimotor and premotor cortex, while speech fluency was temporarily induced using choral and metronome-timed speech. Results showed that this combined treatment reduced the percentage of disfluent speech significantly more than fluency training alone and that this effect persisted up to 6 weeks after the intervention.

Finally, Yada and colleagues [43] hypothesized that the reduction of stuttering severity can be achieved using anodal stimulation to address the underactivation of Broca's Area (BA), WA, and RW and/or using cathodal stimulation to address overactivation in right homolog region of Broca's area (RB). Fifteen patients (18–40 years old) received, while reading passages aloud, either anodal, cathodal, or sham stimulation over one of the language areas (BA, WA) and its right hemisphere homolog (RB, RW), with the second electrode placed over the contralateral supraorbital region. Among the combinations of stimulation sites and polarities, the authors observed a highly selective effect of tDCS, with only cathodal stimulation over RB significantly reducing the frequency of stuttering.

20.7 tDCS in Rett Syndrome

Rett Syndrome is a rare genetic disorder of neurodevelopment, associated with mutations in the MECP2 gene, located on the X chromosome, and characterized by several intellectual, linguistic, and motor disabilities.

In the only study assessing the effect of tDCS in this population of patients, Fabio and colleagues combined the linguistic training with ten consecutive daily sessions (2 mA; 20 minutes) of anodal tDCS over the BA (with the cathode in the contralateral position) in three women with Rett Syndrome [44]. Quantitative EEG measures were recorded before the tDCS, immediately after, and at 1-month follow-up. The results showed a general improvement in language, motor coordination with an increase of functional movements, and an increase in the frequency and power of alpha, beta, and theta EEG bands, which are typically under-represented in Rett Syndrome patients.

20.8   Conclusions

The available literature on the therapeutic effects of tDCS in subjects with neurodevelopmental disorders, mainly children and adolescents, was reviewed in this chapter. The included studies generally indicate an improvement of symptoms and support the use of tDCS as a treatment tool for these disorders, especially when used in combination with cognitive training. Importantly, despite differences in stimulation protocols and study designs, the available data show that patients with different neurodevelopmental disorders well-tolerate treatments, and no significant adverse effects were reported. However, several methodological limitations, such as small sample sizes, inconsistent use of sham protocols, placebo effects, and nonuniform samples, hamper the relevance of the available findings. Furthermore, only short-term measures of clinical response were usually collected. Therefore, further studies, with more representative and uniform samples, with sham conditions and mid/long-term assessments, are needed to clarify the efficacy of the protocols on the intended outcome measures. Finally, a thorough characterization of the patients with neurodevelopmental disorders who might show a greater therapeutic effect is warranted to identify potential predictors of response to tDCS, as indeed was done, for example, for clinical predictors of response of depressed patients [45].

References

1. Sauvaget A, Poulet E, Mantovani A, Bulteau S, Damier P, Moutaud B, et al. The psychiatric neuromodulation unit: implementation and management. J ECT. 2018;34(4):211–9.
2. D'Urso G, Mantovani A, Patti S, Toscano E, de Bartolomeis A. Transcranial direct current stimulation in obsessive-compulsive disorder, posttraumatic stress disorder, and anxiety disorders. J ECT. 2018;34:172–81.
3. American Psychiatric Association. Diagnostic and statistical manual of mental disorders (DSM-5®). San Francisco: American Psychiatric Publication; 2013.
4. Barahona-Corrêa JB, Velosa A, Chainho A, Lopes R, Oliveira-Maia AJ. Repetitive transcranial magnetic stimulation for treatment of autism spectrum disorder: a systematic review and meta-analysis. Front Integr Neurosci. 2018;9:12–27.
5. D'Urso G, Ferrucci R, Bruzzese D, Pascotto A, Priori A, Altamura CA, et al. Transcranial direct current stimulation for autistic disorder. Biol Psychiatry. 2014;76(5):e5–6.
6. D'Urso G, Bruzzese D, Ferrucci R, Priori A, Pascotto A, Galderisi S, et al. Transcranial direct current stimulation for hyperactivity and noncompliance in autistic disorder. World J Biol Psychiatry. 2015;16(5):361–6.

7. Gómez L, Vidal B, Maragoto C, Morales L, Berrillo S, Vera Cuesta H, et al. Non-invasive brain stimulation for children with autism spectrum disorders: a short-term outcome study. Behav Sci. 2017;7(3):63.

8. Amatachaya A, Auvichayapat N, Patjanasoontorn N, Suphakunpinyo C, Ngernyam N, Aree-uea B, et al. Effect of anodal transcranial direct current stimulation on autism: a randomized double-blind crossover trial. Behav Neurol. 2014;2014:173073.

9. Amatachaya A, Jensen MP, Patjanasoontorn N, Auvichayapat N, Suphakunpinyo C, Janjarasjitt S, et al. The short-term effects of transcranial direct current stimulation on electroenceph-alography in children with autism: a randomized crossover controlled trial. Behav Neurol. 2015;2015:928631.

10. Wilson JE, Quinn DK, Wilson JK, Garcia CM, Tesche CD. Transcranial direct current stimula-tion to the right temporoparietal junction for social functioning in autism spectrum disorder: a case report. J ECT. 2018;34(1):e10.

11. Wilson JE, Trumbo MC, Wilson JK, Tesche CD. Transcranial direct current stimulation (tDCS) over right temporoparietal junction (rTPJ) for social cognition and social skills in adults with autism spectrum disorder (ASD). J Neural Transm. 2018;125(12):1857–66.

12. Van Steenburgh JJ, Varvaris M, Schretlen DJ, Vannorsdall TD, Gordon B. Balanced bifron-tal transcranial direct current stimulation enhances working memory in adults with high-functioning autism: a sham-controlled crossover study. Mol Autism. 2017;8(1):40.

13. Rothärmel M, Moulier V, Vasse M, Isaac C, Faerber M, Bendib B, et al. A prospective open-label pilot study of transcranial direct current stimulation in high-functioning autistic patients with a dysexecutive syndrome. Neuropsychobiology. 2019;2:1–11.

14. Schneider HD, Hopp JP. The use of the Bilingual Aphasia Test for assessment and transcranial direct current stimulation to modulate language acquisition in minimally verbal children with autism. Clin Linguist Phon. 2011;25(6–7):640–54.

15. Costanzo F, Menghini D, Casula L, Amendola A, Mazzone L, Valeri G, et al. Transcranial direct current stimulation treatment in an adolescent with autism and drug-resistant catatonia. Brain Stimul. 2015;8(6):1233–5.

16. D'Urso G, Mantovani A, Barbarulo AM, Labruna L, Muscettola G. Brain-behavior relation-ship in a case of successful ECT for drug refractory catatonic OCD. J ECT. 2012;28(3):190–3.

17. Buccelli C, Di Lorenzo P, Paternoster M, D'Urso G, Graziano V, Niola M. Electroconvulsive therapy in Italy: will public controversies ever stop? J ECT. 2016;32(3):207–11.

18. Thomas R, Sanders S, Doust J, Beller E, Glasziou P. Prevalence of attention deficit/hyperactiv-ity disorder: a systematic review and meta-analysis. Pediatrics. 2015;135(4):e994–1001.

19. Prehn-Kristensen A, Munz M, Goder R, Wilhelm I, Korr K, Vahl W, et al. transcranial oscil-latory direct current stimulation during sleep improves declarative memory consolidation in children with attention-deficit/hyperactivity disorder to a level comparable to healthy controls. Brain Stimul. 2014;7(6):793–9.

20. Munz MT, Prehn-Kristensen A, Thielking F, Mölle M, Göder R, Baving L. Slow oscillating transcranial direct current stimulation during non-rapid eye movement sleep improves behav-ioral inhibition in attention-deficit/hyperactivity disorder. Front Cell Neurosci. 2015;9:307.

21. Bandeira ID, Guimaraes RS, Jagersbacher JB, Barretto TL, de Jesus-Silva JR, Santos SN, et al. Transcranial direct current stimulation in children and adolescents with attention deficit/hyperactivity disorder (ADHD): a pilot study. J Child Neurol. 2016;31(7):918–24.

22. Soff C, Sotnikova A, Christiansen H, Becker K, Siniatchkin M. Transcranial direct current stimulation improves clinical symptoms in adolescents with attention deficit hyperactivity dis-order. J Neural Transm (Vienna). 2017;124(1):133–44.

23. Sotnikova A, Soff C, Tagliazucchi E, Becker K, Siniatchkin M. Transcranial direct cur-rent modulates neuronal networks in attention deficit hyperactivity disorder. Brain Topogr. 2017;30(5):656–72.

24. Cachoeira CT, Leffa DT, Mittelstadt SD, Mendes LST, Brunoni AR, Pinto JV, et al. Positive effects of transcranial direct current stimulation in adult patients with attention-deficit/hyper-activity disorder–a pilot randomized controlled study. Psychiatry Res. 2017;2470:28–32.

25. Breitling C, Zaehle T, Dannhauer M, Bonath B, Tegelbeckers J, Flechtner H-H, et al. Improving interference control in ADHD patients with transcranial direct current stimulation (tDCS). Front Cell Neurosci. 2016;10:72.
26. Soltaninejad Z, Nejati V, Ekhtiari H. Effect of anodal and cathodal transcranial direct current stimulation on DLPFC on modulation of inhibitory control in ADHD. J Atten Disord. 2019;23(4):325–32.
27. Nejati V, Salehinejad MA, Nitsche MA, Najian A, Javadi AH. Transcranial direct current stimulation improves executive dysfunctions in ADHD: implications for inhibitory control, interference control, working memory, and cognitive flexibility. J Atten Disord. 2017;1087054717730611.
28. Wang Z, Maia TV, Marsh R, Colibazzi T, Gerber A, Peterson BS. The neural circuits that generate tics in Tourette's syndrome. Am J Psychiatry. 2011;168(12):1326–37.
29. Mrakic-Sposta S, Marceglia S, Mameli F, Dilena R, Tadini L, Priori A. Transcranial direct current stimulation in two patients with Tourette syndrome. Mov Disord. 2008;23(15):2259–61.
30. Carvalho S, Gonçalves ÓF, Soares JM, Sampaio A, Macedo F, Fregni F, et al. Sustained effects of a neural-based intervention in a refractory case of tourette syndrome. Brain Stimul. 2015;8:657–9.
31. D'Urso G, Brunoni AR, Anastasia A, Micillo M, de Bartolomeis A, Mantovani A. Polarity-dependent effects of transcranial direct current stimulation in obsessive-compulsive disorder. Neurocase. 2016;22(1):60–4.
32. D'urso G, Brunoni AR, Mazzaferro MP, Anastasia A, de Bartolomeis A, Mantovani A. Transcranial direct current stimulation for obsessive–compulsive disorder: a randomized, controlled, partial crossover trial. Depress Anxiety. 2016;33(12):1132–40.
33. Ferrer E, Shaywitz BA, Holahan JM, Marchione K, Shaywitz SE. Uncoupling of reading and IQ overtime: empirical evidence for a definition of dyslexia. Psychol Sci. 2010;21:93–101.
34. D'Urso G, Mantovani A, Micillo M, Priori A, Muscettola G. Transcranial direct current stimulation and cognitive-behavioral therapy: evidence of a synergistic effect in treatment-resistant depression. Brain Stimul. 2013;6(3):465–7.
35. Costanzo F, Varuzza C, Rossi S, Sdoia S, Varvara P, Oliveri M, et al. Reading changes in children and adolescents with dyslexia after transcranial direct current stimulation. Neuroreport. 2016;27(5):295–300.
36. Costanzo F, Varuzza C, Rossi S, Sdoia S, Varvara P, Oliveri M, et al. Evidence for reading improvement following tDCS treatment in children and adolescents with Dyslexia. Restor Neurol Neurosci. 2016;34(2):215–26.
37. Costanzo F, Rossi S, Varuzza C, Varvara P, Vicari S, Menghini D. Long-lasting improvement following tDCS treatment combined with a training for reading in children and adolescents with dyslexia. Neuropsychologia. 2019;130:38–43.
38. Rahimi V, Mohamadkhani G, Alaghband-Rad J, Kermani FR, Nikfarjad H, Marofizade S. Modulation of temporal resolution and speech long-latency auditory-evoked potentials by transcranial direct current stimulation in children and adolescents with dyslexia. Exp Brain Res. 2019;237(3):873–82.
39. Heth I, Lavidor M. Improved reading measures in adults with dyslexia following transcranial direct current stimulation treatment. Neuropsychologia. 2015;70:107–13.
40. Wingate ME. A standard definition of stuttering. J Speech Hear Disord. 1964;29:484–9.
41. Chesters J, Watkins KE, Möttönen R. Investigating the feasibility of using transcranial direct current stimulation to enhance fluency in people who stutter. Brain Lang. 2017;164:68–76.
42. Chesters J, Möttönen R, Watkins KE. Transcranial direct current stimulation over left inferior frontal cortex improves speech fluency in adults who stutter. Brain. 2018;141(4):1161–71.
43. Yada Y, Tomisato S, Hashimoto RI. Online cathodal transcranial direct current stimulation to the right homologue of Broca's area improves speech fluency in people who stutter. Psychiatry Clin Neurosci. 2019;73(2):63–9.

44. Fabio RA, Gangemi A, Capri T, Budden S, Falzone A. Neurophysiological and cognitive effects of transcranial direct current stimulation in three girls with Rett syndrome with chronic language impairments. Res Dev Disabil. 2018;76:76–87.
45. D'Urso G, Dell'Osso B, Rossi R, Brunoni AR, Bortolomasi M, Ferrucci R, et al. Clinical predictors of acute response to transcranial direct current stimulation (tDCS) in major depression. J Affect Disord. 2017;219:25–30.

Transcranial Direct Current Stimulation (tDCS) in Anxiety Disorders

21

Carmelo M. Vicario, Mohammad A. Salehinejad, Alessio Avenanti, and Michael A. Nitsche

21.1 Introduction

The interest in using transcranial direct current stimulation (tDCS) as a complementary or alternative tool for the treatment of neurological and psychiatric disorders has been significantly growing since the last decade, as shown by the exponential increase of scientific publications in the field (see [1], for an overview). One key factor for the interest in this noninvasive brain stimulation technique refers to its

C. M. Vicario (✉)
Dipartimento di Scienze Cognitive, Psicologiche, Pedagogiche e degli studi culturali, Università di Messina, Messina, Italy

Department of Psychology and Neurosciences, Leibniz Research Centre for Working Environment and Human Factors, Dortmund, Germany
e-mail: cvicario@unime.it

M. A. Salehinejad
Department of Psychology and Neurosciences, Leibniz Research Centre for Working Environment and Human Factors, Dortmund, Germany

International Graduate School of Neuroscience, Ruhr University Bochum, Bochum, Germany

A. Avenanti
Fondazione Santa Lucia, IRCCS, Rome, Italy

Dipartimento di Psicologia and Centro studi e ricerche in Neuroscienze Cognitive, Università di Bologna, Cesena, Italy

Centro de Investigación en Neuropsicología y Neurociencias Cognitivas, Universidad Católica del Maule, Talca, Chile

M. A. Nitsche
Department of Psychology and Neurosciences, Leibniz Research Centre for Working Environment and Human Factors, Dortmund, Germany

Department of Neurology, University Medical Hospital Bergmannsheil, Bochum, Germany

© Springer Nature Switzerland AG 2020
B. Dell'Osso, G. Di Lorenzo (eds.), *Non Invasive Brain Stimulation in Psychiatry and Clinical Neurosciences*,
https://doi.org/10.1007/978-3-030-43356-7_21

potential to modulate neural activity by acting on synaptic plasticity (e.g., [2]), which is supposed to be abnormal in several brain disorders [2–4]. tDCS has indeed been shown to induce long-term potentiation (LTP) and long-term depression (LTD)–like plasticity in humans (e.g., [5–8]). In line with these premises, therapeutic effects of tDCS have been shown in numerous clinical disorders of the central nervous system in both adult and pediatric populations. For recent reviews in the field, see [9–14].

In the current chapter, we provide an updated overview on the therapeutic effects of tDCS for the treatment of anxiety disorders in adult populations according to the Diagnostic and Statistical Manual of Mental Disorders (DSM-5) classification of anxiety disorders [15]. In particular, we aim to examine the currently available literature on the effects of tDCS for the treatment of specific phobias (SP), social anxiety disorder (SAD), panic disorder (PD), agoraphobia, and generalized anxiety disorder (GAD).

According to recent suggestions (e.g., [16]), one important pathological mechanism in anxiety disorders is maladaptive neuroplasticity. Evidence for altered neuroplasticity is shown by studies documenting hypoactivation of the left dorsolateral prefrontal cortex (DLPFC) (e.g., [17, 18]) and hyperactivation of the right DLPFC in anxiety [19]. In line with these premises, tDCS might represent a useful tool to counteract respective patterns of maladaptive neuroplasticity by modulating pathological hypo/hyperactivation of the DLPFC in respective clinical populations. Moreover, the link between prefrontal regions and subcortical regions involved in threat and fear processing (e.g., amygdala) is another rationale for targeting anxiety through modulation of the DLPFC with tDCS [20]. In fact, functional abnormalities of the amygdala, the key neural region of the "fear circuit," have been documented in several anxiety disorders (see [21] for a review).

Since an extended overview of the neurophysiological foundation and mechanisms of action of tDCS is presented in this book, we are here only providing a brief introduction dedicated to this topic. For a more exhaustive/detailed overview, please see also the following recent reviews in the field (e.g., [8, 22–24]).

21.2   Mechanisms of Action of tDCS

tDCS is a well-established noninvasive brain stimulation tool that allows to stimulate the cerebral cortex via two or more electrodes with opposite polarities (i.e., anodal and cathodal) placed on the scalp and connected with a battery-driven constant current stimulator with a maximum output in the milliampere (mA) range [14]. A relatively weak electrical direct current (usually 1–2 mA) is applied via the electrodes, and a proportion of it enters the brain [6, 7, 25–28]. As a general principle, increases of cortical excitability have been documented during and after stimulation with the anode over the target area. On the other hand, a decreased cortical excitability was found to follow stimulation with the cathode over the respective region [8]. A single stimulation session of up to 15-minutes duration affects cortical excitability for up to 90 minutes [7, 26, 29], and this effect can be further extended by repeated stimulation (i.e., cumulative effects) [5]. The prolonged effects of tDCS on cortical excitability are linked to mechanisms of synaptic modulation, as suggested by pharmacological studies in humans [30] and animal models [2, 3]. Evidence suggests that tDCS induces plasticity of glutamatergic synapses, which is calcium dependent. tDCS after-effects (both anodal and cathodal) are prevented by NMDA receptor block but enhanced by respective receptor agonists [6, 7, 31, 32]. Moreover, GABAergic activity is reduced by both anodal and cathodal tDCS [33], and this reduction might serve as a gating mechanism for tDCS-induced plasticity. Because of calcium dynamics involved in glutamatergic plasticity, nonlinear effects are observed if stimulation intensity and duration extend beyond specific limits. Low calcium enhancement of the postsynaptic neuron induces long-term depression (LTD), whereas high concentration is involved in long-term potentiation (LTP) [34]. Extending calcium concentration further activates counter-regulatory mechanisms antagonizing calcium influx, and reduces or converts plasticity induction [35]. This explains why enhancing the stimulation intensity of cathodal tDCS from 1 to 2 mA converts LTD- into LTP-like plasticity [36, 37, 38], and why extending stimulation duration of anodal tDCS from 13 to 26 minutes results in LTD-like plasticity [5].

21.3   Overview of the Available tDCS Studies in Anxiety Disorders

Before reporting the effects of tDCS on anxiety disorders based on the DSM-5 classification, we start with a focus on the efficacy of this technique to modulate trait anxiety, which is a common aspect of all anxiety disorders [39, 40]. Ironside and coworkers [20] examined the effects of tDCS over the prefrontal cortex (PFC) on the behavioral response to a threatening stimulus (i.e., participants were required to perform an attentional task requiring them to ignore threatening face distractors) in individuals with trait anxiety. Additionally, threat-related activation of the amygdala, which is crucially involved in fear generation, was obtained by functional magnetic resonance imaging (fMRI). In this double-blind, within-subject, randomized clinical trial, eighteen women with high trait anxiety (age mean = 23.1; age range, 18–42 years) were included. High trait anxiety was defined as scoring higher than 45 on the Spielberger State-Trait Anxiety Inventory (STAI), which measures the severity of current symptoms of anxiety and a generalized propensity to be anxious [41]. Trait anxiety was further confirmed using the Structured Clinical Interview for DSM-IV disorders. Following a counterbalanced order, active vs. sham tDCS was applied over the left and right DLPFC (i.e., anodal left / cathodal right DLPFC; more details in Table 21.1), in two single sessions, separate by one month. Immediately after (roughly 7 minutes) the end of tDCS, participants began an fMRI emotional task with fearful or neutral facial expressions, in order to study amygdala activation during performance of attentional control over fearful stimuli. The results showed a reduced influence of threat distractors on task accuracy following tDCS. Active tDCS compared to sham improved performance accuracy under low

Table 21.1 A total of 83 participants were involved in all the examined studies

#	Article	Study type (blinding)	N	age (mean ± SD)	Target electrode site	Return electrode/size	Intensity	Duration	Polarity	Control	Measure	Outcome
Specific phobia (SP)												
1	Palm et al. [53]	Open-label study	N = 8	45.6 ± 12.3	Left DLPFC (F3)	Right supraorbit/7 × 5 cm	2 mA	5 × 30 minutes	Anodal	No control	DHI, VSS, HADS	Reduction of DHI scores, no significant reduction of HADS
Social anxiety disorder (SAD)												
2	Heeren et al. [42]	RCT (double blind)	N = 19	24.16 ± 4.87	Left DLPFC (F3)	Ipsilateral arm/7 × 5 cm	2 mA	25 minutes (single session)	Anodal	Sham	Dot-probe task (online)	Decreased attention bias during anodal tDCS
Panic disorder (PD)												
3	Shiozawa et al. [43]	Case study (follow-up)	N = 1	44	Right DLPFC (F4)	Contralateral deltoid/5 × 5 cm	2 mA	10 × 30 minutes	Cathodal	No control	HAS/BAI	Decrease in HAS, BAI
Generalized anxiety disorder (GAD)												
4	Shiozawa et al. [44]	Case study (45-day follow-up)	N = 1	58	Right DLPFC (F4)	Contralateral deltoid/5 × 5 cm	2 mA	15 × 30 minutes	Cathodal	No control	HRS-A/BAI	Decrease in HRS-A, BAI
5	Movahed et al. [45]	RCT (single blind)	N = 18	28.73 ± 9.6	Right DLPFC (F4)	Contralateral deltoid/7 × 5 cm	2 mA	15 × 30 minutes	Cathodal	Sham	HARS, PSWQ	Decrease in HARS, PSWQ

6	Lin et al. [46]	RCT (single blind) (8 weeks follow-up)	N = 20	44.5 ± 10.2	Right DLPFC (F4)	Left mastoid/7 × 5 cm	2 mA	10 × 20 minutes	Cathodal	Sham	HAMA, HAMD	Decrease in HAMA, HAMD
Trait anxiety												
7	Ironside et al. [20]	RCT (double blind)	N = 16	23.1 ± 3.7	Bilateral DLPFC	Right DLPFC/5 × 5 cm	2 mA	20 minutes (single session)	Right cathodal, left anodal	Sham	Attentional load task (offline in the scanner)	Improved attentional control and changes in the amygdala activity

BAI Beck Anxiety Inventory; *DLPFC* dorsolateral prefrontal cortex, *DHI* Dizziness Handicap Inventory, *HADS* Hospital Anxiety and Depression Scale, *HAMD* Hamilton rating scale for depression, *HAMA – HARS –HAS – HRS-A* Hamilton rating scale for anxiety, *PSWQ* Penn State worry questionnaire, *RCT* randomized controlled trial, *SD* standard deviation, *tDCS* transcranial direct current stimulation, *VSS* Vertigo Symptom Scale

attentional load by reducing vigilance to threat. Importantly, this behavioral improvement was accompanied by reduced amygdala activation and increased cortical activation (of the frontal and parietal regions) in response to fearful face distractors under tDCS. This study is an excellent example for the exploration of neurocognitive mechanisms of tDCS on fear processing. It delivers not only information about the alteration of psychological processes via this intervention, but it also suggests moreover respective physiological mechanisms, including activity reduction of the amygdala, which is relevant for fear induction, by altered dorsolateral prefrontal activity generated by tDCS.

21.3.1 tDCS for the Treatment of Panic Disorder (PD)

PD is classified as an anxiety disorder characterized by recurrent panic attacks with several symptoms such as palpitation, sweating, shaking, nausea, dizziness, derealization, and depersonalization [15]. This disorder is characterized by an alteration of the activity of key frontal and limbic areas, such as the medial prefrontal cortex and the amygdala [48]. Recent imaging studies have documented alterations of an even more extended brain network (e.g., [49]), including sensory regions of the occipital, parietal, and temporal cortices and the insula [48].

For the treatment of PD with tDCS, to date, only a case study performed by Shiozawa et al. [43] is available. In this study, a middle-aged woman was treated with ten stimulation sessions (once daily, five sessions per week, for 2 weeks) of cathodal (2 mA) stimulation over the right DLPFC (for more details, refer to Table 21.1). The Hamilton Anxiety Scale (HAS) showed a significant reduction of anxiety symptoms, as compared to baseline scores. Moreover, this pattern remained stable at the 30 days' follow-up. Although promising, the results shown in this single case report are too preliminary to make any firm conclusion about the therapeutic effectiveness of tDCS for the treatment of PD. Further investigations adopting a double-blind/sham-controlled design are recommended.

21.3.2 tDCS for the Treatment of Social Anxiety Disorder (SAD)

SAD is characterized by marked fear, anxiety, or avoidance of social interactions, including situations in which one is scrutinized, or situations in which one is the focus of the attention [15]. Functional and structural alterations of several neural regions, including the fusiform gyrus, thalamus, amygdala, insula, anterior cingulate cortex (ACC), as well as the striatum and DLPFC [50] have been identified to be involved in this disorder. This indicates that SAD, beyond the involvement of core regions relevant for fear and anxiety, is characterized by pathological alterations in a number of additional regions involved in sensory processing and attentional control [50].

Heeren et al. [42] performed a double-blind within-subject protocol in young female individuals with a DSM-5 diagnosis of SAD. Participants received a single session of anodal (2 mA) or sham tDCS over the left DLPFC (more details are reported in Table 21.1) during conduction of a probe discrimination task assessing Attentional Bias (AB). This task was chosen due to evidence that SAD is associated with and maintained by AB for social threat [42]. The results document a significant decrease in AB for threat during anodal tDCS over the left DLPFC as compared to the respective sham stimulation condition. As for PD, the extremely limited literature in the field does not allow to derive clear conclusions about the therapeutic effectiveness of tDCS for the treatment of SAD. Moreover, the only currently available study [42] provides only indirect evidence for some potential of tDCS for the treatment of SAD, as the authors did not include standard clinical measures aiming to compare SAD symptom severity before and after treatment, but used a surrogate marker. Also here, further investigations adopting a double-blind/sham-controlled design are recommended.

21.3.3 tDCS for the Treatment of Generalized Anxiety Disorder (GAD)

Patients affected by GAD are characterized by persistent and excessive worries about a number of different things such as work, family, or money [15]. In terms of pathologically altered neural activation patterns/-rostral anterior cingulate cortex (sg/rACC) and medial prefrontal cortex (mPFC) has been described consistently, while activity alterations of the amygdala and the hippocampus seem to be more variable in GAD [50].

Shiozawa et al. [44] performed the first tDCS single case study in a middle-aged woman affected by GAD. The authors performed 15 consecutive once-daily cathodal tDCS sessions (except for the weekends) over the right DLPFC (more details are reported in Table 21.1); the anode was placed extracephalically over the contralateral deltoid muscle. Stimulation intensity was 2.0 mA. Anxiety symptoms measured via the HAS and Beck Anxiety Inventory (BAI) significantly improved after 15 days of treatment. This improvement remained stable at follow-ups after 30 and 45 days.

More recently [45], a total of 18 patients affected by GAD (46% females and 64% males) were randomly assigned either to (2 mA) cathodal tDCS ($n = 6$) over the right DLPFC (more details are reported in Table 21.1), pharmacotherapy ($n = 6$), or sham stimulation ($n = 6$) in a sham-controlled, double-blind parallel-group study. Symptoms were measured via the HAS. The intervention resulted in significant improvements of the anxiety index in the tDCS and pharmacotherapy groups, as compared to the sham group. The difference between the active intervention methods was not significant.

Finally, Lin et al. [46] conducted a randomized, placebo-controlled, single-blind study in which the effect of cathodal tDCS over the right DLPFC (with the reference electrode over the contralateral mastoid) was investigated in 20 patients diagnosed with GAD. The patients of the real stimulation group ($n = 10$) received 10 days of stimulation with a current intensity of 2 mA, for 20 min per day. The Hamilton Rating

Scales for Anxiety (HAMA) and depression (HAMD) were evaluated at baseline, 2 weeks, 4 weeks, and 8 weeks after the beginning of treatment. They found a significant improvement of the HAMA scores in the real stimulation group 2, 4, and 8 weeks after the start of the treatment, while no symptom improvement was reported in the group that received sham tDCS. In summary, the available study results suggest the right DLPFC as a potential target for the treatment of GAD via cathodal tDCS. The currently available literature in the field is however limited and does not allow to make exhaustive conclusions about the therapeutic efficacy of this stimulation protocol for the treatment of GAD. Nevertheless, compared to tDCS treatment of PD and SAD, the results provided by Movahed et al. [45] and Lin et al. [46] deliver more definite support for the therapeutic effectiveness of right DLPFC tDCS for the treatment of anxiety disorders, as the authors tested two relatively medium-sized samples ($N = 18$, $N = 20$ respectively), and the respective study designs were blinded. Further investigation adopting double-blind/sham-controlled designs is recommended in this regard. Reasonable next steps to enhance the efficacy of the intervention will also include the implementation of mechanistic studies that focus on optimizing approaches (additional stimulation areas, network stimulation, optimization of duration/intensity), and to embrace a larger multicenter perspective.

21.3.4 tDCS for the Treatment of Agoraphobia

Agoraphobia is an anxiety disorder characterized by marked fear or anxiety of situations such as public transportation, open or enclosed spaces [15]. Neuroimaging research [51] has pointed out an increased activation of the insula and the ventral striatum in patients affected by agoraphobia, compared with healthy controls, during anticipation of agoraphobia-specific stimuli. No studies testing the effects of tDCS for the treatment of agoraphobic patients have been performed so far.

21.3.5 tDCS for the Treatment of Specific Phobias (SP)

SP refers to a clinical condition characterized by marked fear, anxiety or avoidance of specific circumstances/situations, such as animals, environments, and others [15]. Results from neuroimaging studies suggest that SP is characterized by an enhanced activation in the insula, DLPFC ACC, amygdala, and prefrontal/orbitofrontal cortices during the processing of phobia-related situations compared to controls [52].

Palm et al. [53] have recently performed the first open-label pilot tDCS study on 8 adult patients affected by phobic postural vertigo (PPV) to modulate disease-related symptoms (vertigo/dizziness). A 2 mA anodal tDCS was applied over the left DLPFC (more details are reported in Table 21.1), once per day for 5 consecutive days. For the assessment of symptoms, the authors used the Vertigo Symptom Scale (VSS) [54], Dizziness Handicap Inventory (DHI) [55], and the Hospital Anxiety and Depression Scale (HADS) [56]. Overall, the results showed a significant reduction of DHI scores. Moreover, anxiety and depression ratings were reported to be moderately improved, however, not significantly. In summary, as the previous anxiety disorders examined in this chapter, the limited literature in the field does not allow to derive firm conclusions about the therapeutic effectiveness of tDCS for the treatment of SP. Further investigations adopting a double-blind/sham-controlled design, as well as extended stimulation protocols, as conducted for other anxiety disorders (see earlier), are recommended.

21.4   Discussion and Future Directions

In this chapter, we provided an overview of all published studies ($N = 6$) investigating the therapeutic effectiveness of tDCS for the treatment of anxiety disorders. Moreover, we have included a recent study testing the effects of tDCS on trait anxiety [20], which is relevant for all anxiety disorders. Overall, the research examined in this chapter provides preliminary evidence in support of the hypothesis that tDCS is a promising therapeutic approach for the treatment of anxiety disorders. However, the extremely limited number of investigations (a total of seven studies, with no research in agoraphobia performed so far), the absence of double-blind/sham-controlled protocols in 4 out of 6 studies performed in anxiety disorders, and the low number of patients in several studies (3 of 7 studies are single case studies) show serious limitations of the current state of research in the field. DLPFC is the major cortical target in the treatment of anxiety disorders via noninvasive brain stimulation, although other cortical targets might represent valid alternatives according to the available physiological literature in the field (see [14] for a review). For instance, in the 57% of the examined studies (4 on 7), the authors chose the right DLPFC as a target with cathodal tDCS to treat anxiety disorders, while 28% of the studies (2 on 7) conducted anodal tDCS over the left DLPFC ($n = 2$); bilateral stimulation over the DLPFC (i.e., anodal left / cathodal right DLPFC) was conducted in one study. Since benefits were reported in response to all types of protocols, it might be concluded that all of these approaches are effective. This pattern of results is in line with a model proposed in a recent systematic review of our group [14], where we suggested that the stimulation of both the left and right DLPFC with anodal and cathodal tDCS, respectively, might counteract maladaptive plasticity of the cortico-meso-limbic network [57] in anxiety disorders, by acting on the up/downregulation mechanisms subserved by these regions for emotional outcomes [14]. In particular, according to this model, benefits from excitatory stimulation of the left DLPFC would be due to the relevance of this region for downregulation of negative emotion (e.g., [58]), and upregulation of positive emotion (e.g., [4, 59]). On the other hand, benefits from inhibitory stimulation over the right DLPFC would be determined from the relevance of this region for downregulation of reactions to negative emotional stimuli/outcomes, in line with evidence that this region is involved in the upregulation of reactions to negative emotional outcomes [60].

The relevance of prefrontal regions, especially the DLPFC, in anxiety disorders can be discussed at least from two perspectives. The first perspective includes the involvement of the DLPFC in cognitive control of behavior and emotion [61].

"Attentional control" and "cognitive change" are two major types of cognitive regulation of emotions that depend on PFC activity [61]. These regulatory strategies modulate both bottom-up and top-down responses to emotional stimuli, which construct expectations for, select alternative interpretations of, and/or make different judgments about emotional stimuli, including fearful objects and threats. This has been the rationale behind recent tDCS studies that aimed to improve emotion regulation through enhancing cognitive control functions in emotional disorders (e.g., [62, 63]).

The second perspective regards, more specifically, the functional connectivity between prefrontal cortical regions and subcortical areas, which allows modulation of threat-related structures (e.g., the amygdala) [20]. While direct modulation of the activity of subcortical regions is not as feasible as modulation of cortical regions by noninvasive brain stimulation techniques, due to effects of regional stimulation on cerebral networks, including subcortical structures [64], it is possible to target subcortical areas indirectly by cortical stimulation. Indeed, evidence from stimulation of the DLPFC and motor areas suggests that tDCS can alter activation and connectivity in regions distant from the electrodes [64, 65].

In the context of research exploring the relevance of the prefrontal cortex as a neural target for the treatment of anxiety disorders via tDCS, it might be relevant to extend respective investigation to the ventro-medial PFC (vmPFC), whose relevance for the treatment of anxiety disorders has been explored only with transcranial magnetic stimulation (rTMS) so far [66]. The vmPFC is reciprocally connected with the amygdala, which is known to be dysfunctional in anxiety disorders [50, 67]. It has moreover been shown to be directly involved in downregulation of negative affective responses [68], and upregulation of positive (rewarding) outcomes [69], which makes it an interesting target for anxiety modulation. In the same line, stimulation of additional areas, which have been shown to be involved in specific syndromes, might be of interest in future studies. This might also include network stimulation approaches.

Lastly, while in this chapter we only included the application of tDCS in anxiety disorders according to the DSM 5 diagnostic criteria, some tDCS studies are available for effects in post-traumatic stress disorder (PTSD) and obsessive–compulsive disorder (OCD). The results from these parallel research fields further enrich the picture on the effects of tDCS in the treatment of anxiety and anxiety-related disorders (e.g., [70–72]). For example, van't Wout-Frank et al. [72] observed a significant reduction of arousal (i.e., reduced skin conductance response) and a clinically meaningful reduction of symptom severity in PTSD in response to tDCS over the vmPFC.

21.4.1 Maximizing Clinical Efficacy

The research discussed here so far refers to pilot studies that were primarily designed to examine the principal efficacy of tDCS in anxiety disorders, aimed to determine whether conducting further research in the field would be promising. Most of the studies were not designed to optimize tDCS efficacy and draw definite conclusions about the implementation of tDCS for clinical treatment of anxiety disorders. Based on the principally promising results of these pilot studies, the next step would be to design studies for optimizing the stimulation protocols in order to maximize clinical efficacy. In this prospective, future studies are recommended to consider optimization approaches, which we will briefly discuss here. These approaches include: [15] optimizing stimulation parameters (i.e., stimulation area, polarity, intensity, duration, repetition, etc.) and [47] combining tDCS with other techniques.

Parameters of respective stimulation protocols play an important role in the efficacy of tDCS and these should be considered and systematically investigated in future studies. The first important parameter is the stimulation target area, which was already briefly discussed in the previous section. Right DLPFC (4 of 7 studies) and left DLPFC (3 of 7 studies) were the only targeted regions in the discussed studies, which are in line with the suggested up/downregulation model of anxiety disorders [14]. Yet, further studies are required to systematically investigate the effects of unilateral / bilateral stimulation of both right and DLPFC regions, which might enhance efficacy of interventions. Furthermore, other target areas might be attractive candidates. The medial PFC, including the VMPFC, is a potentially important region in regulating emotions and anxiety, but also other areas, as discussed earlier, might be relevant. Another important stimulation parameter is stimulation polarity, which is closely associated with the intended LTP- or LTD-like effects of the target area [6, 7, 26]. In the studies conducted so far, the right DLPFC received cathodal stimulation to reduce excitability, and the left DLPFC anodal stimulation to enhance excitability. The underlying rationale is to counteract respective pathological activity reductions of the left, and enhancements of the right DLPFC, which have been identified in anxiety disorders, and share similarities with respective alterations in depression [73].

In addition to tDCS montage (e.g., stimulation area and polarity, and also electrode size), stimulation intensity, duration, and repetition rate contribute to the efficacy of stimulation protocols. Findings from stimulation studies in other clinical fields (e.g., tinnitus [74], cognitive functions in Parkinson's disease [75], schizophrenia [76]) show that higher intensities of stimulation can result in more effective symptom improvement. However, the relationship between increased intensity and magnitude of the respective effects is not necessarily linear. It was recently shown that different intensities of anodal stimulation have similar effects on motor cortex plasticity at the group level [29], whereas the intensity-dependent effect of cathodal tDCS includes nonlinearities [36, 37, 77]. However, all of the above-mentionend studies were conducted with healthy adults. That said, the transferability of such nonlinear effects on clinical symptoms and cognitive/behavioral performance is not yet clear and needs further investigation. Due to pathologically altered cerebral activity in clinical syndromes, a one-to-one transferability might not be given, and thus titration studies in clinical populations are required to identify the optimal stimulation intensity in anxiety disorders .

Extension of the duration of stimulation sessions and repetitive stimulation are other factors to consider in order to improve the clinical efficacy of tDCS. tDCS studies on motor cortex excitability show that a longer duration of tDCS within a specific time frame is able to prolong induced plasticity in the human motor cortex [6, 7, 26, 78], and that repetition within specific intervals enhances efficacy [5]. However, similarly to what has been observed in terms of stimulation intensity, a nonlinear relation between stimulation duration, repetitive stimulation, and observed effects on cortical excitability should be taken into consideration [5, 36, 37]. Finally, repetition rate is another important parameter to consider in order to enhance clinical efficacy of tDCS. Previous tDCS studies in clinical populations have shown that the efficacy of tDCS over motor and prefrontal regions is boosted by repeated sessions of stimulation [79, 80]. Optimizing stimulation protocols in anxiety disorders by adapting these parameters might improve tDCS efficacy and provide a more realistic picture of its clinical potential. Considering that daily stimulation over 4–6 weeks is required in order to achieve a clinically significant effects of rTMS in depression [81, 82], it might well be that most of the clinical tDCS studies conducted so far are relevantly underpowered.

In addition to the stimulation parameters discussed here, it is important to discuss the combination of tDCS with other standard interventions in anxiety disorders as an additional optimizing strategy. Behavioral, cognitive, and psychological interventions are major treatment approaches in anxiety disorders, which can be combined with tDCS to increase clinical efficacy. Previous studies showed sustained and longer symptom improvement following tDCS combined with cognitive training or psychological interventions in some neuropsychiatric disorders, including depression [47, 83, 84]. The respective sustained improvement of symptoms achieved by such combined therapies can be explained by fostering the formation of new memories induced by therapeutic approaches, which include relearning, enhancement of cognitive control [47], and other processes via tDCS-induced plasticity enhancement. Moreover, the combination of tDCS with pharmacological interventions further boosts the neuroplastic effects of tDCS (for an overview, see [4, 30]), which might have clinical relevance [85, 86].

21.5 Conclusion

In summary, the current state of research suggests that tDCS might be an efficient tool for the treatment of anxiety disorders. However, the low number of high-quality investigations in this field does not allow to make definite conclusions. Future investigations should not only enhance the number of available studies but also take into account approaches that might qualitatively improve the field. These includes (1) double-blind, sham-controlled protocols with a relatively high number of participants; (2) systematic titration of stimulation parameters such as intensity, duration, repetition rate/intervals, and cortical targets for optimization; (3) combination of tDCS with standard therapies such as cognitive-behavioral therapy and/or pharmacotherapy; (4) combination of tDCS with physiological measures, such as functional imaging, including fMRI, EEG, and vegetative parameters (e.g., heart rate and skin conductance), which provide important neurophysiological indices, in addition to the behavioral changes induced via tDCS [22]. Moreover, as suggested in our recent work [14], to specifically test the up/downregulation model mentioned earlier, the exposure to positive/negative emotional stimuli should be systematically included in future investigations in the field.

Declaration of Interests This work was supported by grants from the (1) Alexander von Humboldt Foundation, Germany; (2) The SFB 1280—Extinction learning; (3) BMBF GCBS project (grant 01EE1403C). M.A.S receives support from the Ministry of Science, Research & Technology, Deputy of Scholarship and Students Affairs, Iran, grant number: 95000171. All authors declare no competing interests.

References

1. Krishnan C, Santos L, Peterson MD, Ehinger M. Safety of noninvasive brain stimulation in children and adolescents. Brain Stimul. 2015;8(1):76–87.
2. Kronberg G, Bridi M, Abel T, Bikson M, Parra LC. Direct current stimulation modulates LTP and LTD: activity dependence and dendritic effects. Brain Stimul. 2017;10(1):51–8.
3. Fritsch B, Reis J, Martinowich K, Schambra HM, Ji Y, Cohen LG, Lu B. Direct current stimulation promotes BDNF-dependent synaptic plasticity: potential implications for motor learning. Neuron. 2010;66(2):198–204.
4. Nitsche MA, Müller-Dahlhaus F, Paulus W, Ziemann U. The pharmacology of neuroplasticity induced by non-invasive brain stimulation: building models for the clinical use of CNS active drugs. J Physiol. 2012;590(19):4641–62.
5. Monte-Silva K, Kuo MF, Hessenthaler S, Fresnoza S, Liebetanz D, Paulus W, Nitsche MA. Induction of late LTP-like plasticity in the human motor cortex by repeated non-invasive brain stimulation. Brain Stimul. 2013;6(3):424–32.
6. Nitsche MA, Fricke K, Henschke U, Schlitterlau A, Liebetanz D, Lang N, Henning S, Tergau F, Paulus W. Pharmacological modulation of cortical excitability shifts induced by transcranial direct current stimulation in humans. J Physiol. 2003;553(Pt 1):293–301.
7. Nitsche MA, Liebetanz D, Antal A, Lang N, Tergau F, Paulus W. Modulation of cortical excitability by weak direct current stimulation – technical, safety and functional aspects. Suppl Clin Neurophysiol. 2003;56:255–76.
8. Stagg CJ, Nitsche MA. Physiological basis of transcranial direct current stimulation. Neuroscientist. 2011;17(1):37–53.
9. Kuo MF, Paulus W, Nitsche MA. Therapeutic effects of non-invasive brain stimulation with direct currents (tDCS) in neuropsychiatric diseases. Neuroimage. 2014;85(Pt 3):948–60.
10. Rivera-Urbina GN, Nitsche MA, Vicario CM, Molero-Chamizo A. Applications of transcranial direct current stimulation in children and pediatrics. Rev Neurosci. 2017;28(2):173–84.
11. Salehinejad MA, Wischnewski M, Nejati V, Vicario CM, Nitsche MA. Transcranial direct current stimulation in attention-deficit hyperactivity disorder: a meta-analysis of neuropsychological deficits. PLoS One. 2019;14(4):e0215095.
12. Vicario CM, Nitsche MA. Non-invasive brain stimulation for the treatment of brain diseases in childhood and adolescence: state of the art, current limits and future challenges. Front Syst Neurosci. 2013;7:94.
13. Vicario CM, Nitsche MA. Transcranial direct current stimulation: a remediation tool for the treatment of childhood congenital dyslexia? Front Hum Neurosci. 2013;7:139.
14. Vicario CM, Salehinejad MA, Felmingham K, Martino G, Nitsche MA. A systematic review on the therapeutic effectiveness of non-invasive brain stimulation for the treatment of anxiety disorders. Neurosci Biobehav Rev. 2019;96:219–31.
15. American Psychiatric Association: Diagnostic and Statistical Manual of Mental Disorders, Fifth Edition. Washington, DC: American Psychiatric Association Publishing; 2013.

16. Månsson KN, Salami A, Frick A, Carlbring P, Andersson G, Furmark T, Boraxbekk CJ. Neuroplasticity in response to cognitive behavior therapy for social anxiety disorder. Transl Psychiatry. 2016;6:e727.
17. Etkin A, Wager TD. Functional neuroimaging of anxiety: a meta-analysis of emotional processing in PTSD, social anxiety disorder, and specific phobia. Am J Psychiatry. 2007;164(10):1476–88.
18. Nishimura Y, Tanii H, Fukuda M, Kajiki N, Inoue K, Kaiya H, Nishida A, Okada M, Okazaki Y. Frontal dysfunction during a cognitive task in drug-naive patients with panic disorder as investigated by multi-channel near-infrared spectroscopy imaging. Neurosci Res. 2007;59(1):107–12.
19. Prasko J, Horácek J, Záleský R, Kopecek M, Novák T, Pasková B, Skrdlantová L, Belohlávek O, Höschl C. The change of regional brain metabolism (18FDG PET) in panic disorder during the treatment with cognitive behavioral therapy or antidepressants. Neuro Endocrinol Lett. 2004;25(5):340–8.
20. Ironside M, Browning M, Ansari TL, et al. Effect of prefrontal cortex stimulation on regulation of amygdala response to threat in individuals with trait anxiety: a randomized clinical trial. JAMA Psychiat. 2019;76(1):71–8.
21. Adolphs R. Fear, faces, and the human amygdala. Curr Opin Neurobiol. 2008;18(2):166–72.
22. Polanía R, Nitsche MA, Ruff CC. Studying and modifying brain function with non-invasive brain stimulation. Nat Neurosci. 2018;21(2):174–87.
23. Woods AJ, Antal A, Bikson M, Boggio PS, Brunoni AR, Celnik P, Cohen LG, Fregni F, Herrmann CS, Kappenman ES, Knotkova H, Liebetanz D, Miniussi C, Miranda PC, Paulus W, Priori A, Reato D, Stagg C, Wenderoth N, Nitsche MA. A technical guide to tDCS, and related non-invasive brain stimulation tools. Clin Neurophysiol. 2016;127(2):1031–48.
24. Stagg CJ, Antal A, Nitsche MA. Physiology of transcranial direct current stimulation. J ECT. 2018;34(3):144–52.
25. Nitsche MA, Cohen LG, Wassermann EM, Priori A, Lang N, Antal A, Paulus W, Hummel F, Boggio PS, Fregni F, Pascual-Leone A. Transcranial direct current stimulation: state of the art 2008. Brain Stimul. 2008;1(3):206–23.
26. Nitsche MA, Paulus W. Excitability changes induced in the human motor cortex by weak transcranial direct current stimulation. J Physiol. 2000;527(Pt 3):633–9.
27. Opitz A, Paulus W, Will S, Antunes A, Thielscher A. Determinants of the electric field during transcranial direct current stimulation. Neuroimage. 2015;109:140.
28. Opitz A, Falchier A, Yan CG, Yeagle EM, Linn GS, Megevand P, Thielscher A, Deborah AR, Milham MP, Mehta AD, Schroeder CE. Spatiotemporal structure of intracranial electric fields induced by transcranial electric stimulation in humans and nonhuman primates. Sci Rep. 2016;6:31236.
29. Jamil A, Batsikadze G, Kuo H-I, et al. Systematic evaluation of the impact of stimulation intensity on neuroplastic after-effects induced by transcranial direct current stimulation. J Physiol. 2017;595(4):1273–88.
30. Nitsche MA, Koschack J, Pohlers H, Hullemann S, Paulus W, Happe S. Effects of frontal transcranial direct current stimulation on emotional state and processing in healthy humans. Front Psych. 2012;3:58.
31. Nitsche MA, Liebetanz D, Schlitterlau A, Henschke U, Fricke K, Frommann K, Lang N, Henning S, Paulus W, Tergau F. GABAergic modulation of DC stimulation-induced motor cortex excitability shifts in humans. Eur J Neurosci. 2004;19(10):2720–6.
32. Nitsche MA, Seeber A, Frommann K, Klein CC, Rochford C, Nitsche MS, Fricke K, Liebetanz D, Lang N, Antal A, Paulus W, Tergau F. Modulating parameters of excitability during and after transcranial direct current stimulationof the human motor cortex. J Physiol. 2005;568(Pt 1): 291–303.
33. Stagg CJ, Best JG, Stephenson MC, O'Shea J, Wylezinska M, Kincses ZT, Morris PG, Matthews PM, Johansen-Berg H. Polarity-sensitive modulation of cortical neurotransmitters by transcranial stimulation. J Neurosci. 2009;29;5202–6.
34. Lisman JE. Three Ca2+ levels affect plasticity differently: the LTP zone, the LTD zone and no man's land. J Physiol. 2001;532(Pt 2):28.

35. Misonou H, Mohapatra DP, Park EW, Leung V, Zhen D, Misonou K, Anderson AE, Trimmer JS. Regulation of ion channel localization and phosphorylation by neuronal activity. Nat Neurosci. 2004;7(7):711–8.
36. Batsikadze G, Moliadze V, Paulus W, Kuo MF, Nitsche MA. Partially non-linear stimulation intensity-dependent effects of direct current stimulation on motor cortex excitability in humans. J Physiol. 2013;591(7):1987–2000.
37. Batsikadze G, Paulus W, Kuo MF, Nitsche MA. Effect of serotonin on paired associative stimulation-induced plasticity in the human motorcortex. Neuropsychopharmacology. 2013;38(11):2260–7.
38. Mosayebi Samani M, Agboada D, Kuo MF, Nitsche MA. Probing the relevance of repeated cathodal transcranial direct current stimulation over the primary motor cortex for prolongation of after-effects. J Physiol. 2020;598(4):805-16.
39. Sandi C, Richter-Levin G. From high anxiety trait to depression: a neurocognitive hypothesis. Trends Neurosci. 2009;32(6):312–20.
40. Weger M, Sandi C. High anxiety trait: a vulnerable phenotype for stress-induced depression. Neurosci Biobehav Rev. 2018;87:27–37.
41. Julian LJ. Measures of anxiety: State-Trait Anxiety Inventory (STAI), Beck Anxiety Inventory (BAI), and Hospital Anxiety and Depression Scale-Anxiety (HADS-A). Arthritis Care Res (Hoboken). 2011;63(Suppl 11):S467–S72.
42. Heeren A, Billieux J, Philippot P, De Raedt R, Baeken C, de Timary P, Maurage P, Vanderhasselt MA. Impact of transcranial direct current stimulation on attentional bias for threat: a proof-of-concept study among individuals with social anxiety disorder. Soc Cogn Affect Neurosci. 2017;12(2):251–60.
43. Shiozawa P, da Silva M, Cordeiro Q. Transcranial direct current stimulation (tDCS) for panic disorder: a case study. J Depress Anxiety. 2014;3:3.
44. Shiozawa P, Leiva AP, Castro CD, da Silva ME, Cordeiro Q, Fregni F, Brunoni AR. Transcranial direct current stimulation for generalized anxiety disorder: a case study. Biol Psychiatry. 2014;75(11):e17–8.
45. Movahed FS, Goradel JA, Pouresmali A, Mowlaie M. Effectiveness of transcranial direct current stimulation on worry, anxiety, and depression in generalized anxiety disorder: a randomized, single-blind pharmacotherapy and sham-controlled clinical trial. Iran J Psychiatry Behav Sci. 2018;12:e11071.
46. Lin Y, Zhang C, Wang Y. A randomized controlled study of transcranial direct current stimulation in treatment of generalized anxiety disorder. Brain Stimul. 2019;12(2).403.
47. Bajbouj M, Aust S, Spies J, et al. PsychotherapyPlus: augmentation of cognitive behavioral therapy (CBT) with prefrontal transcranial direct current stimulation (tDCS) in major depressive disorder—study design and methodology of a multicenter double-blind randomized placebo-controlled trial. Eur Arch Psychiatry Clin Neurosci. 2018;268(8):797–808.
48. Lai CH. Fear network model in panic disorder: the past and the future. Psychiatry Investig. 2019;16(1):16–26.
49. Sobanski T, Wagner G. Functional neuroanatomy in panic disorder: Status quo of the research. World J Psychiatry. 2017;7(1):12–33.
50. Duval ER, Javanbakht A, Liberzon I. Neural circuits in anxiety and stress disorders: a focused review. Ther Clin Risk Manag. 2015;11:115–26.
51. Wittmann A, Schlagenhauf F, Guhn A, Lueken U, Gaehlsdorf C, Stoy M, Bermpohl F, Fydrich T, Pfleiderer B, Bruhn H, Gerlach AL, Kircher T, Straube B, Wittchen HU, Arolt V, Heinz A, Ströhle A. Anticipating agoraphobic situations: the neural correlates of panic disorder with agoraphobia. Psychol Med. 2014;44(11):2385–96.
52. Linares IM, Trzesniak C, Chagas MH, Hallak JE, Nardi AE, Crippa JA. Neuroimaging in specific phobia disorder: a systematic review of the literature. Braz J Psychiatry. 2012;34(1):101–11. Review.
53. Palm U, Kirsch V, Kübler H, Sarubin N, Keeser D, Padberg F, Dieterich M. Transcranial direct current stimulation (tDCS)for treatment of phobic postural vertigo: an open label pilot study. Eur Arch Psychiatry Clin Neurosci. 2019;269(2):269–72.

54. Yardley L, Masson E, Verschuur C, Haacke N, Luxon L. Symptoms, anxiety and handicap in dizzy patients: development of the vertigo symptom scale. J Psychosom Res. 1992;36(8):731–41.
55. Jacobson GP, Newman CW. The development of the dizziness handicap inventory. Arch Otolaryngol Head Neck Surg. 1990;116:424–7.
56. Zigmond AS, Snaith RP. The Hospital anxiety and depression scale. Acta Psychiatr Scand. 1983;67:361–70.
57. Banks SJ, Eddy KT, Angstadt M, Nathan PJ, Phan KL. Amygdala-frontal connectivity during emotion regulation. Soc Cogn Affect Neurosci. 2007;2(4):303–12.
58. Peña-Gómez C, Vidal-Piñeiro D, Clemente IC, Pascual-Leone Á, Bartrés-Faz D. Downregulation of negative emotional processing by transcranial direct current stimulation: effects of personality characteristics. PLoS One. 2011;6(7):e22812.
59. Vanderhasselt MA, De Raedt R, Brunoni AR, Campanhã C, Baeken C, Remue J, Boggio PS. tDCS over the left prefrontal cortex enhances cognitive control for positive affective stimuli. PLoS One. 2013;8(5):e62219.
60. De Raedt R, Leyman L, Baeken C, Van Schuerbeek P, Luypaert R, Vanderhasselt MA, Dannlowski U. Neurocognitive effects of HF-rTMS over the dorsolateral prefrontal cortex on the attentionalprocessing of emotional information in healthy women: an event-related fMRI study. Biol Psychol. 2010;85(3):487–95.
61. Ochsner KN, Gross JJ. The cognitive control of emotion. Trends Cogn Sci. 2005;9(5):242–9.
62. Brunoni AR, Tortella G, Benseñor IM, Lotufo PA, Carvalho AF, Fregni F. Cognitive effects of transcranial direct current stimulation in depression: results from the SELECT-TDCS trial and insights for further clinical trials. J Affect Disord. 2016;202:46–52.
63. Salehinejad MA, Ghanavai E, Rostami R, Nejati V. Cognitive control dysfunction in emotion dysregulation and psychopathology of major depression (MD): evidence from transcranial brain stimulation of the dorsolateral prefrontal cortex (DLPFC). J Affect Disord. 2017;210:241–8.
64. Polanía R, Paulus W, Nitsche MA. Modulating cortico-striatal and thalamo-cortical functional connectivity with transcranial direct current stimulation. Hum Brain Mapp. 2012;33(10):2499–508.
65. Weber MJ, Messing SB, Rao H, Detre JA, Thompson-Schill SL. Prefrontal transcranial direct current stimulation alters activation and connectivity in cortical and subcortical reward systems: a tDCS-fMRI study. Hum Brain Mapp. 2014;35(8):3673–86.
66. Paes F, Baczynski T, Novaes F, Marinho T, Arias-Carrión O, Budde H, Sack AT, Huston JP, Almada LF, Carta M, Silva AC, Nardi AE, Machado S. Repetitive Transcranial Magnetic Stimulation (rTMS) to treat social anxiety disorder: casereports and a review of the literature. Clin Pract Epidemiol Ment Health. 2013;9:180–8.
67. Herry C, Ciocchi S, Senn V, Demmou L, Müller C, Lüthi A. Switching on and off fear by distinct neuronal circuits. Nature. 2008;454(7204):600–6.
68. Diekhof EK, Geier K, Falkai P, Gruber O. Fear is only as deep as the mind allows: a coordinate-based meta-analysis of neuroimagingstudies on the regulation of negative affect. Neuroimage. 2011;58(1):275–85.
69. Hutcherson CA, Plassmann H, Gross JJ, Rangel A. Cognitive regulation during decision making shifts behavioral control between ventromedialand dorsolateral prefrontal value systems. J Neurosci. 2012;32(39):13543–54.
70. Brunelin J, Mondino M, Bation R, Palm U, Saoud M, Poulet E. Transcranial direct current stimulation for obsessive-compulsive disorder: a systematic review. Brain Sci. 2018;8(2):37.
71. Gowda SM, Narayanaswamy JC, Hazari N, et al. Efficacy of pre-supplementary motor area transcranial direct current stimulation for treatment resistant obsessive compulsive disorder: a randomized, double blinded, sham controlled trial. Brain Stimul. 2019;12:922–9.
72. van't Wout-Frank M, Shea MT, Larson VC, Greenberg BD, Philip NS. Combined transcranial direct current stimulation with virtual reality exposure for posttraumatic stress disorder: feasibility and pilot results. Brain Stimul. 2019;12(1):41–3.

73. Grimm S, Beck J, Schuepbach D, et al. Imbalance between left and right dorsolateral pre-frontal cortex in major depression is linked to negative emotional judgment: an fMRI study in severe major depressive disorder. Biol Psychiatry. 2008;63(4):369–76.
74. Shekhawat GS, Sundram F, Bikson M, et al. Intensity, duration, and location of high-definition transcranial direct current stimulation for tinnitus relief. Neurorehabil Neural Repair. 2016;30(4):349–59.
75. Boggio PS, Ferrucci R, Rigonatti SP, et al. Effects of transcranial direct current stimulation on working memory in patients with Parkinson's disease. J Neurol Sci. 2006;249(1):31–8.
76. Hoy KE, Arnold SL, Emonson MRL, Daskalakis ZJ, Fitzgerald PB. An investigation into the effects of tDCS dose on cognitive performance over time in patients with schizophrenia. Schizophr Res. 2014;155(1):96–100.
77. Mosayebi Samani M, Agboada D, Jamil A, Kuo M-F, Nitsche MA. Titrating the neuroplastic effects of cathodal transcranial direct current stimulation (tDCS) over the primary motor cortex. Cortex. 2019;119:350–61.
78. Nitsche MA, Paulus W. Sustained excitability elevations induced by transcranial DC motor cortex stimulation in humans. Neurology. 2001;57(10):1899–901.
79. Fregni F, Boggio PS, Nitsche MA, Rigonatti SP, Pascual-Leone A. Cognitive effects of repeated sessions of transcranial direct current stimulation in patients with depression. Depress Anxiety. 2006;23(8):482–4.
80. Ho K-A, Taylor JL, Chew T, et al. The effect of Transcranial Direct Current Stimulation (tDCS) electrode size and current intensity on motor cortical excitability: evidence from single and repeated sessions. Brain Stimul. 2016;9(1):1–7.
81. McClintock SM, Reti IM, Carpenter LL, et al. Consensus recommendations for the clinical application of Repetitive Transcranial Magnetic Stimulation (rTMS) in the treatment of depression. J Clin Psychiatry. 2018;79(1). pii: 16cs10905.
82. O'Reardon JP, Solvason HB, Janicak PG, Sampson S, Isenberg KE, Nahas Z, McDonald WM, Avery D, Fitzgerald PB, Loo C, Demitrack MA, George MS, Sackeim HA. Efficacy and safety of transcranial magnetic stimulation in the acute treatment of major depression: a multisite randomized controlled trial. Biol Psychiatry. 2007;62(11):1208–16.
83. Nejati V, Salehinejad MA, Shahidi N, Abedin A. Psychological intervention combined with direct electrical brain stimulation (PIN-CODES) for treating major depression: a pre-test, post-test, follow-up pilot study. Neurol Psychiatry Brain Res. 2017;25:15–23.
84. Segrave RA, Arnold S, Hoy K, Fitzgerald PB. Concurrent cognitive control training augments the antidepressant efficacy of tDCS: a pilot study. Brain Stimul. 2014;7(2):325–31.
85. Brunoni AR, Valiengo L, Baccaro A, et al. The sertraline vs electrical current therapy for treating depression clinical study: results from a factorial, randomized, controlled trial. JAMA Psychiat. 2013;70(4):383–91.
86. Valiengo L, Benseñor IM, Goulart AC, et al. The sertraline versus electrical current therapy for treating depression clinical study (select-TDCS): results of the crossover and follow-up phases. Depress Anxiety. 2013;30(7):646–53.

tES in Dementia: From Pathophysiology to Treatment

22

Arianna Menardi, Bradmon Manor,
and Emiliano Santarnecchi

Modern societies are currently facing a rapid growth of their older adults' population as a function of increased life expectancies and overall greater wellbeing. Consequently, fast therapeutic advances in the treatment of aging-related pathologies are also becoming necessary. Pharmacological interventions and cognitive stimulation approaches remain the leading standards in the field, despite being characterized by potentially serious side-effects and the necessity of longstanding commitment, respectively. In recent years, noninvasive brain stimulation (NIBS) has been proven useful in boosting cognitive and motor performances in healthy young adults, leading to the query of whether similar beneficial effects could be translated to older age

A. Menardi
Padova Neuroscience Center, Department of Neuroscience,
University of Padova, Padova, Italy

Siena Brain Investigation and Neuromodulation Laboratory,
University of Siena School of Medicine, Siena, Italy

B. Manor
Hinda and Arthur Marcus Institute for Aging Research, Hebrew Senior Life,
Boston, MA, USA

Harvard Medical School, Boston, MA, USA
e-mail: bradmanor@hsl.harvard.edu

E. Santarnecchi (✉)
Siena Brain Investigation and Neuromodulation Laboratory,
University of Siena School of Medicine, Siena, Italy

Harvard Medical School, Boston, MA, USA

Berenson-Allen Center for Non-invasive Brain Stimulation,
Beth Israel Deaconess Medical Center, Boston, MA, USA
e-mail: esantarn@bidmc.harvard.edu

© Springer Nature Switzerland AG 2020
B. Dell'Osso, G. Di Lorenzo (eds.), *Non Invasive Brain Stimulation
in Psychiatry and Clinical Neurosciences*,
https://doi.org/10.1007/978-3-030-43356-7_22

individuals as well. Compared to young, older adults are known to undergo substantial structural and functional reorganizations of their brains, exacerbated in the presence of dementia, which are strongly influenced by genetic and environmental factors. Substantial differences in brain functioning are detected since the beginning of the aging curve as a matter of a progressive substantial decrease in gray matter volume and white matter tracts, as well as in a preponderant loss of hemispheric specificity (Hemispheric Asymmetry Reduction in Older Adults, HAROLD [1]) and a progressive more effortful cognitive processing, requiring greater frontal lobe involvement compared to younger individuals (Posterior to Anterior Shift in Aging, PASA [2]). Although cognitive decay accompanies normal aging, its progressive worsening can limit individuals' independence, first resulting in a diagnosis of Mild Cognitive Impairment (MCI) and subsequently dementia. The most common forms of neurodegenerative diseases include Alzheimer's Disease (AD) and Frontotemporal Dementia (FTD), followed by other conditions such as Parkinson's Disease (PD) and Dementia with Lewy Bodies (DLB). Although each differs clinically, certain shared elements exist that make dementia an interesting target for transcranial electrical stimulation (tES). First of all, cortical atrophy generally starts in a limited region of the brain and progressively propagates toward the surrounding tissues. As an example, the entorhinal cortex is where AD is believed to start, followed by the hippocampi and temporal lobes, until when the whole neocortex becomes affected. PD, on the other hand, is characterized by loss of dopaminergic neurons starting in the substantia nigra and progressively involving frontostriatal pathways. This leads to a second important aspect, which is the presence of proteinopathy, meaning an excessive accumulation of—and failure to clear—altered proteins. Examples of such proteins include amyloid-β plaques, tau neurofibrillary tangles, and Lewy Bodies aggregates, whose combination and presence is shared across dementia's types. As the protein cascade hypothesis is nowadays believed not to be the only mechanism contributing to neurodegeneration, substantial interest is directed toward the role of glial activation and neuroinflammation as new therapeutic targets [3]. A third and last element binding different forms of dementia seems to be the occurrence of cortical atrophy along defined pathways that mirror the topography of networks in the brain. In AD, a gradual disaggregation of the Default Mode Network (DMN) is observed along a posterior-ventral and anterior-dorsal gradient [4], which not only mirrors the pattern of decay reported by other clinical biomarkers (e.g., amyloidosis and hippocampal atrophy) [5], but also shows a significant correlation with the emergent symptomatology [4]. Concomitantly, greater Salience Network (SN) activity is observed [6], whereas the opposite pattern (decreased SN activity and enhanced DMN activity) characterizes FTD [3].

Each of the aforementioned features of dementia represents a critical target and an important starting point for therapeutic and rehabilitative strategies. tES is a useful tool in this direction, as its induced electrical field is less focal compared to that of other techniques, such as Transcranial Magnetic Stimulation (TMS), making it suitable for the targeting of broader cortical regions and brain networks. Moreover, recent results have demonstrated that its repeated application may be efficacious in increasing plasma levels of amyloid-β, which are lower in AD patients compared to healthy controls [7]. Brain stimulation interventions have therefore been developed with the intent to induce more young-like brain functional patterns or to reduce excessive cortical excitability seen in older patients. In doing so, tES has come particularly helpful as it can be used to facilitate depolarization (excitatory effect) or hyperpolarization (inhibitory effect) of the resting membrane potentials of neurons, therefore modulating neuronal firing. Compared to other NIBS techniques, such as TMS, tES is at a lower risk of inducing adverse events, such as epileptic seizures, which can arise in individuals with pathologically higher cortical excitability. Finally, devices are relatively flexible and allow stimulation to be carried out while comfortably at home or during sleep, easing the administration of intervention therapies (see Fig. 22.1). As more evidence is collected on the use of tES as a therapeutic tool in the aging population, the introduction of the concept of *perturbation-based biomarkers* is also foreseen. Altered response patterns to external perturbations might indeed highlight abnormal brain responses, which could in turn ease the discrimination between normal versus pathological functional decay. In this sense, the use of NIBS techniques may become fundamental to detect brain dysfunctions before cognitive symptoms become overt.

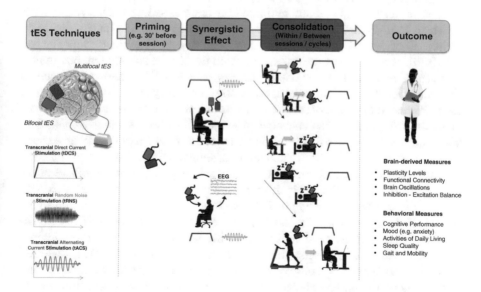

Fig. 22.1 tES application modalities and measurable outcomes. (Left) Different electrode montages can be applied to deliver different current shapes. (Center) The versatility of tES protocols is shown, allowing stimulation to be carried out in various settings, such as before, during, or after cognitive-motor training or in resting-state scenarios, including sleep. (Right) Quantitative outcome measures, for which positive effects have been reported following tES, are listed

22.1 tES and Cognition

22.1.1 Healthy Aging

Functional rearrangements occurring along the aging curve progressively result in a reduction in hemispheres' specialization (HAROLD model [1]), accompanied by a greater need of recruiting frontal regions to carry out a task at hand (PASA model [2]). Both models are at least partly believed to represent compensatory strategies by the brain, which might in turn represent the target of modulatory approaches by means of tES. As such, most stimulation protocols have been ideated either to (1) aid compensatory mechanisms (for example, stimulating frontal regions to boost their role in sustaining task execution) or by (2) contrasting functional shifts, trying to restore young-like cortical recruitment patterns (for example, inhibiting excessive frontal involvement or reducing the cortical hyperexcitability seen in old age). For instance, left and right anterior temporal lobe stimulation has been applied to improve proper names recall in young subjects and elderly adults. Greater improvement was seen when the truthful neural substrate was stimulated in the young group, whereas older adults benefitted more when the opposite (left) lobe was targeted [8], suggesting that stimulation of the nondominant hemisphere could aid compensatory mechanisms that are in action to support task's request, with higher benefits for the aged group. By means of an opposite approach, semantic word generation was ameliorated in healthy older adults by inhibiting the excessive frontal hyperactivity, which in turn promoted the establishment of more young-like patterns of brain activity, as evidenced by resting-state functional Magnetic Resonance Imaging (rs-fMRI) [9]. Irrespective of the rationale behind the chosen stimulation, one important aspect reported in older adults' studies concerns the timeframe needed to observe a significant effect. Indeed, especially in memory consolidation protocols, improvement in the recall of previously learnt information has been reported in the hours following, rather than concomitantly, the stimulation. As an example, older adults showed a less steep forgetting curve 1 week after a series of learning sessions where they received sham or anodal transcranial Direct Current Stimulation (a-tDCS), whereas learning rate was not affected [10], suggesting an offline effect on consolidation. Similarly, significant improvement in a free-recall task was observed in the 48 h following a-tDCS, with no substantial effect on immediate recall [11]. In a prior study, the same authors tested the effects of a-tDCS administered during a reminder session of a previously learnt list of words, resulting in a significant reduction in the forgetting rate from 3 to 30 days after [12]. Repeated stimulation sessions over multiple days combined with an active cognitive training (e.g., memory training) also induced beneficial effects up to 4 weeks following the end of stimulation, whereas immediate positive effects were detected only as a function of the cognitive training per se, with no contribution of a-tDCS [13]. Interestingly, transfer effects on cognitive functions outside the targeted one were detected, which equally persisted in the weeks following the stimulation [13]. On the other hand, no difference in the effects of sham tDCS or a-tDCS at 1 or 2 mA was reported on the performance at a visual n-back task assessed during and after

35 min from stimulation [14]. One possible interpretation suggested by the authors is that repeated sessions may be needed to induce significant cognitive effects in older participants. Furthermore, prior work has highlighted how tES effects on elderly adults might occur in the hours following stimulation, opposed to the immediate effects detectable in young individuals. Therefore, the timeline of stimulation and subsequent effects on cognition should always be carefully considered.

Finally, although memory and language impairments represent the most common complaints during aging, many other behaviors become affected that contribute in diminishing individuals' autonomy in daily life. Few examples include difficulties in dual-task execution, planning, and decision making. As such, the possibility to intervene on those aspects could substantially improve later-life quality, for example for what concerns economic and monetary decisions. As an example, the left Dorsolateral Prefrontal Cortex (DLPFC) has been made a target to facilitate concurrent execution of different tasks, resulting in a significant reduction of the cognitive costs required by each task in the dual assignment condition, but not in a single task condition, also proving the specificity of the stimulation [15]. Further, a-tDCS applied over the right DLPFC significantly improved older adults' error awareness, which was replicated in a separate experiment [16].

This preliminary yet promising evidence warrants future studies carefully designed to determine the extent to which noninvasive approaches are useful in offsetting, or at least delaying, age-related cognitive decline. These studies should consider *customizing stimulation targets* based upon individual or population characteristics, which often differ substantially across age groups. Prior studies reporting positive results following the stimulation of a given cortical target, for a given intensity and duration, with a given effect upon a cognitive measure of interest, might not necessarily translate into benefit for a demographically different population. As an example, a-tDCS over the right DLPFC with the cathodal electrode placed over the left DLPFC was successful in substantially decreasing gambling risks among young adults, whereas the identical montage led to a worsening of the same behavior in older adults [17, 18].

Second, even within the same demographic population, substantial differences in the effects of tES can be driven by *interindividual differences in baseline cognitive performances*. For example, individuals already disadvantaged, who show lower performances on a task, have been reported to benefit less from stimulation compared to their higher-level counterpart. One study proved how older subjects, who showed less lateralized spatial attention at baseline, were negatively affected in their performance following left posterior parietal cortex stimulation in respect to sham [19]. On the other hand, stimulation of the right homologous area had a positive effect in the higher-performing group [19]. Through a similar rationale, left and right DLPFC stimulation yielded better performances on a visual and verbal working memory task in highly educated older adults, whereas an opposite, detrimental effect was reported for the less educated group [20]. Those findings highlight the need to consider interindividual differences, which might explain diverse compensatory capacities in the recruitment of brain regions, in line with the notion of the impact of the Cognitive Reserve on individuals' functional characterization [21].

22.1.2 Mild Cognitive Impairment

Mild Cognitive Impairment (MCI) represents an intermediate stage between healthy aging and dementia, characterized by a decrease in cognitive performance compared to a prior level of functioning, which is however not severe enough to affect the independence of the individual in the activities of daily living (ADL) [22]. MCI patients have a high epidemiological impact as they represent 7–24% of all individuals over the age of 65 [23], and 10–15% of older adults with MCI are diagnosed with dementia every year [24, 25]. To date, NIBS approaches have attempted to (1) identify those individuals with MCI who will worsen into dementia, so that early preventative measures can be taken, and (2) intervene against further cognitive decay in this population in order to maximize quality of life and minimize the risk of related disorders, such as depression and anxiety, which often arise from the acknowledgment of one's own mental decline.

The identification of the ones, among those patients, for which MCI will just represent a transitory phase before a formal diagnosis of dementia, has been proven particularly difficult. Electrophysiological, neuroimaging, and neuropsychological approaches are routinely promoted in clinical practice to characterize structural and functional profiles of the individual [26, 27], but still represent expensive and unsure tools, with high levels of uncertainty especially for borderline patients [28, 29]. However, an important advancement in this direction has been made in recent years thanks to the characterization of brain oscillatory activity and its relationship with cognitive decline [30]. Indeed, altered oscillatory activity and decreased cognitive performances have been linked by prior studies [31], both of them being related to the accumulation of amyloid-β [32, 33], the main protein alteration seen in Alzheimer's Disease (AD). In particular, the oscillatory activity might appear preserved in a resting condition and altered instead during task execution, with limits of the many biases that can affect task execution (instructions' comprehension, tiredness, compliance, etc.) [30]. Nevertheless, tACS can be applied to induce brain oscillation passively, mimicking oscillatory patterns associated with cognitive processing [34–36]. Based on this rationale, the authors have therefore applied tACS at the gamma frequency band, which plays an important role in ensuring transmission across cortical regions and networks [37], and which prior studies have linked with cognitive processes in aging [38–40]. Interestingly, healthy old adults and most MCI patients positively responded to tACS, resulting in an increase in the gamma band as assessed both immediately and 1 hour after the end of stimulation [30]. Furthermore, the gamma after-effects significantly correlated with increased performance at several neuropsychological tasks, such as motor learning, verbal fluency, digit span, and attentive matrices [30]. On the other hand, no significant effect was observed in the AD population; at a 2-year follow-up, MCI patients who also failed to respond to stimulation had converted into AD [30]. One hypothesis is that the reduced capacity of tACS to modulate underlying oscillatory activity could represent an early detector of dysfunctional connectivity between DLPFC and the Dorsomedial Prefrontal Cortex (DMPFC) [30], i.e., sites where tACS was applied in the aforementioned study, thus providing a first evidence of the applicability of *perturbation-based biomarkers* to detect the presence of—and to monitor—brain diseases.

As for the possibility to actively improve cognitive performances, few other studies have been carried out in recent years showing promising results in this direction. In particular, 20–30 minutes of a-tDCS over the bilateral DLPFC have been successful in ameliorating subjective perceptions of cognitive functioning when compared to sham [41], as well as in improving memory strategies [41] and recall, both immediate and delayed, with beneficial effects persisting up to 1-month follow-up [42]. Interestingly, the combined use of neuroimaging techniques, such as positron emission tomography (PET) and rs-fMRI, has revealed tDCS-induced functional rearrangements, resulting in increased regional metabolism [41] of relevant areas and effective reduction of frontal hyperactivity [43], thus counteracting typical pathological functional shifts.

Apart from overt cognitive decay, other aspects of daily life become affected during the aging course, contributing to the core of dementia-related symptoms. Among those, sleep patterns are readily altered at the MCI stage [44]. In particular, slow-sleep oscillations and thalamocortical spindles play an important role in memory consolidation, such as that disruption of their temporal coupling is suggested to cause the early amnestic symptomatology [45] and to possibly contribute in the MCI to dementia conversion [46, 47]. Based on this rationale, slow-wave oscillations tDCS (so-tDCS) applied during daytime nap in a population of MCI patients was successful in targeting the coupling between slow oscillations and spindle activity, promoting their functional synchronization in the EEG spectra and amplifying both their power [44]. As a consequence, visual declarative memory also improved in the MCI patients [44].

Together, available studies of tES in healthy older adults and in those suffering from MCI have shown promise in targeting neural substrates responsible for age-related changes in cognition. Moreover, tES may be used to directly stimulate and improve the function of cortical regions responsible for a given behavior, or promote compensatory activity of surrounding neural substrates. Hyperactivity and over-recruitment of frontal areas are commonly reported in older adults and might represent compensatory strategies by the brain, which suppression may be desirable to reintroduce young-like patterns and better functional outputs [43].

Worth mentioning is also the feasibility of tailoring tES interventions based on the individual's habits, enabling the administration of rehabilitative protocols in more ecological environments. Few studies have provided evidences regarding the combined use of tES and cognitive rehabilitation [48], as well as its noninvasiv use during well-established and routinely behaviors, like daytime naps [44] in the older adults. This approach may open the road for future interventions to be carried out directly at home, outside the laboratory environment.

22.1.3 Dementia

The use of tES is not limited to the quality enrichment of normal aging, or in the prevention of the MCI symptomatology, but rather it has proven useful at the level of dementia too, a disease stage characterized by substantial cortical atrophy and altered functionality that severely limits the independence of the individual in the activities of daily living. Due to the many facets of dementia's pathological profile, it is not surprising that the mechanisms of action of tES have also been studied over multiple domains [49] (see Fig. 22.2). From its effects on the membrane potential, to the synaptic level, and up to the induced modulation of the brain oscillatory activity and functional connectivity, several studies have reported and commented upon the efficacy of tES [49]. At the level of mere neuronal excitability, alterations in the membrane potential result in abnormal profiles of hypo- versus hyperactivated cortical regions. With respect to AD pathology, the progressive

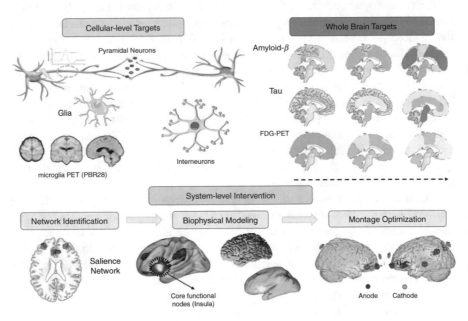

Fig. 22.2 tES levels of intervention. tES could be applied to modulate a range of hierarchically organized levels, from synaptic coupling between neurons (moderating membrane's potential and neurotransmitters release), up to larger-scale functional networks. At the cellular level, excitatory effects can be induced through the stimulation of pyramidal neurons, whereas inhibitory effects are achievable by targeting inhibitory interneurons. Particular interest is nowadays directed toward the potential use of tES in modulating neuroinflammation through microglia targeting. At the whole brain level, pathological targets include physiological mechanisms that might counteract amyloid-β and tau protein levels increase and the associated metabolic decrease as measured via FDG-PET imaging. At the system level, modern devices allow multisite stimulation, enabling the targeting of specific cortical networks. Such technological advances represent a substantial improvement from previous bifocal approaches, whereby large rectangular sponges were applied on the scalp to target broad and unspecific underlying cortical sites

accumulation of amyloid-β has been held responsible for this [50]. In particular, temporoparietal regions [51] have been observed to show slow-wave activity in contrast with the hyperexcitability of the motor cortex [52] and overall greater global cortical excitability [53], which has led to the rationale of applying a-tDCS to increase the activity of the former and cathodal tDCS (c-tDCS) to downregulate the latter. Rebalancing the underlying activity of cortical circuits appears crucial for the restoring of cognitive functioning in AD [54]. Nowadays, it is possible through the established role of tDCS modulating depolarization and hyperpolarization of the neural membranes [55]. Similarly, at synaptic level, the study of the effects of tES on dementia-related alterations has mainly focused on glutamatergic and GABAergic alterations, i.e., the main excitatory and inhibitory neurotransmitters of the brain. tDCS after-effects closely resemble long-term potentiation (LTP) and long-term depression (LTD) at the synaptic level [56], the former being considered responsible for learning and memory processes, which are altered in dementia. In animal models of AD, disruption of LTP was closely related to N-methyl-D-Aspartate (NMDA) receptors disruption in the hippocampus by the accumulation of amyloid-β [57]. Considering that tDCS LTP-like effects are also partly dependent on the NMDA receptors, its use in actively contrasting their disruption and in promoting cortical plasticity is therefore expected. In particular, glutamatergic alteration correlates with cognitive decline in patients [58], who might otherwise benefit from a-tDCS application. Indeed, increased glutamate and glutamine levels were reported in the right parietal cortex following stimulation over the same region [59], proving the specificity of tDCS in targeting molecular patterns that might prompt behavior ural improvements in pathological samples. Apart from the study of amyloid-induced alterations at neurotransmitters' levels, new approaches are considering tau aggregates and glial activation (an expression of neuroinflammation) as potential targets of interest. Not surprisingly, all those underlying alterations at neuronal and synaptic level sum up in much broader deviations from normality in the brain oscillatory activity and functional connectivity patterns. As already mentioned in the introduction, resting-state networks are progressively altered in various forms of dementia, showing patterns of disaggregation that mirror the spreading of the corresponding proteinopathy and cortical atrophy [4–6]. Similarly, altered temporal oscillatory activity has been reported across different brain regions, such as between frontal and parietal regions or between frontal and hippocampal structures in AD [60, 61]. In this sense, the use of tES has mostly been directed toward promoting their functional recoupling, favoring regional synchronization at least momentarily.

The main aim of any stimulation protocol is improving individual cognitive functioning in order to promote activities of daily living. As such, traditional targets include bilateral or unilateral prefrontal cortices (especially DLPFC) and temporal lobes, as neural substrates of language, executive functional deficits, and memory impairments, respectively. Within AD pathology, a-tDCS applied at home daily for 6 months was successful in boosting global cognitive performances and language abilities, preventing executive functions decay at a marginal level [62]. The authors further reported those changes in cognitive functioning to be accompanied by a preserved glucose regional metabolism in the inferior/middle temporal gyrus for the active group, compared to the metabolic decrease observed in the sham group [62]. Similarly, both a-tDCS and c-tDCS applied over 10 sessions helped improve global cognitive performance at the Mini Mental State Examination (MMSE) in 34 AD patients, with an effect on Performance Intelligent Quotient (p-IQ) at the Wechsler Adult Intelligence Scale (WAIS) for c-tDCS [63]. The induced cognitive changes were further paralleled by a decrease in the P300 latency, an EEG Event-Related Potential (ERP) component known to be pathologically increased in this group of patients [63]. Complex quantitative EEG rearrangements following tES have also been described in other studies. One recent investigation has reported that the tDCS-induced increase in the high-frequency power over temporoparietal regions was positively associated with improvement at the MMSE, partially reversing the abnormal EEG patterns seen in AD [64]. Loss of phase coherence is also commonly reported in AD, as a result of both connection loss between cortical regions and atrophy. In this study, coherence resulted higher after tDCS, positively correlating also with better performances in a word recognition test [64]. Overall, those studies provide evidence of the metabolic and electrophysiological changes that accompany pathological aging and that can be partially addressed by means of noninvasive stimulation. Most importantly, those studies prove how tES induces functional changes that rely on measurable neural changes. Prior researches have also reported increased recognition memory [65], persisting up to 4 weeks [66]. In a single case study, tES combined with traditional cognitive therapy helped to maintain spared cognitive functioning for longer time, promoting patient's stability up to 3 months [67]. Nevertheless, caution is highly recommended as negative findings have also been reported, possibly due to the greater severity of the population tested and their reduced number [68].

Apart from the pervasive memory impairments, language skills are also impoverished both in AD and FTD, and even more in an FTD variant, known as Primary Progressive Aphasia (PPA). Anomic spells frequently characterize the early stages of those pathologies, contributing to the diminished communication efficiency. Interestingly, tDCS, administered during a picture-naming training, was reported to be efficacious in improving naming capacities in 10 anomic AD and FTD patients, with generalized benefits to also untrained items, as well as in other neuropsychological tasks, such as digit span [69]. Real stimulation, compared to sham, guaranteed the effects to remain for at least 2 weeks after the end of the training [69]. In a sample of PPA patients, a similar stimulation protocol also successfully increased performance over trained items, with a slower rate of decline for those same items in the 6 months following stimulation, but with no effects over untrained ones [70]. On the other hand, generalization over untrained material was reported in a different study where tES was combined with language therapy, once again suggesting the greater synergic effects of combined interventions [71, 72]. Interestingly, a prior study had linked improved performance in naming with greater gray matter volume over the left fusiform gyrus, left middle and right inferior temporal gyri, such as that greater baseline volume over those regions was predictive of greater performance gains following stimulation [73]. Since regional volume loss is among the first characteristics of neurodegeneration, those findings prompt toward the need of addressing cognitive functions as early as possible to maximize patients' improvement [73]. Although language-related processes and communication skills have been the most targeted aspects of cognition in FTD and PPA patients (see also [74, 75]), very recent applications of tES were capable of addressing other important weakened functions, such as behavioral dyscontrol and the inability to predict others' responses from the perspective of an impaired Theory of Mind [76, 77]. Both studies are of great importance as personality changes, disinhibition, and misbehavior have a severe effect not only on patient him/herself, but represent a substantial cause of distress for family members and caregivers too.

Finally, one last application for tES interventions has focused on other forms of dementia that since the earliest stages are characterized by the presence of motor-related disorders, as observed in Parkinson's Disease (PD) and Dementia with Lewy Bodies (DLB). In one of the first studies, a-tDCS over the primary motor cortex (M1) of PD patients had a significant effect on motor functions, as assessed by the Parkinson's Disease Rating Scale, whereas no effect was reported when c-tDCS was applied or when DLPFC was targeted instead [78]. Similarly to what was reported for AD and FTD patients, a-tDCS applied to prefrontal regions in patients with PD was successful in improving working memory [79], attention [80], and phonemic fluency, which was accompanied by greater connectivity in verbal fluency networks as assessed by rs-fMRI [81]. Subsequent investigation assessing verbal fluency in PD patients also observed an improved response following a-tDCS combined with physical therapy, which persisted at 3-month follow-up [82]. Parkinson's Disease Cognitive Rating Scale scores also increased following a-tDCS, allowing PD patients with MCI to score within the normal range following stimulation [82].

22.2   tES and Cognitive-Motor Function

Cognitive decline associated with both biological aging and disease has direct, deleterious effects on motor control with often profound functional implications. In particular, standing, walking, turning, and transferring call upon numerous cognitive-motor brain networks involved in the planning, execution, and adaptation of full-body movements. This high-level control is amplified when our daily activities require us to navigate complex, ever-changing environments, often while completing additional tasks like reading, talking, or making decisions. Cognitive impairment, and in particular executive dysfunction, is in fact a strong independent risk factor for balance decline [83], gait instability [84], ADL disability [85], and falls [86] in older adults. Those with dementia, for example, are five times more likely to suffer from falls and their morbid consequences as compared to older adults living with intact cognitive functions [87, 88]. Thus, in addition to the potential of promoting traditional cognitive outcomes, tES aimed at enhancing the functionality of cognitive-motor brain networks holds promise as a strategy to offset age- and dementia-related declines in cognitive-motor control—especially those that disrupt safe navigation and threaten functional independence.

The potential for NIBS to reduce falls in older adults has not been examined to date. Preliminary yet promising evidence, however, suggest that tES may improve the cortical control of walking (i.e., gait) and standing (i.e., posture) in older adults without overt neurological disease. Limited evidence also suggests that it may be beneficial to mobility in those with MCI or Parkinson's disease. The majority of this evidence comes from published studies using tDCS with the intent of facilitating the excitability of either the prefrontal or motor cortices. Available work has examined both the acute effects of a single session of stimulation and/or the longer-term effects of multiple sessions over several consecutive weeks.

Zhou and colleagues have published a series of studies suggesting that a-tDCS, designed to target the left DLPFC, acutely improves the control of standing and walking—especially in "dual-task" situations. Participants of each study completed two visits during which dual-task performance was assessed immediately before and after a-tDCS or sham stimulation. The dual-task paradigm involved trials of standing and walking both with and without simultaneous performance of a serial subtraction cognitive task. In healthy young adults [89], in healthy older adults [15], and in very old adults presenting with mild cognitive impairment [90], dual tasking resulted in a significant "cost" (i.e., performance decrement) to both gait and standing postural control. In each cohort, a-tDCS, as compared to sham, significantly reduced the dual-task cost to several metrics of gait and postural control, when tested in the 30 min following stimulation.

Building upon this work, the same group recently published a pilot double-blinded randomized sham-controlled trial of a 2-week, 10-session a-tDCS intervention in very old adults without overt illness or disease, yet who presented with both slow gait and mild-to-moderate executive dysfunction. tDCS, compared to sham, resulted in dual-task gait postural control improvements that persisted throughout a 2-week follow-up period. Moreover, the a-tDCS group exhibited clinically meaningful improvements in global cognitive function as measured by the Montreal Cognitive Assessment (MoCA).

While the foregoing preliminary evidence indicates that tDCS targeting prefrontal regions may improve the dual-task gait and balance performance, the effects of tDCS targeting the motor cortex or other brain regions or networks with known involvement in mobility in aging are still largely unexplored. In one of few other studies, Kaminski et al. [91] examined whether tDCS designed to facilitate the excitability of the primary motor cortex (M1) facilitated learning of a dynamic balance task in 30 healthy older adults. Participants received a single session of tDCS or sham stimulation while completing a balance training task. The researchers reported that both the group receiving tDCS and the group receiving sham stimulation learned from training, yet that tDCS did not influence the level of task learning. Thus, while tES may augment certain aspects of gait and balance in older adults, additional research is needed to determine optimal targets and dosage, if such interventions should be paired with other evidence-based balance and mobility programs, and ultimately, if improvements in gait and balance translate into increased safety and improve ADL performance in older adults with MCI or AD.

Beyond MCI and AD, tES appears to have positive impact on cognitive-motor symptoms in patients with Parkinson's disease. The available evidence is heterogeneous in both intervention characteristics and outcome measures [92], and potential interactions between tDCS and parkinsonian medications remain poorly understood [93]. Nevertheless, tES, aimed at modulating the excitability of primary motor and/or prefrontal brain regions, appears to improve functional outcomes in this population. Lattari et al. [94], for example, examined the effects of a single session of a-tDCS targeting the left DLPFC in a double-blinded, sham-controlled, within-subject, crossover study in 17 individuals with PD. The intervention and all study assessments were completed with participants in the "on-medication" state. a-tDCS, compared to sham, led to acute improvements in whole-body mobility as measured by the Berg Balance Scale, the Dynamic Gait Index, and the Timed Up-and-Go (TUG). Similarly, Hadoush et al. [95] reported that a 10-session a-tDCS intervention aimed at facilitating bilateral motor and prefrontal excitability, as compared to an inactive sham, led to improved balance and reduced fear of falling in patients with idiopathic Parkinson's disease. Recently, Dagan et al. [96] reported the immediate after-effects of a single session of "multitarget" tDCS designed to simultaneously facilitate the excitability of the left DLPFC and the leg regions of the bilateral M1. This stimulation significantly reduced the severity of "freezing of gait," as compared to stimulation targeting M1 alone or an active sham control. These promising immediate after-effects of tDCS on freezing of gait—a complex symptom theorized to arise from abnormalities in both cognitive and motor brain functions—warrant investigation of the longer-term effects of multisession tES interventions on this and other cognitive-motor symptoms in patients who suffer from PD, with and without concomitant cognitive dysfunction.

22.3   Future Perspectives

Literature studies provide a rationale for the use of tES interventions in the aging process, suggesting a plausible role of stimulation in boosting individual performances, from motor to higher-order cognitive functioning. Nevertheless, substantial improvement is still needed to augment protocol efficiency. First of all, (1) *target selection* represents a critical aspect, as most approaches rely on stimulating prefrontal cortices (especially left DLPFC) based on their known involvement in higher-order cognitive processes, and relying on the rationale that prior studies had used it too, but substantially failing to consider interindividual topological differences and networks' structure. Furthermore, this approach limits the application of stimulation to a single region, while it is known that several cortical nodes constitute the frontoparietal network, and therefore the goodness of the task execution is more likely determined by their combined contribution. Therefore, recent technological advances have started promoting the use of *multifocal* stimulation, whereby a genetic algorithm is used to determine electrode arrangements on the scalp to produce a desired electrical field, maximizing the chances of stimulating the targeted cortical network, while minimizing unspecific cortical effects [97, 98]. So far, motor network stimulation by means of eight separate electrodes was proven more efficient in increasing cortical excitability of the left M1 compared to the traditional bifocal approach, doubling its effects [97].

As stimulation approaches move toward a better spatial tailoring, (2) *more time-dynamic tuning of the delivered electrical currents* is also foreseen. Indeed, state-dependent effects are known to widely drive stimulation efficacy. Very recently, a-tDCS effects over DLPFC-mediated executive functions were observed to be largely determined by underlying electrophysiological phenomena, such as that the individuals who benefitted more from stimulation were the ones with the lower amplitude at baseline [99]. Continuous monitoring of the underlying brain states could therefore be very informative to determine when to best deliver the electrical pulse, acknowledging that neural populations might be modulated with a different degree depending on their current state [99]. Based on this, *closed-loop approaches* have started to emerge in the literature, where the simultaneous registration of the individual EEG activity is used to tune the current delivery from the stimulation device. As predictive algorithms are used to determine the forthcoming neural oscillation to be targeted, thus automatizing the process of stimulation, closed-loop approaches have the potential to be applied under various conditions, for example during sleep. (3) *Sleep modulation* particularly suits neurodegenerative studies, where difficulties in memory consolidation are a hallmark. Based on the rationale that slow-wave oscillations, observed at the scalp level during sleep, reflect large-scale synchronization between cortical and subcortical regions, promoting the consolidation of short-term memory into long-term memory, closed-loop tACS has been successfully applied in healthy subjects to improve memory performances [100]. Furthermore, a strict relationship seems to exist between AD proteinopathy and the quality and duration of sleep, such as that cerebrospinal levels of tau and amyloid-β are associated with poorness in slow-wave sleep in patients [101]. The use of tES during sleep seems therefore a promising tool to address both the mechanisms of protein clearance and those of memory consolidation, with the potential to lead to *home-based therapy*, posing a new challenge for future studies.

Finally, tACS stimulation has gained renewed interest in recent years for the possibility of (4) *targeting gamma oscillations*, which are fast EEG oscillations occurring around 40 Hz. Prior animal work has demonstrated that the induction of gamma activity via optogenetics or sensory stimulation reduces amyloid-β plaques [102], and that impaired coupling between (fast) gamma and (slow) theta oscillations over frontal regions was not only associated with impaired working memory performances, but it occurred in AD and MCI patients even before overt behavioral symptoms (for a review, see [103]). Furthermore, failure to respond to tACS applied at the gamma frequency band correctly discriminated between MCI patients designated to convert into AD 2 years later and those who did not [30], proving tACS gamma to be a potential useful *perturbation-based biomarker* in predicting MCI to AD conversion.

22.4   Summary

To date, various tES interventions have been proven effective in targeting spared functions in older adults, boosting performance levels at both cognitive and motor tasks and their concomitant execution (dual-task). Evidence on the effectiveness of tES is corroborated by the corresponding changes in neuroimaging, electroencephalographic, and metabolic data recorded before and after stimulation, or compared across active and sham stimulation cohorts. As more evidence will be gathered in future years, the use of tES should be promoted in patients' care routine, considering its potential use as a therapeutic tool and as a biomarker of disease progression. Future technological advances will further enable us to gain better understanding of the underlying neuropathological mechanisms of dementia, and address innovative therapeutic targets, hoping to further improve everyday medical care.

References

1. Cabeza R. Hemispheric asymmetry reduction in older adults: the HAROLD model. Psychol Aging. 2002;17(1):85–100.
2. Davis SW, Dennis NA, Daselaar SM, Fleck MS, Cabeza R. Qué PASA? The posterior–anterior shift in aging. Cereb Cortex. 2008;18(5):1201–9.
3. Calsolaro V, Edison P. Neuroinflammation in Alzheimer's disease: current evidence and future directions. Alzheimers Dement. 2016;12(6):719–32.
4. Jones DT, Knopman DS, Gunter JL, Graff-Radford J, Vemuri P, Boeve BF, et al. Cascading network failure across the Alzheimer's disease spectrum. Brain. 2016;139(2):547.
5. Buckner RL. Molecular, structural, and functional characterization of Alzheimer's disease: evidence for a relationship between default activity, amyloid, and memory. J Neurosci. 2005;25(34):7709–17.
6. Zhou J, Greicius MD, Gennatas ED, Growdon MF, Jang JY, Rabinovici GD, et al. Divergent network connectivity changes in behavioural variant frontotemporal dementia and Alzheimer's disease. Brain. 2010;133(5):1352.
7. Khedr EM, Salama RH, Hameed MA, Elfetoh NA, Seif P. Therapeutic role of transcranial direct current stimulation in Alzheimer disease patients: double-blind, placebo-controlled clinical trial. Neurorehabil Neural Repair. 2019;33(5):384–94.
8. Ross LA, McCoy D, Wolk DA, Coslett HB, Olson IR. Improved proper name recall in aging after electrical stimulation of the anterior temporal lobes. Front Aging Neurosci. 2011;3:16.
9. Meinzer M, Lindenberg R, Antonenko D, Flaisch T, Floel A. Anodal transcranial direct current stimulation temporarily reverses age-associated cognitive decline and functional brain activity changes. J Neurosci. 2013;33(30):12470–8.
10. Floel A, Suttorp W, Kohl O, Kurten J, Lohmann H, Breitenstein C, et al. Non-invasive brain stimulation improves object-location learning in the elderly. Neurobiol Aging. 2012;33(8):1682–9.
11. Sandrini M, Manenti R, Brambilla M, Cobelli C, Cohen LG, Cotelli M. Older adults get episodic memory boosting from noninvasive stimulation of prefrontal cortex during learning. Neurobiol Aging. 2016;39:210–6.
12. Sandrini M, Brambilla M, Manenti R, Rosini S, Cohen LG, Cotelli M. Noninvasive stimulation of prefrontal cortex strengthens existing episodic memories and reduces forgetting in the elderly. Front Aging Neurosci. 2014;6:289.

13. Jones KT, Stephens JA, Alam M, Bikson M, Berryhill ME. Longitudinal neurostimulation in older adults improves working memory. PLoS One. 2015;10(4):e0121904.
14. Nilsson J, Lebedev AV, Lövdén M. No significant effect of prefrontal tDCS on working memory performance in older adults. Front Aging Neurosci. 2015;7:230.
15. Manor B, Zhou J, Jor'dan A, Zhang J, Fang J, Pascual-Leone A. Reduction of dual-task costs by noninvasive modulation of prefrontal activity in healthy elders. J Cogn Neurosci. 2015;28(2):275–81.
16. Harty S, Robertson IH, Miniussi C, Sheehy OC, Devine CA, McCreery S, et al. Transcranial direct current stimulation over right dorsolateral prefrontal cortex enhances error awareness in older age. J Neurosci. 2014;34(10):3646–52.
17. Fecteau S, Knoch D, Fregni F, Sultani N, Boggio P, Pascual-Leone A. Diminishing risk-taking behavior by modulating activity in the prefrontal cortex: a direct current stimulation study. J Neurosci. 2007;27(46):12500–5.
18. Boggio PS, Campanhã C, Valasek CA, Fecteau S, Pascual-Leone A, Fregni F. Modulation of decision-making in a gambling task in older adults with transcranial direct current stimulation. Eur J Neurosci. 2010;31:593–7.
19. Learmonth G, Thut G, Benwell CSY, Harvey M. The implications of state-dependent tDCS effects in aging: behavioural response is determined by baseline performance. Neuropsychologia. 2015;74:108–19.
20. Berryhill ME, Jones KT. tDCS selectively improves working memory in older adults with more education. Neurosci Lett. 2012;521(2):148–51.
21. Stern Y. What is cognitive reserve? Theory and research application of the reserve concept. J Int Neuropsychol Soc. 2002;8(3):448–60.
22. Portet F, Ousset PJ, Visser PJ, Frisoni G, Nobili F, Scheltens P, et al. Mild cognitive impairment (MCI) in medical practice: a critical review of the concept and new diagnostic procedure. Report of the MCI Working Group of the European Consortium on Alzheimer's disease. J Neurol Neurosurg Psychiatry. 2006;77(6):714–8.
23. Langa KM, Levine DA. The diagnosis and management of mild cognitive impairment: a clinical review. JAMA. 2014;312(23):2551–61.
24. Petersen RC, Doody R, Kurz A, Mohs RC, Morris JC, Rabins PV, et al. Current concepts in mild cognitive impairment. Arch Neurol. 2001;58(12):1985–92.
25. Petersen RC, Caracciolo B, Brayne C, Gauthier S, Jelic V, Fratiglioni L. Mild cognitive impairment: a concept in evolution. J Intern Med. 2014;275(3):214–28.
26. Drago V, Babiloni C, Bartrés-Faz D, Caroli A, Bosch B, Hensch T, et al. Disease tracking markers for Alzheimer's disease at the prodromal (MCI) stage. J Alzheimers Dis. 2011;26(s3):159–99.
27. Bertè F, Lamponi G, Calabrò RS, Bramanti P. Elman neural network for the early identification of cognitive impairment in Alzheimer's disease. Funct Neurol. 2014;29(1):57–65.
28. Vega JN, Newhouse PA. Mild cognitive impairment: diagnosis, longitudinal course, and emerging treatments. Curr Psychiatry Rep. 2014;16(10):490.
29. Hugo J, Ganguli M. Dementia and cognitive impairment: epidemiology, diagnosis, and treatment. Clin Geriatr Med. 2014;30(3):421.
30. Naro A, Corallo F, De Salvo S, Marra A, Di Lorenzo G, Muscarà N, et al. Promising role of neuromodulation in predicting the progression of mild cognitive impairment to dementia. J Alzheimers Dis. 2016;53(4):1375–88.
31. Yener GG, Başar E. Sensory evoked and event related oscillations in Alzheimer's disease: a short review. Cogn Neurodyn. 2010;4(4):263–74.
32. Sheng M, Sabatini BL, Sudhof TC. Synapses and Alzheimer's disease. Cold Spring Harb Perspect Biol. 2012;4(5):a005777.
33. Uhlhaas PJ, Singer W. Neural synchrony in brain disorders: relevance for cognitive dysfunctions and pathophysiology. Neuron. 2006;52(1):155–68.
34. Santarnecchi E, Muller T, Rossi S, Sarkar A, Polizzotto NR, Rossi A, et al. Individual differences and specificity of prefrontal gamma frequency-tACS on fluid intelligence capabilities. Cortex. 2016;75:33–43.

35. Hoy KE, Bailey N, Arnold S, Windsor K, John J, Daskalakis ZJ, et al. The effect of γ-tACS on working memory performance in healthy controls. Brain Cogn. 2015;101:51–6.
36. Cabral-Calderin Y, Anne Weinrich C, Schmidt-Samoa C, Poland E, Dechent P, Bähr M, et al. Transcranial alternating current stimulation affects the BOLD signal in a frequency and task-dependent manner: effect of tACS on the BOLD signal. Hum Brain Mapp. 2016;37(1):94–121.
37. Abuhassan K, Coyle D. Employing neuronal networks to investigate the pathophysiological basis of abnormal cortical oscillations in Alzheimer's disease - IEEE Conference Publication. In: Annual international conference of the IEEE Engineering in Medicine and Biology Society (IEEE), 2011. p. 2065–8.
38. Missonnier P, Herrmann FR, Michon A, Fazio-Costa L, Gold G, Giannakopoulos P. Early disturbances of gamma band dynamics in mild cognitive impairment. J Neural Transm. 2010;117(4):489–98.
39. Moretti DV, Frisoni G, Fracassi C, Pievani M, Geroldi C, Binetti G, et al. MCI patients' EEGs show group differences between those who progress and those who do not progress to AD. Neurobiol Aging. 2011;32(4):563–71.
40. Park JY, Lee KS, An SK, Lee J, Kim J-J, Kim KH, et al. Gamma oscillatory activity in relation to memory ability in older adults. Int J Psychophysiol. 2012;86(1):58–65.
41. Yun K, Song I-U, Chung Y-A. Changes in cerebral glucose metabolism after 3 weeks of non-invasive electrical stimulation of mild cognitive impairment patients. Alzheimers Res Ther. 2016;8(1):49.
42. Murugaraja V, Shivakumar V, Sivakumar PT, Sinha P, Venkatasubramanian G. Clinical utility and tolerability of transcranial direct current stimulation in mild cognitive impairment. Asian J Psychiatr. 2017;30:135–40.
43. Meinzer M, Lindenberg R, Phan MT, Ulm L, Volk C, Floel A. Transcranial direct current stimulation in mild cognitive impairment: behavioral effects and neural mechanisms. Alzheimers Dement. 2015;11(9):1032–40.
44. Ladenbauer J, Ladenbauer J, Külzow N, de Boor R, Avramova E, Grittner U, et al. Promoting Sleep oscillations and their functional coupling by transcranial stimulation enhances memory consolidation in mild cognitive impairment. J Neurosci. 2017;37(30):7111–24.
45. Westerberg CE, Mander BA, Florczak SM, Weintraub S, Mesulam M-M, Zee PC, et al. Concurrent impairments in sleep and memory in amnestic mild cognitive impairment. J Int Neuropsychol Soc. 2012;18(3):490.
46. Wang G, Grone B, Colas D, Appelbaum L, Mourrain P. Synaptic plasticity in sleep: learning, homeostasis and disease. Trends Neurosci. 2011;34(9):452–63.
47. Ju Y-ES, Lucey BP, Holtzman DM. Sleep and Alzheimer disease pathology—a bidirectional relationship. Nat Rev Neurol. 2014;10(2):115.
48. Gonzalez PC, Fong KNK, Chung RCK, Ting K-H, Law LLF, Brown T. Can transcranial direct-current stimulation alone or combined with cognitive training be used as a clinical intervention to improve cognitive functioning in persons with mild cognitive impairment and dementia? A systematic review and meta-analysis. Front Hum Neurosci. 2018;12:416.
49. Hansen N. Action mechanisms of transcranial direct current stimulation in Alzheimer's disease and memory loss. Front Psychiatry. 2012;3:48.
50. Blanchard BJ, Thomas VL, Ingram VM. Mechanism of membrane depolarization caused by the Alzheimer Aβ1–42 peptide. Biochem Biophys Res Commun. 2002;293(4):1197–203.
51. Fernandez A, Maestù F, Amo C, Gil P, Fehr T, Wienbruch C, et al. Focal temporoparietal slow activity in Alzheimer's disease revealed by magnetoencephalography. Biol Psychiatry. 2002;52(7):764–70.
52. Di Lazzaro V, Oliviero A, Pilato F, Saturno E, Dileone M, Marra C, et al. Motor cortex hyper-excitability to transcranial magnetic stimulation in Alzheimer's disease. J Neurol Neurosurg Psychiatry. 2004;75(4):555–9.
53. Rossini P, Rossi S, Babiloni C, Polich J. Clinical neurophysiology of aging brain: From normal aging to neurodegeneration. Prog Neurobiol. 2007;83(6):375–400.

54. Ardolino G, Bossi B, Barbieri S, Priori A. Non-synaptic mechanisms underlie the after-effects of cathodal transcutaneous direct current stimulation of the human brain. J Physiol. 2005;568(2):653–63.
55. Nitsche MA, Paulus W. Excitability changes induced in the human motor cortex by weak transcranial direct current stimulation. J Physiol. 2000;527(3):633–9.
56. Paulus W. Outlasting excitability shifts induced by direct current stimulation of the human brain. Suppl Clin Neurophysiol. 2004;57:708–14.
57. Yamin G. NMDA receptor–dependent signaling pathways that underlie amyloid β-protein disruption of LTP in the hippocampus. J Neurosci Res. 2009;87(8):1729–36.
58. Parameshwaran K, Dhanasekaran M, Suppiramaniam V. Amyloid beta peptides and glutamatergic synaptic dysregulation. Exp Neurol. 2008;210(1):7–13.
59. Clark VP, Coffman BA, Trumbo MC, Gasparovic C. Transcranial direct current stimulation (tDCS) produces localized and specific alterations in neurochemistry: a 1H magnetic resonance spectroscopy study. Neurosci Lett. 2011;500(1):67–71.
60. Montez T, Poil S-S, Jones BF, Manshanden I, Verbunt JPA, van Dijk BW, et al. Altered temporal correlations in parietal alpha and prefrontal theta oscillations in early-stage Alzheimer disease. Proc Natl Acad Sci U S A. 2009;106(5):1614–9.
61. Grady CL, Furey ML, Pietrini P, Horwitz B, Rapoport SI. Altered brain functional connectivity and impaired short-term memory in Alzheimer's disease. Brain. 2001;124(4):739–56.
62. Im JJ, Jeong H, Bikson M, Woods AJ, Unal G, Oh KJ, et al. Effects of 6-month at-home transcranial direct current stimulation on cognition and cerebral glucose metabolism in Alzheimer's disease. Brain Stimul. 2019;12(5):1222–8.
63. Khedr EM, Gamal NFE, El-Fetoh NA, Khalifa H, Ahmed EM, Ali AM, et al. A double-blind randomized clinical trial on the efficacy of cortical direct current stimulation for the treatment of Alzheimer's disease. Front Aging Neurosci. 2014;6:275.
64. Marceglia S, Mrakic-Sposta S, Rosa M, Ferrucci R, Mameli F, Vergari M, et al. Transcranial direct current stimulation modulates cortical neuronal activity in Alzheimer's disease. Front Neurosci. 2016;10:134.
65. Ferrucci R, Mameli F, Guidi I, Mrakic-Sposta S, Vergari M, Marceglia S, et al. Transcranial direct current stimulation improves recognition memory in Alzheimer disease. Neurology. 2008;71(7):493–8.
66. Boggio PS, Ferrucci R, Mameli F, Martins D, Martins O, Vergari M, et al. Prolonged visual memory enhancement after direct current stimulation in Alzheimer's disease. Brain Stimul. 2012;5(3):223–30.
67. Penolazzi B, Bergamaschi S, Pastore M, Villani D, Sartori G, Mondini S. Transcranial direct current stimulation and cognitive training in the rehabilitation of Alzheimer disease: a case study. Neuropsychol Rehabil. 2014;25(6):799–817.
68. Bystad M, Grønli O, Rasmussen ID, Gundersen N, Nordvang L, Wang-Iversen H, et al. Transcranial direct current stimulation as a memory enhancer in patients with Alzheimer's disease: a randomized, placebo-controlled trial. Alzheimers Res Ther. 2016;8:13.
69. Roncero C, Kniefel H, Service E, Thiel A, Probst S, Chertkow H. Inferior parietal transcranial direct current stimulation with training improves cognition in anomic Alzheimer's disease and frontotemporal dementia. Alzheimers Dement. 2017;3(2):247–53.
70. Hung J, Bauer A, Grossman M, Hamilton RH, Coslett HB, Reilly J. Semantic feature training in combination with Transcranial Direct Current Stimulation (tDCS) for progressive anomia. Front Hum Neurosci. 2017;11:253.
71. Tsapkini K, Frangakis C, Gomez Y, Davis C, Hillis AE. Augmentation of spelling therapy with transcranial direct current stimulation in primary progressive aphasia: preliminary results and challenges. Aphasiology. 2014;28(8–9):1112–30.
72. Tsapkini K, Webster KT, Ficek BN, Desmond JE, Onyike CU, Rapp B, et al. Electrical brain stimulation in different variants of primary progressive aphasia: a randomized clinical trial. Alzheimers Dement. 2018;4:461–72.

73. Cotelli M, Manenti R, Paternicò D, Cosseddu M, Brambilla M, Petesi M, et al. Grey matter density predicts the improvement of naming abilities after tDCS intervention in agrammatic variant of primary progressive aphasia. Brain Topogr. 2016;29(5):738–51.

74. Gervits F, Ash S, Coslett HB, Rascovsky K, Grossman M, Hamilton R. Transcranial direct current stimulation for the treatment of primary progressive aphasia: an open-label pilot study. Brain Lang. 2016;162:35–41.

75. Wang J, Wu D, Chen Y, Yuan Y, Zhang M. Effects of transcranial direct current stimulation on language improvement and cortical activation in nonfluent variant primary progressive aphasia. Neurosci Lett. 2013;549:29–33.

76. Cotelli M, Adenzato M, Cantoni V, Manenti R, Alberici A, Enrici I, et al. Enhancing theory of mind in behavioural variant frontotemporal dementia with transcranial direct current stimulation. Cogn Affect Behav Neurosci. 2018;18(6):1065–75.

77. Ferrucci R, Mrakic-Sposta S, Gardini S, Ruggiero F, Vergari M, Mameli F, et al. Behavioral and neurophysiological effects of Transcranial Direct Current Stimulation (tDCS) in fronto-temporal dementia. Front Behav Neurosci. 2018;12:235.

78. Fregni F, Boggio PS, Santos MC, Lima M, Vieira AL, Rigonatti SP, et al. Noninvasive cortical stimulation with transcranial direct current stimulation in Parkinson's disease. Mov Disord. 2006;21(10):1693–702.

79. Boggio PS, Ferrucci R, Rigonatti SP, Covre P, Nitsche MA, Pascual-Leone A, et al. Effects of transcranial direct current stimulation on working memory in patients with Parkinson's disease. J Neurol Sci. 2006;249(1):31–8.

80. Elder GJ, Firbank MJ, Kumar H, Chatterjee P, Chakraborty T, Dutt A, et al. Effects of transcranial direct current stimulation upon attention and visuoperceptual function in Lewy body dementia: a preliminary study. Int Psychogeriatr. 2016;28(2):341.

81. Pereira JB, Junqué C, Bartrés-Faz D, Martì MJ, Sala-Llonch R, Compta Y, et al. Modulation of verbal fluency networks by transcranial direct current stimulation (tDCS) in Parkinson's disease. Brain Stimul. 2013;6(1):16–24.

82. Manenti R, Brambilla M, Benussi A, Rosini S, Cobelli C, Ferrari C, et al. Mild cognitive impairment in Parkinson's disease is improved by transcranial direct current stimulation combined with physical therapy. Mov Disord. 2016;31:715–24.

83. Muir-Hunter SW, Clark J, McLean S, Pedlow S, Hemmen AV, Odasso MM, et al. Identifying balance and fall risk in community-dwelling older women: the effect of executive function on postural control. Physiother Can. 2014;66(2):179.

84. Yogev-Seligmann G, Hausdorff JM, Giladi N. The role of executive function and attention in gait. Mov Disord. 2008;23(3):329–42.

85. Johnson JK, Lui L-Y, Yaffe K. Executive function, more than global cognition, predicts functional decline and mortality in elderly women. J Gerontol A Biol Sci Med Sci. 2007;62(10):1134–41.

86. Mirelman A, Herman T, Brozgol M, Dorfman M, Sprecher E, Schweiger A, et al. Executive function and falls in older adults: new findings from a five-year prospective study link fall risk to cognition. PLoS One. 2012;7(6):e40297.

87. Shaw FE. Falls in older people with dementia. Geriatr Aging. 2003;6(7):37–40.

88. Pellfolk T, Gustafsson T, Gustafson Y, Karlsson S. Risk factors for falls among residents with dementia living in group dwellings. Int Psychogeriatr. 2009;21(1):187–94.

89. Zhou J, Hao Y, Wang Y, Jor'dan A, Pascual-Leone A, Zhang J, et al. Transcranial direct current stimulation reduces the cost of performing a cognitive task on gait and postural control. Eur J Neurosci. 2014;39(8):1343–8.

90. Manor B, Zhou J, Harrison R, Lo O-Y, Travison TG, Hausdorff JM, et al. Transcranial direct current stimulation may improve cognitive-motor function in functionally limited older adults. Neurorehabil Neural Repair. 2018;32(9):788–98.

91. Kaminski E, Hoff M, Rjosk V, Steele CJ, Gundlach C, Sehm B, et al. Anodal transcranial direct current stimulation does not facilitate dynamic balance task learning in healthy old adults. Front Hum Neurosci. 2017;11:16.

92. Lafaucheur J-P, Antal A, Ayache SS, Benninger DH, Brunelin J, Cogiamanian F, et al. Evidence-based guidelines on the therapeutic use of transcranial direct current stimulation (tDCS). Clin Neurophysiol. 2017;128(1):56–92.
93. Rektorova I, Anderkova L. Noninvasive brain stimulation and implications for nonmotor symptoms in Parkinson's disease. Int Rev Neurobiol. 2017;134:1091–110.
94. Lattari E, Costa SS, Campos C, de Oliveira AJ, Machado S, Maranhao Neto GA. Can transcranial direct current stimulation on the dorsolateral prefrontal cortex improves balance and functional mobility in Parkinson's disease? Neurosci Lett. 2017;636:165–9.
95. Hadoush H, Al-Jarrah M, Khalil H, Al-Sharman A, Al-Ghazawi S. Bilateral anodal transcranial direct current stimulation effect on balance and fearing of fall in patient with Parkinson's disease. NeuroRehabilitation. 2018;42(1):63–8.
96. Dagan M, Herman T, Harrison R, Zhou J, Giladi N, Ruffini G, et al. Multitarget transcranial direct current stimulation for freezing of gait in Parkinson's disease. Mov Disord. 2018;33(4):642–6.
97. Fischer DB, Fried PJ, Ruffini G, Ripolles O, Salvador R, Banus J, et al. Multifocal tDCS targeting the resting state motor network increases cortical excitability beyond traditional tDCS targeting unilateral motor cortex. Neuroimage. 2017;157:34–44.
98. Ruffini G, Fox MD, Ripolles O, Cavaleiro Miranda P, Pascual-Leone A. Optimization of multifocal transcranial current stimulation for weighted cortical pattern targeting from realistic modeling of electric fields. Neuroimage. 2014;89:216–25.
99. Dubreuil-Vall L, Chau P, Ruffini G, Widge AS, Camprodon JA. tDCS to the left DLPFC modulates cognitive and physiological correlates of executive function in a state-dependent manner. Brain Stimul. 2019;12:1456–63.
100. Jones AP, Choe J, Bryant NB, Robinson CSH, Ketz NA, Skorheim SW, et al. Dose-dependent effects of closed-loop tACS delivered during slow-wave oscillations on memory consolidation. Front Neurosci. 2018;12:867.
101. Liguori C, Romigi A, Nuccetelli M, Zannino S, Sancesario G, Martorana A, et al. Orexinergic system dysregulation, sleep impairment, and cognitive decline in Alzheimer disease. JAMA Neurol. 2014;71(12):1498–505.
102. Iaccarino HF, Singer AC, Martorell AJ, Rudenko A, Gao F, Gillingham TZ, et al. Gamma frequency entrainment attenuates amyloid load and modifies microglia. Nature. 2016;540(7632):230–5.
103. Rajji TK. Impaired brain plasticity as a potential therapeutic target for treatment and prevention of dementia. Expert Opin Ther Targets. 2018;23:21–8.

Neuropsychological, Emotional, and Cognitive Investigations with Transcranial Direct Current Stimulation (TDCS)

23

Philipp A. Schroeder and Christian Plewnia

The application of transcranial brain stimulation in research on the neural implementations of human cognition, emotion, and action offers unique insights for cognitive and affective neuroscience: By manipulating brain activity, the main rationale of experimental studies permits causal inferences between neurophysiological effects in targeted brain regions and behavioral outcomes [1, 2]. In cognitive investigations, however, neurophysiological effects are not directly observable and must be estimated from other research or concurrent imaging [3, 4]. In the last two decades, neuropsychological, emotional, and cognitive research has grown thanks to tDCS and is now available to a large group of researchers from different disciplines.

In this chapter, the focus is on subthreshold transcranial direct current stimulation (tDCS), but we emphasize the potential of other brain stimulation methods such as electrical stimulation with alternating currents (tACS) or random noise (tRNS), (repetitive) transcranial magnetic stimulation (TMS), invasive deep brain stimulation (DBS), or transcranial focused ultrasound stimulation (tFUS) [2, 5]. Offering an exhaustive guide for choosing between the existing methods is beyond the scope of this chapter. On behalf of tDCS (and transcranial electric stimulation in general), adverse sensations usually diminish to a negligible degree after some minutes of stimulation, no distracting noise would influence normally occurring behavior, and tDCS configurations can usually comply with task requirements, including

P. A. Schroeder
Department of Psychology, Clinical Psychology and Psychotherapy, University of Tübingen, Tübingen, Germany
e-mail: philipp.schroeder@uni-tuebingen.de

C. Plewnia (✉)
Department of Psychiatry and Psychotherapy, Neurophysiology and Interventional Neuropsychiatry, University of Tübingen, Tübingen, Germany
e-mail: christian.plewnia@uni-tuebingen.de

relatively free movement. Credible placebo conditions can be established with sham tDCS, by eliciting comparable tactile sensations, in the beginning and end of a stimulation session, to control for expectation effects [6]. The subtle neurophysiological effects of weak direct currents in tDCS stipulate a neuromodulatory perspective and require the extensive consideration of any cortical activities concurrent to its application.

To date, tDCS can be considered a flexible and powerful research tool, which was readily integrated in research on human cognition and emotion. What is more often neglected, however, are assumptions on the neural effects of tDCS in any brain region. In our experience, it is insufficient to consider tDCS as a manipulation of a static system, sometimes refined by considering global electric field distributions and/or general neurophysiological models, with questionable relevance for the behaving individual of interest. Rather, it is important to consider the behavioral and biological context in which brain stimulation is applied: Enhancement of neural activity is not equivocal to behavioral improvement, plasticity is subject to homeostatic processes, and (epi-)genetic factors critically influence the outcome of the intervention. In this chapter, we describe possible applications of tDCS interventions for research in neuropsychological, emotional, and cognitive field. Emerging principles for research in those areas are highlighted, and paradigmatic studies are explored. Finally, we suggest and comment on future directions regarding technical and design-specific developments in the field.

23.1 tDCS for Neuropsychological Investigations

To appreciate the potential of tDCS for neuropsychological investigation, it is mandatory to consider its neurophysiological effects first. As a neuromodulation tool, tDCS on its own cannot disrupt brain activity, elicit action potentials, or induce virtual lesions; instead, tDCS will always *modulate* ongoing brain activity and thereby interact with processes that are currently present in the active brain state. The most established neurophysiological account of tDCS effects assumes polarity-specific changes in cortical excitability. This account was primarily corroborated by changes in motor-evoked potentials during and after tDCS of the primary motor cortex [7, 8], by altered tactile discrimination during and after tDCS of sensorimotor cortex [9], and altered motion discrimination during and after tDCS of visual cortices [10]. Alternative but related accounts for stimulation effects include general induction of neuroplasticity, altered signal-to-noise ratio, or stochastic resonance [1]. In any of these accounts, the neurophysiological outcome of tDCS is dependent on current flow relative to neuron orientation [11]. At a larger spatial scale, an overall effect in a brain region targeted by tDCS is better characterized by more or less likely spontaneous firing due to the subtle shift of resting membrane potentials than by the transient activation or deactivation of functional tissue [7, 12]. Nonlinearities in stimulation effects—e.g., polarity asymmetry or intensity dependence—are present even in basic neurophysiological readouts, and increases in current intensity (or switching the tDCS polarity) do not necessarily encompass higher (or inverse) neural effects [13, 14]. As long as their sources are not fully understood, nonlinearities complicate essential assumptions on dosage, stimulation intensity, duration, and other technical parameters.

In the cognitive domain, studies can be particularly sensitive to nonlinear tDCS effects because polarity asymmetry may render anodal or cathodal tDCS ineffective for a task [15, 16]. In our latest analysis on polarity-specific modulations of spatial-numerical associations ($N = 144$), the effect size for anodal tDCS was remarkably lower (Cohen's $d = 0.2$) than the effect size for cathodal tDCS (Cohen's $d = 0.5$), which is often mirror-inverted in favor of anodal tDCS for other cognitive functions. Several interpretations of this asymmetric pattern are plausible, e.g., activity thresholds for a cognitive operation could be directionally resistant, and thus physiologically restrain impairment but support enhancement, including the complementary activation of distant network parts to sustain global activity levels. It is likely that compensatory cognitive processes—possibly along with crosscortical regulation networks—are readily available to maintain the most important functional cognitive states. Moreover, heterogeneities of cortical areas, which differently respond to anodal vs. cathodal tDCS, may shape or play into the different net outcomes of stimulation interactions [17]. For instance, anodal and cathodal tDCS appear to act on different (but related) neurotransmitter concentrations (GABA and glutamate) [18], which again could be involved in cognitive tasks to different extents. However, more fundamental research is required to clarify these hypotheses.

Timing is another critical aspect. In addition to the neuromodulatory effects during stimulation, after-effects of tDCS can indicate prolonged neuromodulation due to neuroplasticity. In neurophysiological studies, excitability increases from anodal tDCS were found to outlast up to 1 hour after stimulation [7, 19]. The exact neuroplastic mechanisms underlying after-effects are likely subject to rather complex interactions between LTP-/LTD-like effects, neurochemical modulations, and compensatory and homeostatic regulation [14]. Certainly, it has to be assumed that tDCS effect before, during, and after a specific cognitive or behavioral process is based on different mechanisms. However, it has been shown, for example, in mouse-brain slices, that synaptic coactivation is essential to induce lasting neuroplastic effects [20]. Accordingly, it has been suggested that tDCS can be functionally targeted by the concurrent task-related activation of networks, inputs, and their intersections with superimposed electric fields [21]. This can be achieved by directing behavior on the task with instruction and feedback parameters: when numerical decisions were explicit in the magnitude comparison task, polarity-specific tDCS effects were found. However, when font color of the identical number symbols was evaluated with the same key presses, behavioral effects vanished [22]. Task difficulty is relevant as well: the working memory n-back task, for instance, was paired with anodal tDCS in a 1-back and a more demanding 3-back version to examine differential effects of the combined intervention on another complex task, but only the 3-back variant induced transfer enhancements significant to sham tDCS [23]. In a delayed memory task, stimulation effects emerged in the most active instruction for pictures cued to be remembered, compared to pictures instructed irrelevant or to forget [24]. Moreover, in a combined fMRI-tDCS study, Hauser et al. [25] described blood-oxygen-level-dependent (BOLD) activation changes underneath the cathode in the inferior prefrontal cortex, but effects were observed only for novel subtractions and not for repeated subtraction operations. This result shows task-induced activity dependence also on a neural level, and the imaging result nicely illustrates the effect of cathodal tDCS on neural tissue, when combined with a respective task [25]. Regarding the timing of stimulation for enhancement of task performance in neuropsychiatric patients, a meta-analysis found greater improvements in post-stimulation accuracy if a task was performed concurrently with the application of tDCS [26]. Nevertheless, recent findings indicate better effects of "offline" stimulation, i.e., before task performance [27]. As brain state can be greatly influenced by instructions, tasks, and expectations, both online and offline studies should consider the "default" neural and behavioral activity during stimulation even if afterward offline performance is of foremost interest. Together, these observations render a very clear recommendation to use the most active task instructions, but also to consider task activations an instrumental aspect of any stimulation protocol.

Individual influences can further shape neuromodulation outcomes due to differences in state-dependent activations in a task, e.g., persons recruiting different strategies based on their experience or resources [28]. Similarly, different physiological reactions may influence stimulation protocols, e.g., by altered neurophysiological activations in smoking vs. nonsmoking schizophrenia patients [29, 30]. Based on the notion that task-relevant dopaminergic signaling may vary in its efficiency due to the genetic profile, also complex interactions between genotype (particularly COMT Val108/158Met) and brain stimulation effects on cognition were observed [31]. Precisely, the COMT Val108/158Met polymorphism is related to prefrontal dopamine, and Met/Met allele carriers, but not Val/Met or Val/Val carriers, were susceptible to online tDCS in set shifting [32] and response inhibition [33]. Conversely, consumption of L-tyrosine, as an experimental manipulation of dopamine levels, modulated effects of tDCS in the n-back task [34]. The nonlinear polarity-specific interactions between dopamine and tDCS relate to neuroplasticity, e.g., long-term potentiation and deprivation, and the dopamine dependence of the cognitive and motor systems [35, 36]. Notably, no interaction between offline bilateral tDCS and COMT polymorphism emerged in the assessment of the n-back task in a recent study [37], highlighting the need for further confirmatory and exploratory research on stimulation genetics.

Adverse sensations are usually minimal but still require systematic assessment and reporting of adverse effects in any stimulation condition [38]. Moreover, it is of utter importance in tDCS research to control for expectation and placebo effects. A recent study showed effects of a powerful vs. fake tDCS framing in the instruction on craving and consumption of snacks, without any effect of the actual active vs. sham tDCS protocol [39]. Careful wording of instructions must be used in combination with control of blinding in participants and examiners to minimize expectation effects. Standard tDCS designs that investigate comparisons between sham and real stimulation will require identical configurations and comparable sensations during sham tDCS, which should be assessed accordingly. Moreover, it is preferable to use double-blind protocols to counteract placebo and expectation effects.

23.2   tDCS for Cognitive Research

Only shortly after the rediscovery of excitability changes by tDCS in the motor cortex, first studies described that tDCS could modulate perception [40], implicit motor learning [41], and working memory [42]. Despite the promising results, updated meta-analytic perspectives on tDCS enhancements of working memory performance with anodal tDCS provided mixed results, and several inconsistencies regarding powerful study designs and optimal parameters remain open [43]. Selecting stimulation targets exclusively based on previous neuroimaging results may not always provide sufficient motivation for tDCS studies. Negative findings could not be refuted according to neurocognitive theories (even if the absence of evidence was rated in Bayesian analyses), since tDCS produces subthreshold modulations, crosscortical effects, and compensatory mechanisms. Despite the relatively simple administration, the interpretation of both positive and negative tDCS results thereby remains a challenge, even if basic requirements such as adequate research design and sample size, challenging and motivating task parameters, as well as sufficiently homogenous participant samples are fulfilled [44]. Regarding various technical parameters, such as return electrode placement, electrode size and shape, attachment method, intensity and timing, there is no standardization in sight, and interpretations should consider the exact configuration decisions.

Theoretical models in cognitive psychology are mostly informed by results from behavioral studies (and corroborated by computational models) and describe the underlying mechanisms that constitute human cognition, e.g., the structure and functionality of working memory. Its neural implementation is not necessarily of foremost interest for models of cognition, and experimental manipulations are at the core of the discipline. Usually, the parameters of the task are manipulated and changes in behavioral assessments are evaluated; however, if brain activity is manipulated directly by tDCS, effects in controlled assessments can already provide novel insights into underlying processes. This primary quality of a controlled manipulation already allows for inferences when combined with behavioral recordings. Moreover, whenever the causal contribution of brain regions, in terms of excitability, relative activity, and neural plasticity, is of interest to a cognitive model, tDCS-induced modulation of the target region in comparison with a placebo or control stimulation can be administered. As we argue in the following, the possible contribution of tDCS in different research designs can go beyond the causality of brain-behavior associations. For example, by contrasting different tasks during the same tDCS protocol, it was possible to reject the hypothesis of a single shared cognitive mechanism underlying implicit processing of numerical and ordinal sequences, which reacted differently to anodal tDCS [16]. Results from those two studies showed opposite responses to the identical tDCS configuration in two tasks, which was incompatible with a unique underlying cognitive mechanism [16, 22].

Practically, manifold neural processes are required to solve a cognitive task, which may require a more fine-grained perspective. To elucidate specific processes in cognition, behavioral negative control tasks should be implemented, along with specific investigations to increase the exploratory power of tDCS studies and exclude trivial effects, e.g., due to higher response speed or better visual acuity, dependent on the targeted brain regions [2]. In our studies on implicit spatial–numerical associations, neither general response speed nor interference processing in explicit conflict tasks explained the results [22, 45]. Another possibility is the inspection of theoretically unrelated parameters from the same task, e.g., responses to control stimuli or general responding irrespective of a predefined contrast. For instance, in a study on response inhibition, the relevant and predefined measure was modulated by tDCS, but control analyses on responses not specifically associated with the inhibition component led to the functional specificity of this tDCS effect [46]. Nevertheless, the selection of appropriate control tasks may be considered as delicate as the design of appropriate active control training groups, and studies with closely matched task parameters can allow for more fine-grained interpretations in the future.

To date, numerous cognitive tasks have been challenged with tDCS over brain regions that were correlated with neuroimaging changes, e.g., attention, learning and memory, decision making, and many more [47]. Neurocognitive theories can be supplemented by varying either task or stimulation parameters in controlled research designs. For example, a central assumption in the discussion on hemispheric specialization of working memory components was addressed by the study of Ruf et al. [48], who applied anodal or sham tDCS either to the left or right hemisphere concurrently to a verbal or spatial adaptive n-back training throughout three training sessions. Working memory training led to greater improvements when it was combined with tDCS of the respective hemisphere, i.e., left-verbal or right-spatial [48]. Their result provides causal evidence for the hemispheric specialization of working memory training and has direct implications for according interventions. Critically, not all cognitive functions appear to be lateralized, and another tDCS study targeting different hemispheres and areas observed similarly modulated adjustments of cognitive control across both hemispheres in prefrontal, but not motor, regions [49]. Pitting effects of different brain regions against each other entails empirical assertions on the practical focality of a specific tDCS intervention, but is also a necessary argumentation to underscore neurocognitive theories.

23.3   tDCS for Emotional Research

Emotional processing includes widespread activity networks across central and peripheral nervous systems [50]. Since conventional tDCS reaches cortical regions, direct emotional reactions in the limbic system, which may curtail higher-order processing, would escape neurophysiological modulation effects. However, as regulation of emotional processing due to emotional control in prefrontal regions is in continuous dialogue with limbic structures [51, 52], an indirect route is available by targeting prefrontal regions with tDCS and triggering emotional systems with according tasks or materials.

Manifold aspects of emotional experience can be considered, and we can only focus on selected aspects here. Emotion regulation, for instance, is a highly relevant ability related to the voluntary control of affective reactions and strategic handling of them with emotional experience. Reappraisal can enhance or diminish the experience of emotional stimuli, which was more extreme in both directions following excitation of the right prefrontal cortex with anodal tDCS [53]. In a study on appraisal of affective picture and craving cues, anodal tDCS to the left dlPFC reduced negative affect [54]. Emotional responses can also influence working memory and the modulation of negative emotion processing by anodal or cathodal tDCS, thereby indirectly improving performance in depressed patients or impairing performance in healthy controls, respectively [55]. Affect regulation, appraisal, and emotional memory are approximated in these tasks by explicit request of up- or downregulation, evaluation, or retrieval of a nonemotional memory trace; different versions of emotional tasks, stimuli, and regulation strategies may respond to prefrontal stimulation and amend to the understanding of fronto-limbic emotional networks.

The modal process model of emotion includes attention as mandatory precursor for appraisal and response (and subsequent emotion regulation) [56]. In absence of an emotional task, importantly, emotional experience was apparently not influenced by tDCS per se; however, emotional face recognition speed was enhanced by anodal tDCS [57]. In the social context, facial emotion recognition is sometimes required despite restricted information, and correctly inferring other's mental state from eye regions has been found central for social intelligence. A widely used instrument to assess emotional recognition capabilities asks volunteers for classification of another's emotional state according to image extracts of eye regions [58]. Here, cathodal tDCS to the left inferior frontal cortex was found to reduce reaction time without changing response correctness, potentially by means of an improved signal-to-noise ratio [59].

Emotional reactions are elicited in laboratory settings by using negative stimuli, or by confronting participants with annoying and stressful tasks. The Paced-Auditory Serial Addition Task (PASAT) is an adaptive continuous addition task well known for its capacity to induce negative mood in participants. If the task is combined with anodal tDCS of prefrontal regions to increase the capacity to downregulate emotional processing, e.g., in subcortical regions, an overall reduction of negative emotional reactivity to the task was observed in healthy male participants [60].

This very general model of emotional control is currently being employed in several directions. Firstly, and further advancing the proposition that deficient emotional control can be regained by using the PASAT as a training [61], several studies are combining emotional control training with tDCS. Results from the study will also compare different electrode configurations and intensity modulations. Next, the direct physiological effects of tDCS on emotional control will be elucidated by measurement of electrocortical potentials [62].

Recent attempts augmented the PASAT by inducing more difficult processing, e.g., in subtraction [63]. Moreover, the PASAT can be combined with the n-back working memory task to challenge participants even more, and allow for higher training intensity. First results with the 2-back PASAT combined with healthy volunteers reproduced an improvement of cognitive control over negative emotions but also implied a stabilization of positive affect in contrast to the sham stimulation [64].

A further promising window into the widespread and interactive components of emotional processing is the concurrent assessment of peripheral signals: in one of our studies probing emotional control of working memory, we assessed skin conductance responses to negative, neutral, and positive emotional stimuli during sham and anodal tDCS. With the tested pictures, increased electrodermal responses were attenuated during anodal stimulation regardless of the negative content [65]. Other physiological measurements can be utilized by assessing heart rate variability or pupil dilation [66]. The possibility of artifacts must be considered, particularly for electric signatures of peripheral as well as central neurophysiology [4]. For a nice illustration, a standardized protocol for eliciting stress—the trier social stress test— can be considered, which consists of a fictive job interview and mental arithmetic in front of an evaluation committee. Following 20 minutes of tDCS to right medial frontal areas, a study assessed endocrine physiology (cortisol levels in saliva), behavioral reports, and fMRI effects in the stress protocol, and thereby documented polarity-dependent modulations in stress responses [67].

23.4   Future Directions and Challenges

The combinations of tDCS with cognitive tasks reveal far less trivial results than often assumed. Powerful and theoretically motivated research designs are well suited to provide novel insights into the neural underpinnings of cognitive processing, but also into the working mechanisms of subthreshold brain stimulation. The complex interaction between stimulation parameters, task requirements, and the individual genetic and neurophysiological makeup challenge the interpretation of tDCS effects on cognitive and emotional processes. Therefore, it is essential to consider the interindividual variability and include individual measures of brain functions to better understand and predict the interactions between electrical stimulation, emotion, and behavior [28].

Preregistration of study analyses and outcomes is a welcome quality enhancement to improve reporting standards and to contribute to the solid understanding of relatively fragile and malleable tDCS effects on cognition and emotion in the future, as reports of null findings cast doubt on the efficacy of tDCS for modulating cognitive functions. For instance, a controversial quantitative review on 271 single-session tDCS studies found no support for reliable modulations of cognition [68]. Although their bold conclusions were attenuated by several methodological problems and conceptual shortcomings [69, 70], including the fact that little-to-none direct study replications with identical technical implementation exist, tDCS effectivity is a recurring theme in contemporary neuroscience research. This becomes especially apparent when considering also commercial devices for cognitive enhancement with opaque placement and DC generation implementations that produce detrimental performance in standardized tests [71].

Given its interventional character, tDCS can be considered a potential treatment in neurological and mental rehabilitation, although it must be highlighted that magnetic brain stimulation methods (e.g., TMS or TBS) at the moment draw on more and more solid evidence [72]. Here, beneficial aspects of tDCS may be practical elements (portability, acceptance) or a targeted and controlled integration into concurrent treatments such as psychotherapy [73]. Combinations with imaging methods are increasingly utilized and will be required to understand the crosscortical effects of neuromodulation on neurophysiology in proximal and distal brain regions.

On the technical side, two major developments can be identified: transcranial electric stimulation using different current forms, and more targeted stimulation using advanced electrode configurations. The latter development includes the application of more focal multielectrode configurations, and is often referred to as high-definition tDCS, which induced polarity-dependent and efficient excitability changes in primary motor cortex [19, 74]. Regarding the modulation of behavior, conventional and HD-tDCS over rIFC induced comparable changes in response inhibition [75] and other indices of cognitive control [49]. Another class of electric stimulation uses alternating currents to induce oscillations (tACS). It is important to highlight that the neurophysiological mechanism of tACS is bluntly different and draws on the idea of coupling brain oscillation frequencies, which can be related to cognitive processes and which would entrain to artificially introduced alternating currents [76, 77].

23.5 Conclusions

Cognitive and emotional processes recruit cerebral regions, which can be modulated by tDCS in subtle and various ways. Beyond causal inferences, the careful manipulations of both technical stimulation and task situation parameters allow for systematic investigation of fundamental principles underlying different facets of human behavior. Integration of stimulation paradigms within cognitive paradigms, training, and neurophysiological assessments can further our understanding of the biological implementations of cognition and emotion. When targeted at dysfunctional networks and abnormal behavior, tDCS can provide novel rehabilitation perspectives and amend the available therapeutic instruments. Moreover, this knowledge will further pave the way for individualized, tolerable, and effective treatments of emotional and behavioral disorders.

References

1. Fertonani A, Miniussi C. Transcranial electrical stimulation: what we know and do not know about mechanisms. Neuroscientist. 2017;23(2):109–23. https://doi.org/10.1177/1073858416631966.
2. Polanía R, Nitsche MA, Ruff CC. Studying and modifying brain function with non-invasive brain stimulation. Nat Neurosci. 2018;21:174–87. https://doi.org/10.1038/s41593-017-0054-4.

3. Driver J, Blankenburg F, Bestmann S, Vanduffel W, Ruff CC. Concurrent brain-stimulation and neuroimaging for studies of cognition. Trends Cogn Sci. 2009;13(7):319–27. https://doi.org/10.1016/j.tics.2009.04.007.
4. Woods AJ, Bikson M, Chelette K, Dmochowski J, Dutta A, Esmaeilpour Z, et al. Transcranial direct current stimulation integration with magnetic resonance imaging, magnetic resonance spectroscopy, near infrared spectroscopy imaging, and electroencephalography. In: Knotkova H, Nitsche MA, Bikson M, Woods AJ, editors. Practical guide to transcranial direct current stimulation: principles, procedures and applications. Cham: Springer; 2019. p. 293–345. https://doi.org/10.1007/978-3-319-95948-1_11.
5. Legon W, Sato TF, Opitz A, Mueller J, Barbour A, Williams A, Tyler WJ. Transcranial focused ultrasound modulates the activity of primary somatosensory cortex in humans. Nat Neurosci. 2014;17(2):322–9. https://doi.org/10.1038/nn.3620.
6. Gandiga PC, Hummel FC, Cohen LG. Transcranial DC stimulation (tDCS): a tool for double-blind sham-controlled clinical studies in brain stimulation. Clin Neurophysiol. 2006;117(4):845–50. https://doi.org/10.1016/j.clinph.2005.12.003.
7. Nitsche MA, Paulus W. Excitability changes induced in the human motor cortex by weak transcranial direct current stimulation. J Physiol. 2000;527(Pt 3):633–9. https://doi.org/10.1111/j.1469-7793.2000.t01-1-00633.x.
8. Priori A, Berardelli A, Rona S, Accornero N, Manfredi M. Polarization of the human motor cortex through the scalp. Neuroreport. 1998;9(10):2257–60. https://doi.org/10.1097/00001756-199807130-00020.
9. Rogalewski A, Breitenstein C, Nitsche MA, Paulus W, Knecht S. Transcranial direct current stimulation disrupts tactile perception. Eur J Neurosci. 2004;20(1):2001–4. https://doi.org/10.1111/j.1460-9568.2004.03450.x.
10. Antal A, Nitsche MA, Kruse W, Kincses TZ, Hoffmann K-P, Paulus W. Direct current stimulation over V5 enhances visuomotor coordination by improving motion perception in humans. J Cogn Neurosci. 2004;16(4):521–7. https://doi.org/10.1162/089892904323057263.
11. Bikson M, Inoue M, Akiyama H, Deans JK, Fox JE, Miyakawa H, Jefferys JGR. Effects of uniform extracellular DC electric fields on excitability in rat hippocampal slices in vitro. J Physiol. 2004;557(Pt 1):175–90. https://doi.org/10.1113/jphysiol.2003.055772.
12. Miniussi C, Harris JA, Ruzzoli M. Modelling non-invasive brain stimulation in cognitive neuroscience. Neurosci Biobehav Rev. 2013;37(8):1702–12. https://doi.org/10.1016/j.neubiorev.2013.06.014.
13. Batsikadze G, Moliadze V, Paulus W, Kuo M-F, Nitsche MA. Partially non-linear stimulation intensity-dependent effects of direct current stimulation on motor cortex excitability in humans. J Physiol. 2013;591(7):1987–2000. https://doi.org/10.1113/jphysiol.2012.249730.
14. Jamil A, Batsikadze G, Kuo H-I, Labruna L, Hasan A, Paulus W, Nitsche MA. Systematic evaluation of the impact of stimulation intensity on neuroplastic after-effects induced by transcranial direct current stimulation. J Physiol. 2017;595(4):1273–88. https://doi.org/10.1113/JP272738.
15. Jacobson L, Koslowsky M, Lavidor M. tDCS polarity effects in motor and cognitive domains: a meta-analytical review. Exp Brain Res. 2012;216(1):1–10. https://doi.org/10.1007/s00221-011-2891-9.
16. Schroeder PA, Nuerk H-C, Plewnia C. Switching between multiple codes of SNARC-like associations: two conceptual replication attempts with anodal tDCS in sham-controlled crossover design. Front Neurosci. 2017;11:654. https://doi.org/10.3389/fnins.2017.00654.
17. Bestmann S, de Berker AO, Bonaiuto J. Understanding the behavioural consequences of non-invasive brain stimulation. Trends Cogn Sci. 2015;19(1):13–20. https://doi.org/10.1016/j.tics.2014.10.003.
18. Stagg CJ, Best JG, Stephenson MC, O'Shea J, Wylezinska M, Kincses ZT, et al. Polarity-sensitive modulation of cortical neurotransmitters by transcranial stimulation. J Neurosci. 2009;29(16):5202–6. https://doi.org/10.1523/JNEUROSCI.4432-08.2009.

19. Kuo H-II, Bikson M, Datta A, Minhas P, Paulus W, Kuo M-FF, Nitsche MA. Comparing cortical plasticity induced by conventional and high-definition 4 × 1 ring tDCS: a neurophysiological study. Brain Stimul. 2013;6(4):644–8. https://doi.org/10.1016/j.brs.2012.09.010.
20. Fritsch B, Reis J, Martinowich K, Schambra HM, Ji Y, Cohen LG, Lu B. Direct current stimulation promotes BDNF-dependent synaptic plasticity: potential implications for motor learning. Neuron. 2010;66(2):198–204. https://doi.org/10.1016/j.neuron.2010.03.035.
21. Bikson M, Rahman A. Origins of specificity during tDCS: anatomical, activity-selective, and input-bias mechanisms. Front Hum Neurosci. 2013;7:688. https://doi.org/10.3389/fnhum.2013.00688.
22. Schroeder PA, Nuerk H-C, Plewnia C. Prefrontal neuromodulation reverses spatial associations of non-numerical sequences, but not numbers. Biol Psychol. 2017;128:39–49. https://doi.org/10.1016/j.biopsycho.2017.07.008.
23. Gill J, Shah-basak PP, Hamilton R. It's the thought that counts: examining the task-dependent effects of transcranial direct current stimulation on executive function. Brain Stimul. 2015;8(2):253–9. https://doi.org/10.1016/j.brs.2014.10.018.
24. Zwissler B, Sperber C, Aigeldinger S, Schindler S, Kissler J, Plewnia C. Shaping memory accuracy by left prefrontal transcranial direct current stimulation. J Neurosci. 2014;34(11):4022–6. https://doi.org/10.1523/JNEUROSCI.5407-13.2014.
25. Hauser TU, Rütsche B, Wurmitzer K, Brem S, Ruff CC, Grabner RH. Neurocognitive effects of transcranial direct current stimulation in arithmetic learning and performance: a simultaneous tDCS-fMRI study. Brain Stimul. 2016;9(6):850–8. https://doi.org/10.1016/j.brs.2016.07.007.
26. Dedoncker J, Brunoni AR, Baeken C, Vanderhasselt M-A. A systematic review and meta-analysis of the effects of transcranial direct current stimulation (tDCS) over the dorsolateral prefrontal cortex in healthy and neuropsychiatric samples: influence of stimulation parameters. Brain Stimul. 2016;9(4):501–17. https://doi.org/10.1016/j.brs.2016.04.006.
27. Friehs MA, Frings C. Offline beats online: transcranial direct current stimulation timing influences on working memory. Neuroreport. 2019;30(12):795–9.
28. Krause B, Cohen Kadosh R. Not all brains are created equal: the relevance of individual differences in responsiveness to transcranial electrical stimulation. Front Syst Neurosci. 2014;8:25. https://doi.org/10.3389/fnsys.2014.00025.
29. Brunelin J, Hasan A, Haesebaert F, Nitsche MA, Poulet E. Nicotine smoking prevents the effects of frontotemporal transcranial direct current stimulation (tDCS) in hallucinating patients with schizophrenia. Brain Stimul. 2015;8(6):1225–7. https://doi.org/10.1016/j.brs.2015.08.002.
30. Thirugnanasambandam N, Grundey J, Adam K, Drees A, Skwirba AC, Lang N, et al. Nicotinergic impact on focal and non-focal neuroplasticity induced by non-invasive brain stimulation in non-smoking humans. Neuropsychopharmacology. 2011;36(4):879–86. https://doi.org/10.1038/npp.2010.227.
31. Wiegand A, Nieratschker V, Plewnia C. Genetic modulation of transcranial direct current stimulation effects on cognition. Front Hum Neurosci. 2016;10:651. https://doi.org/10.3389/fnhum.2016.00651.
32. Plewnia C, Zwissler B, Längst I, Maurer B, Giel KE, Krüger R. Effects of transcranial direct current stimulation (tDCS) on executive functions: influence of COMT Val/Met polymorphism. Cortex. 2013;49(7):1801–7. https://doi.org/10.1016/j.cortex.2012.11.002.
33. Nieratschker V, Kiefer C, Giel KE, Krüger R, Plewnia C. The COMT Val/Met polymorphism modulates effects of tDCS on response inhibition. Brain Stimul. 2015;8(2):283–8. https://doi.org/10.1016/j.brs.2014.11.009.
34. Jongkees BJ, Sellaro R, Beste C, Nitsche MA, Kühn S, Colzato LS. L-Tyrosine administration modulates the effect of transcranial direct current stimulation on working memory in healthy humans. Cortex. 2017;90:103–14. https://doi.org/10.1016/j.cortex.2017.02.014.
35. Fresnoza S, Stiksrud E, Klinker F, Liebetanz D, Paulus W, Kuo MF, Nitsche MA. Dosage-dependent effect of dopamine D2 receptor activation on motor cortex plasticity in humans. J Neurosci. 2014;34(32):10701–9. https://doi.org/10.1523/JNEUROSCI.0832-14.2014.

36. Monte-Silva K, Liebetanz D, Grundey J, Paulus W, Nitsche MA. Dosage-dependent non-linear effect of l-dopa on human motor cortex plasticity. J Physiol. 2010;588(18):3415–24. https://doi.org/10.1113/jphysiol.2010.190181.

37. Jongkees BJ, Loseva AA, Yavari FB, Nitsche MA, Colzato LS. The COMT Val 158 Met polymorphism does not modulate the after-effect of tDCS on working memory. Eur J Neurosci. 2019;49(2):263–74. https://doi.org/10.1111/ejn.14261.

38. Brunoni AR, Amadera J, Berbel B, Volz MS, Rizzerio BG, Fregni F. A systematic review on reporting and assessment of adverse effects associated with transcranial direct current stimulation. Int J Neuropsychopharmacol. 2011;14(8):1133–45. https://doi.org/10.1017/S1461145710001690.

39. Ray MK, Sylvester MD, Helton A, Pittman BR, Wagstaff LE, McRae TR, et al. The effect of expectation on transcranial direct current stimulation (tDCS) to suppress food craving and eating in individuals with overweight and obesity. Appetite. 2019;136(2019):1–7. https://doi.org/10.1016/j.appet.2018.12.044.

40. Antal A, Nitsche MA, Paulus W. External modulation of visual perception in humans. Neuroreport. 2001;12(16):3553–5. https://doi.org/10.1097/00001756-200111160-00036.

41. Nitsche MA, Schauenburg A, Lang N, Liebetanz D, Exner C, Paulus W, Tergau F. Facilitation of implicit motor learning by weak transcranial direct current stimulation of the primary motor cortex in the human. J Cogn Neurosci. 2003;15(4):619–26. https://doi.org/10.1162/089892903321662994.

42. Fregni F, Boggio PS, Nitsche MA, Bermpohl F, Antal A, Feredoes E, et al. Anodal transcranial direct current stimulation of prefrontal cortex enhances working memory. Exp Brain Res. 2005;166(1):23–30. https://doi.org/10.1007/s00221-005-2334-6.

43. Hill AT, Fitzgerald PB, Hoy KE. Effects of anodal transcranial direct current stimulation on working memory: a systematic review and meta-analysis of findings from healthy and neuropsychiatric populations. Brain Stimul. 2016;9(2):197–208. https://doi.org/10.1016/j.brs.2015.10.006.

44. Berryhill ME, Peterson DJ, Jones KT, Stephens JA. Hits and misses: leveraging tDCS to advance cognitive research. Front Psychol. 2014;5:800. https://doi.org/10.3389/fpsyg.2014.00800.

45. Schroeder PA, Pfister R, Kunde W, Nuerk H-C, Plewnia C. Counteracting implicit conflicts by electrical inhibition of the prefrontal cortex. J Cogn Neurosci. 2016;28(11):1737–48. https://doi.org/10.1162/jocn.

46. Friehs MA, Frings C. Pimping inhibition: anodal tDCS enhances stop-signal reaction time. J Exp Psychol Hum Percept Perform. 2018;44(12):1933–45. https://doi.org/10.1037/xhp0000579.

47. Coffman BA, Clark VP, Parasuraman R. Battery powered thought: enhancement of attention, learning, and memory in healthy adults using transcranial direct current stimulation. Neuroimage. 2014;85:895–908. https://doi.org/10.1016/j.neuroimage.2013.07.083.

48. Ruf SP, Fallgatter AJ, Plewnia C. Augmentation of working memory training by transcranial direct current stimulation (tDCS). Sci Rep. 2017;7(1):876. https://doi.org/10.1038/s41598-017-01055-1.

49. Gbadeyan O, McMahon K, Steinhauser M, Meinzer M. Stimulation of dorsolateral prefrontal cortex enhances adaptive cognitive control: a high-definition transcranial direct current stimulation study. J Neurosci. 2016;36(50):12530–6. https://doi.org/10.1523/JNEUROSCI.2450-16.2016.

50. Damasio AR, Everitt BJ, Bishop D. The somatic marker hypothesis and the possible functions of the prefrontal cortex [and discussion]. Philos Trans R Soc B Biol Sci. 1996;351(1346):1413–20.

51. Miller EK, Cohen JD. An integrative theory of prefrontal cortex function. Annu Rev Neurosci. 2001;24:167–202. https://doi.org/10.1146/annurev.neuro.24.1.167.

52. Ochsner KN, Gross JJ. The cognitive control of emotion. Trends Cogn Sci. 2005;9(5):242–9. https://doi.org/10.1016/j.tics.2005.03.010.

53. Feeser M, Prehn K, Kazzer P, Mungee A, Bajbouj M. Transcranial direct current stimulation enhances cognitive control during emotion regulation. Brain Stimul. 2014;7(1):105–12. https://doi.org/10.1016/j.brs.2013.08.006.

54. Pripfl J, Lamm C. Focused transcranial direct current stimulation (tDCS) over the dorsolateral prefrontal cortex modulates specific domains of self-regulation. Neurosci Res. 2015;91:41–7. https://doi.org/10.1016/j.neures.2014.09.007.
55. Plewnia C, Schroeder PA, Wolkenstein L. Targeting the biased brain: non-invasive brain stimulation to ameliorate cognitive control. Lancet Psychiatry. 2015;2(4):351–6. https://doi.org/10.1016/S2215-0366(15)00056-5.
56. Gross JJ, Thompson R. Emotion regulation: conceptual foundations. In: Gross JJ, editor. Handbook of emotion regulation. New York: Guildford Press; 2007. p. 3–24.
57. Nitsche MA, Koschack J, Pohlers H, Hullemann S, Paulus W, Happe S. Effects of frontal transcranial direct current stimulation on emotional state and processing in healthy humans. Front Psych. 2012;3:58. https://doi.org/10.3389/fpsyt.2012.00058.
58. Baron-Cohen S, Wheelwright S, Hill J, Raste Y, Plumb I. The "'Reading the Mind in the Eyes'" test revised version: a study with normal adults, and adults with Asperger syndrome or high-functioning autism. J Child Psychol Psychiatry Allied Discip. 2001;42:241–51.
59. Klimm N, Ehlis A-C, Plewnia C. EP 26. Reduction of excitability in the left inferior frontal gyrus by cathodal tDCS facilitates emotion recognition. Clin Neurophysiol. 2016;127(9):e244–5. https://doi.org/10.1016/j.clinph.2016.05.081.
60. Plewnia C, Schroeder PA, Kunze R, Faehling F, Wolkenstein L. Keep calm and carry on: improved frustration tolerance and processing speed by transcranial direct current stimulation (tDCS). PLoS One. 2015;10(4):e0122578. https://doi.org/10.1371/journal.pone.0122578.
61. Siegle GJ, Ghinassi F, Thase ME. Neurobehavioral therapies in the 21st century: summary of an emerging field and an extended example of cognitive control training for depression. Cognit Ther Res. 2007;31(2):235–62. https://doi.org/10.1007/s10608-006-9118-6.
62. Faehling F, Plewnia C. Controlling the emotional bias: performance, late positive potentials, and the effect of anodal transcranial direct current stimulation (tDCS). Front Cell Neurosci. 2016;10(June):1–13. https://doi.org/10.3389/fncel.2016.00159.
63. Pope PA, Miall RC. Task-specific facilitation of cognition by cathodal transcranial direct current stimulation of the cerebellum. Brain Stimul. 2012;5(2):84–94. https://doi.org/10.1016/j.brs.2012.03.006.
64. Wiegand A, Sommer A, Nieratschker V, Plewnia C. Improvement of cognitive control and stabilization of affect by prefrontal transcranial direct current stimulation (tDCS). Sci Rep. 2019;9:6797. https://doi.org/10.1038/s41598-019-43234-2.
65. Schroeder PA, Ehlis A-C, Wolkenstein L, Fallgatter AJ, Plewnia C. Emotional distraction and bodily reaction: modulation of autonomous responses by anodal tDCS to the prefrontal cortex. Front Cell Neurosci. 2015;9:482. https://doi.org/10.3389/fncel.2015.00482.
66. Schestatsky P, Simis M, Freeman R, Pascual-Leone A, Fregni F. Non-invasive brain stimulation and the autonomic nervous system. Clin Neurophysiol. 2013;124(9):1716–28. https://doi.org/10.1016/j.clinph.2013.03.020.
67. Antal A, Fischer T, Saiote C, Miller R, Chaieb L, Wang DJJ, et al. Transcranial electrical stimulation modifies the neuronal response to psychosocial stress exposure. Hum Brain Mapp. 2014;35(8):3750–9. https://doi.org/10.1002/hbm.22434.
68. Horvath JC, Forte JD, Carter O. Quantitative review finds no evidence of cognitive effects in healthy populations from single-session transcranial direct current stimulation (tDCS). Brain Stimul. 2015;8(3):535–50. https://doi.org/10.1016/j.brs.2015.01.400.
69. Antal A, Keeser D, Priori A, Padberg F, Nitsche MA. Conceptual and procedural shortcomings of the systematic review "evidence that transcranial direct current stimulation (tDCS) generates little-to-no reliable neurophysiologic effect beyond MEP amplitude modulation in healthy human subjects: a systematic review" by Horvath and co-workers. Brain Stimul. 2015;8:27–31. https://doi.org/10.1016/j.brs.2015.05.010.
70. Price AR, Hamilton RH. A re-evaluation of the cognitive effects from single-session transcranial direct current stimulation. Brain Stimul. 2015;8(3):663–5.
71. Steenbergen L, Sellaro R, Hommel B, Lindenberger U, Kühn S, Colzato LS. "Unfocus" on focus: commercial tDCS headset impairs working memory. Exp Brain Res. 2015;234(3):637–43. https://doi.org/10.1007/s00221-015-4391-9.

72. Lefaucheur JP, André-Obadia N, Antal A, Ayache SS, Baeken C, Benninger DH, et al. Evidence-based guidelines on the therapeutic use of repetitive transcranial magnetic stimulation (rTMS). Clin Neurophysiol. 2014;125(11):2150–206. https://doi.org/10.1016/j.clinph.2014.05.021.
73. Bajbouj M, Aust S, Spies J, Herrera-Melendez AL, Mayer SV, Peters M, et al. PsychotherapyPlus: augmentation of cognitive behavioral therapy (CBT) with prefrontal transcranial direct current stimulation (tDCS) in major depressive disorder—study design and methodology of a multicenter double-blind randomized placebo-controlled tria. Eur Arch Psychiatry Clin Neurosci. 2018;268(8):797–808. https://doi.org/10.1007/s00406-017-0859-x.
74. Datta A, Bansal V, Diaz J, Patel J, Reato D, Bikson M. Gyri-precise head model of transcranial direct current stimulation: improved spatial focality using a ring electrode versus conventional rectangular pad. Brain Stimul. 2009;2(4):201–7, 207.e1. https://doi.org/10.1016/j.brs.2009.03.005.
75. Hogeveen J, Grafman J, Aboseria M, David A, Bikson M, Hauner KK. Effects of high-definition and conventional tDCS on response inhibition. Brain Stimul. 2016;9(5):720–9. https://doi.org/10.1016/j.brs.2016.04.015.
76. Helfrich RF, Schneider TR, Rach S, Trautmann-Lengsfeld SA, Engel AK, Herrmann CS. Entrainment of brain oscillations by transcranial alternating current stimulation. Curr Biol. 2014;24(3):333–9. https://doi.org/10.1016/j.cub.2013.12.041.
77. Polanía R, Nitsche MA, Korman C, Batsikadze G, Paulus W. The importance of timing in segregated theta phase-coupling for cognitive performance. Curr Biol. 2012;22(14):1314–8. https://doi.org/10.1016/j.cub.2012.05.021.

Clinical Drivers for Personalization of Transcranial Current Stimulation (tES 3.0)

Giulio Ruffini, Juilien Modolo, Roser Sanchez-Todo, Ricardo Salvador, and Emiliano Santarnecchi

24.1 Introduction

The brain is a complex, plastic, electrical *network* operating at multiple scales. There is a growing body of evidence suggesting that large-scale networks underlie both integration and differentiation processes that are fundamental for information processing. For instance, putatively simple cognitive tasks such as object recognition have been shown to involve networks that include the bilateral occipital, the left temporal, and the left/right frontal regions [1]. Neuropsychiatric disorders ultimately result from network dysfunctions that may arise from the abnormality in one or more isolated brain regions but produce alterations in larger brain networks (see [2–4]). Because of these observations, networks are natural targets of therapeutic interventions [5].

Interest in *neuromodulation* has increased in recent decades and it is now considered a promising tool for the management of conditions that range from psychiatric diseases to chronic neuropathic pain and epilepsy. Transcranial electrical current

G. Ruffini · R. Sanchez-Todo · R. Salvador
Neuroelectrics Corporation, Cambridge, MA, USA
e-mail: giulio.ruffini@neuroelectrics.com;
roser.sanchez@neuroelectrics.com; ricardo.salvador@neuroelectrics.com

J. Modolo
Univ Rennes, INSERM, LTSI—U1099, Rennes, France
e-mail: julien.modolo@inserm.fr

E. Santarnecchi (✉)
Berenson-Allen Center for Non-invasive Brain Stimulation,
Beth Israel Deaconess Medical Center, Boston, MA, USA

Harvard Medical School, Boston, MA, USA
e-mail: esantarn@bidmc.harvard.edu

© Springer Nature Switzerland AG 2020
B. Dell'Osso, G. Di Lorenzo (eds.), *Non Invasive Brain Stimulation in Psychiatry and Clinical Neurosciences*,
https://doi.org/10.1007/978-3-030-43356-7_24

stimulation (tES[1]) or transcranial current stimulation (tCS), as it is also known, is a safe [6], tolerable, noninvasive brain stimulation technique. Its origins follow the history of the discovery of electricity itself. Work in the twentieth century using low-intensity currents culminated in the investigation of weak direct and alternating currents by Nitsche and Paulus [7], who demonstrated that by applying a direct current through the scalp, the excitability of brain tissue can change up to 40%, as revealed by transcranial magnetic stimulation (TMS).

By passing electrical currents through the scalp and into the brain, tES generates *electric fields* that can alter brain function by coupling to neurons. A weak electric field can shift the neuronal membrane operating point, in a way that will make the cell more or less excitable, or, equivalently, more or less likely to fire given some inputs. This means that an electric field can immediately alter the way that the exposed part of the brain processes information, leading to longer-term changes through plasticity. Thus, by shifting the operating point of neurons, tES electric fields can affect the way parts of the brain participate in tasks (motor, cognitive, or others), and through *plasticity mechanisms*, contribute to its rewiring. tES comprises a number of *different techniques*: transcranial direct current stimulation (tDCS), alternating current stimulation (tACS), and random noise stimulation (tRNS) [8]. While other temporal waveforms are possible, the common elements of tES are the weak character of currents (typically below 2 mA) and spectral support below a few hundred Hertz (extremely low frequencies, <300 Hz). In tACS, the stimulation currents have a sinusoidal time dependence (as in AC current). Amplitude, frequency, and relative phases across stimulation electrodes can be controlled. tACS stimulation may provide a powerful way to couple to the oscillatory behavior of the brain, which is at present an active research field in basic and clinical neuroscience. In tRNS, a less explored tES modality, the stimulation current is varied randomly. Its main effects appear to be excitatory.

tES is similar, in terms of physical principles, to *transcranial magnetic stimulation (TMS)*, or electroconvulsive therapy (ECT), as all operate through the induction of electric fields in the brain. However, compared to TMS and ECT, in tES the generated electric fields are orders of magnitude weaker (see Figs. 24.1 and 24.2). *TMS* creates quite strong and brief electric field pulses that actually cause neuron firing (action potentials). A repetitive TMS (rTMS) session for depression delivers 3000 TMS pulses each ~0.2 ms wide, which sum to ~1 second of total effective stimulation (rounded, the precise number depends on pulse shape) with a peak field strength of ~150 V/m. Multiplying time of effective application and peak electric field gives a rough measure of dose of of 150 V·s/m that can be compared to other stimulation

---

[1] Abbreviations used: *ASL* arterial spin labeling, *BCM* Bienenstock, Cooper, and Munro plasticity theory, *CSF* cerebrospinal fluid, *ECT* electroconvulsive therapy, *EEG* electroencephalography, *EN* epileptogenic network, *fMRI* functional MRI, *GM* grey matter, *HBM* hybrid brain model, *MEG* magnetoencephalography, *MRI* magnetic resonance imaging, *NIRS* near-infrared spectroscopy, *NMM* neural mass model, *SEEG* stereographic EEG, *tACS* transcranial alternating current, *tDCS* transcranial direct current, *tCS* transcranial current stimulation, same as *tES* transcranial electrical stimulation, *tRNS* transcranial random noise stimulation, *STDP* Spike Timing Dependent Plasticity, *TMS* transcranial magnetic stimulation, *WM* white matter

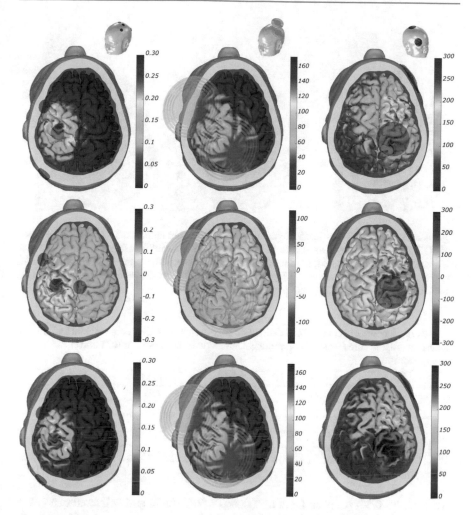

Fig. 24.1 Electric field distribution in the cortical surface induced by tDCS (left column), TMS (central column), and ECT (right column). The top row shows the magnitude of the E-field, the middle row the normal component (positive/negative when the E-field is directed in/out of the cortical surface) and the bottom row the magnitude of the tangential component of the E-field. Typical electrodes/coils and stimulation intensities were used to calculate the E-field: multichannel montage with PiSTIM electrodes (1 cm radius, cylindrical Ag/AgCl electrodes) with a total injected current of 1.0 mA in the tDCS model; Magstim's 70 mm figure-8 coil at 67.7 A/µs for the TMS calculations (the value reported in the literature for the RMT using this coil, [9]); bipolar montage (frontoparietal right unilateral, FP-RUL configuration) with 5 cm diameter cylindrical electrodes and a 800 mA current in the ECT model. All E-field values are reported in V/m. The head model in which the simulations were run is common for all cases

techniques. *ECT* generates strong peak electric fields of about 400 V/m with current of ~800 mA [10] applied over timescales of about a few tenths of a second, with delivered charges of the order of a few hundred mC. *tES* induces weak electric fields that gently modify neuronal oscillations during relatively long times (20 minutes or

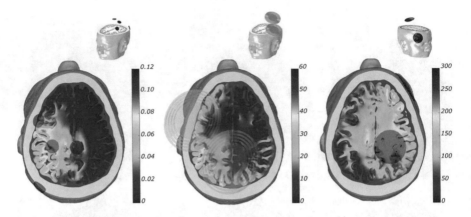

Fig. 24.2 Magnitude of the electric field induced by tDCS (left column), TMS (central column), and ECT (right column) in an axial slice cutting through the GM and WM. The location of the slice with respect to the coil/electrodes is shown in the figures' insets. The parameters of the electrodes and coil are the same as described in Fig. 24.1. All *E*-field values are reported in V/m. The head model in which the simulations were run is common for all cases

Table 24.1 A comparison of different stimulation dose metrics based on peak field and time of application – but not area – using representative numbers in each case (for ECT and rTMS as used in depression)

Metric (units)	tES	rTMS	ECT
Peak field in cortex, E_{peak} (V/m)	0.5	150	400
Injected current (mA)	1	-	800
Summed pulse Duration, T (s)	1200	1	0.2
Charge delivered, Q (mC)	1200	–	160
Amplitude-duration, $E_{peak} \times T$ (V s/m)	600	150	80

more), with ~0.5 V/m peak field, or a dose of 600 V s/m and delivered charges of the order of 1200 mC [11]. In all cases, multiple sessions are employed for therapeutic results. See Table 24.1 for a comparison of dosing between these techniques. To note that, since the therapeutic mechanisms of action are not well understood for any of them, our dosing comparison remains indicative.

Traditionally, tES has been applied using two large sponge electrodes on the scalp. However, newer systems use several small, EEG-like electrodes. Aided by realistic *modeling*, *multielectrode tES* can be used to produce controlled, precise electric fields in the brain, resulting in more specific electric field distributions and less variable effects [8, 12, 13]. tES is naturally combined with the measurement of *EEG* since both technologies rely on the electrical nature of the human brain. EEG can be used to study changes induced by tES, comparing the effects across groups or pre- and poststimulation. Similarly, tES is also often combined with fMRI, ASL, and NIRS, for example, for the study of brain networks pre-, during- and post-stimulation.

Research with tES includes basic neurophysiology and cognitive neuroscience. Basic research with tES (and its combination with other techniques) has the goal of deciphering the way the human brain works. By altering the operating points of neural networks, information can be gathered on fundamental mechanisms. This provides the means for realizing causal studies rather than correlation-based ones. *Clinical applications* of tES have been studied for almost two decades. The most mature ones are in fibromyalgia, major depression without drug resistance and in addictions/cravings (with probable efficacy, Level B evidence [14]), but many others are being developed, including epilepsy, chronic neuropathic pain, tinnitus, major depression with drug resistance, brain cancer, and cognitive remediation in neurodegeneration. Clinical applications of tES rely, mostly, on its plastic effects (those that remain after treatment is over). Under the hypothesis that brain function depends on its connectivity, neuromodulation aims to rewire the brain to achieve therapeutic effects.

Today, tES montages are *optimized* on the assumption that the effects can be directly quantified from the measurement of the electric field on the cortex, as we discuss more in-depth below. However, we know that such "passive electrical" physical models cannot fully describe the complex physiological phenomena that underlie brain function and stimulation effects (the physics of *life*). As neuroscience moves from a correlation-based science to a model-driven one, *computational models of the brain* (physics of electric fields and of their interaction with complex, active neuronal networks) will play a key role in the development of novel mechanistic understanding and computational optimization strategies for brain stimulation.

In this chapter, we will focus on the treatment of *disorders with oscillatory signatures*. On the one hand, *epilepsy* is characterized by hypersynchronous oscillations stemming from the hyperactivation of one or more foci. Drug-resistant epilepsies represent not only a considerable challenge for the health care system but also a tremendous burden at the individual, family, and community levels. They are characterized by an epileptogenic network (EN) interconnecting distant brain areas located in one of the two hemispheres. There is a large body of evidence suggesting that patient-specific ENs [15] are responsible for the generation and spread of seizures through synchronization processes that interconnect neuronal assemblies with altered excitability [16]. Such networks are the potential targets for therapy. *Depression* manifests alterations in the alpha (~10 Hz) [17–19] and gamma frequency EEG bands [20]. Similarly, patients with *PTSD* also display alterations in the alpha and gamma band, characterized by intrinsic sensory hyperactivity (i.e., suppressed posterior alpha power, localized to the visual cortex—cuneus and precuneus) and increased gamma activity in the prefrontal lobe as compared to patients with generalized anxiety disorder and healthy control subjects [21]. Finally, patients with *schizophrenia* [22, 23] *and autism spectrum disorder (ASD)* [24, 25] as well as neurodegenerative disorders such as *Alzheimer's disease (AD)* and *frontotemporal dementia (FTD)* [26], all present disturbances in the gamma frequency band, with additional involvement of slower frequencies (e.g., theta) and their coupling. These disturbances often manifest themselves in different systems or networks and arise from different neuropathological substrates. Models able to incorporate the complex physiology of the healthy brain—and its variation when pathology arises—are needed to develop disease-modifying therapies.

We discuss below how hybrid models can be used to represent such pathologies to develop *in silico* treatment optimization strategies through the combination of tES and drugs. When informed by the relevant patient data, such models can, for instance, define individual stimulation frequency in tACS, taking into account (1) individual brain anatomy and cortical folding, (2) the location of cortical and subcortical oscillators, (3) cortical columnar organization and the corresponding layer-specific generators for activity in different frequency bands, (4) layer-to-layer interplay supporting cross-frequency coupling (e.g., theta-gamma coupling), (5) distribution/location of inhibitory and excitatory neuronal populations (e.g., GABAergic interneurons targeted via gamma-tACS in the case of AD and Schizophrenia), and many other features currently not accessible via canonical modeling work. Here, we comment on some of the efforts currently being made in this direction, supporting the adoption of hybrid models by the clinical community.

As we will see, the use of HBMs enables what may be called *tES 3.0*, where tES 1.0 refers to the early use of sponges, with bipolar montages and targets defined on electrode space, and tES 2.0 to the current use of multielectrode systems with targets defined by the electrical field on the cortex [27]. tES 3.0 is the unfolding vision of EEG-guided multielectrode systems with personalized hybrid-model-driven targeting and optimization.

24.2 Realistic Physical Modeling of Passive Tissues

The electric field (abbreviated as E-field) induced in the brain by tES is the mechanistic link to the concurrent effects of stimulation [8]. Although some *in vivo* techniques are available to measure the E-field, they either require invasive methods [28, 29] or rely on complex setups, which currently cannot be implemented in any practical manner [30, 31]. The only method currently available to predict the E-field distribution in the brain with a high spatial resolution is numerical modeling of Maxwell's equations in conductive media. Modeling approaches for tES have matured over the last few years, now offering the possibility of generating subject-specific models of the distribution of the E-field in the brain for any montage [13]. These models can also be combined with optimization algorithms, to guide montage design in order to target specific regions or networks more efficiently.

The distribution of the E-field in the head is governed by well-known equations that apply to electrostatic phenomena: the E-field (in units of volts per meter, V/m) can be obtained by taking the gradient of the electrostatic potential (Φ in units of volts, V), which obeys Laplace's equation [32]. These equations can be solved analytically for simple head geometries, like concentric spheres [32], but not for more complex shapes. For the latter, numerical techniques such as the finite element (FE) method—a method that is commonly used in tES E-field calculations [13, 33]—need to be employed.

Different pipelines are available to generate head models and obtain the solution with FE analysis [13, 34, 35], but they all follow essentially the same basic steps (see Fig. 24.3). The first step is creating a realistic geometric representation of the head tissues. This is usually done by relying on structural MRIs of the subjects, which are then segmented into the most important tissues (Fig. 24.3a): scalp, skull (sometimes with representations of air sinuses and separation between spongy and compact bone, [36]), cerebrospinal fluid (CSF, including the ventricles), gray matter (GM), and white matter (WM). Most pipelines rely on at least a T1-weighted MRI, which should not have any type of crop and offer enough neck coverage to guarantee accurate calculations for lower electrode positions [37]. Guidelines for optimizing the MRI sequences for segmentation purposes are available and it is crucial to follow them, as they minimize misclassifications of tissues during segmentation, which can impact E-field predictions [38]. These segmented tissue masks are then used to create triangulated surfaces of the different tissues. The latter renders the tissue interfaces as smooth, which is realistic from an anatomical perspective [39]. In the FE method, this geometry is then further discretized into smaller shapes called finite elements (usually tetrahedra) comprising the finite element mesh. At this stage, realistic representations of the electrodes are also added to the head model [40] (Fig. 24.3a). The FE method calculates Φ within each finite element based on the values at the vertices of the finite elements (nodes of the mesh). The E-field can then be derived from the gradient of Φ. This calculation requires knowledge about the currents in each electrode, as well as the electrical properties of the tissues (Fig. 24.3b). Biological tissues in the low-frequency range (i.e., below 1 kHz) can be represented as linear (ohmic) materials characterized by their electrical conductivity (σ in Siemens per meter, S/m). To date, there is still a wide range of electrical conductivity values reported in literature [41], and their estimation is an active area of research. One important property of the linear nature of biological tissues is that no phase differences arise between the waveform of the injected scalp current (in the case of tACS and tRNS) and that of the E-field in the tissues. This notion has been confirmed in *in-vivo* recordings [28]. Certain tissues, like white matter, have anisotropic conductivity profiles due to

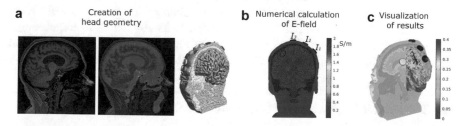

a Creation of head geometry   **b** Numerical calculation of E-field   **c** Visualization of results

Fig. 24.3 Typical steps involved in the creation of a head model for tES calculations. (**a**) Creation of the head model geometry from the anatomical data (T1w-MRI). (**b**) Numerical calculations of the E-field, which requires the specification of the electrical conductivities of each tissue (in units of S/m) and the currents of the electrodes. (**c**) Visualization of the E-field distribution in both the cortical surface (the magnitude of the E-field is shown in the figure, in V/m) and as a vector plot in a coronal slice through the WM and GM. Anodes are shown in red and cathodes in blue

constraints imposed by the alignment of fibers in charge flow in the brain [42]. This can also be included in the model, provided that diffusion-weighted MRIs are available for the subject being modeled [43].

The results of these calculations can be visualized as maps of the spatial distribution of the E-field displayed on the cortical surface (see Fig. 24.3c). Since the E-field is a vector, either the magnitude or a component of the field along a specific direction is normally displayed. Regarding the E-field components, most published studies focus on the component normal to the cortical surface (E_n), which is thought to be the most determinant one to predict the polarization of pyramidal cells, which are aligned perpendicularly to the cortical surface [13, 27, 44]. These field values can also be averaged over cortical patches. Since it is likely that many neurons are affected by the E-field distribution of tES, these surface averaged values may be more appropriate to quantify the effects of a specific montage. In some studies, current density values (J, in units of Ampères per meter squared, A/m^2) are presented, instead of the electric field [45]. This is another vector which, for isotropic tissues, is defined as the product of the electrical conductivity by the electric field vector. The range of values of J (or E) is uncorrelated with the ratio of injected current by the electrode surface area, which is also mistakenly referred to as current density [46].

Computational head models have been used to study the basic properties of the E-field distribution in tES [12, 47], alternative electrode designs [48], or the influence of head lesions in the E-field distribution [49, 50]. These studies usually model the E-field distribution induced by specific montages used in trials in a retrospective manner. In recent years, however, models have also been combined with optimization algorithms to guide montage design [27, 51]. These optimization approaches take as input a target region in which a target E-field value is specified. The optimization algorithm then determines the montage, involving a pool of many electrodes in predefined positions (like the ones of the 10–10 EEG system, [52]) that better approximates the target E-field distribution. These optimization algorithms are typically combined with multichannel montages containing many small electrodes to generate more controllable E-field distributions [12, 47]. The optimization procedure can be conducted in a personalized way, using the computational head models created for each subject in the study. This is particularly important given the considerable intersubject variability in the E-field distribution due to anatomical differences [53]. Optimization-based montage design is ideally suited to target single ROIs as well as distributed brain networks, with the target maps being generated from the functional data, such as resting-state fMRI networks or the EEG data [54].

24.3 Physiological tES Models Across Scales

Since tES, depending on the montage used, can induce an electric field in the brain that can span across several brain regions, it is an absolute requirement to evaluate the effects of this electric field on neural elements. One major challenge is to understand and integrate how tES-induced electric field interacts with brain tissue at different spatial scales, from the single neuron or synapse level, to the large-scale circuit level. Progress on that issue is especially important since understanding the fundamental mechanisms of tES might involve identifying the repercussions from the effects at one level (cellular) to the other (network). A related issue is understanding how an electric field of low magnitude (on the order of 1 V/m) can modulate brain tissue activity despite not being able to induce spiking (see [55] for a review). In order to understand how modulation of activity at the cellular level induces deregulations of oscillatory activity at the network level, which are associated with some neurological disorders, these issues need to be addressed.

At the single-cell level, it has been shown that the tES-induced electric field depolarizes the neuron membrane by approximately 0.2 mV per V/m of the *in situ* electric field [56]. Assuming a maximal value of an *in situ* electric field of 1 V/m, this implies that the membrane of neurons is depolarized by 0.2 mV, which is significantly lower than the depolarization required to induce spiking (on the order of 20 mV). These weak membrane perturbations may be seen to affect the function of dendrites, soma, axon hillock, and axon terminals in different ways. For example, modulation of cell firing patterns will be affected by polarization at the soma and axon hillock, while at axon terminals synaptic release may be affected. A few modeling studies have proposed that such global, weak polarization changes can impact spike timing and phase synchronization in local networks through nonlinear network-amplification effects [57]. Those cellular-scale results have direct implications to understand tES effects: spike timing is indeed crucial in the induction of synaptic plasticity changes, for example, through the Spike Timing Dependent Plasticity (STDP) rule [58]. It has been suggested that changes in spike timing of a few milliseconds, accumulated over several minutes, might induce gradual changes in synaptic weights due to the properties and asymmetry of the STDP rule, in line with the reported lasting effects of tES [59]. Furthermore, phase synchronization of firing in networks is a more subtle, but important effect, since it may explain changes in the amplitude of spontaneous, endogenous oscillations following tES [60]. Increasing/decreasing the phase synchronization of spiking from numerous neurons would result in an increase/decrease of the endogenous oscillation by modulation of coherence. Interestingly, support for this idea has emerged from experimental recordings in animals and humans [61–63].

A few studies have also investigated the brain-scale effects of tES. For example, a modeling study investigating the effects of alpha-frequency tES on simulated whole-brain activity and associated scalp EEG [64], pointed at a maximal effect of tES when the stimulation frequency was the same as the endogenous oscillation (alpha frequency), with an effect rapidly fading when the difference between the endogenous and stimulation frequencies increased. Therefore, one challenge and opportunity of tES seems that it can only modulate endogenous oscillations (and not induce *de novo* activity, since tES cannot induce spiking), possibly by matching the stimulation frequency close to the endogenous frequency and entraining activity. This could greatly improve the design of tES by targeting specific rhythms associated with the desired function. Overall, it appears that candidate mechanisms of tES have been identified at several scales, which could explain at least partly the reported effects in animals and humans. However, a unified model of the tES mechanism is still lacking, a major challenge that could be addressed through the use of hybrid brain models (HBMs), which are reviewed in the next section.

24.4   The Architecture of HBMs

Today, model-driven optimization for multichannel transcranial stimulation is based on the physical features of the subject's brain, such as head geometry (extracted from MRI images) and tissue conductivities, as mentioned in previous sections. Nevertheless, there is a clear need to expand the horizon of optimization to more sophisticated models that also represent physiological information of the subject. In this section, we will explain how to combine the physical and physiological data of the individual brain in order to create a personalized computational model and design more refined personalized optimization strategies—in other words, how to design a Hybrid Brain Model.

In the framework where the brain is represented as a network, coupled mathematical differential equations (either ordinary or partial) can be used to describe the spatiotemporal dynamics of brain activity and traveling waves [65], at the level of one node or of larger-scale networks, corresponding to multiple coupled nodes. Traditionally, two main classes of models have been used to derive these differential equations. On the one hand, spiking neuron models such as the Hodgkin-Huxley model [66] describe the detailed dynamics of individual neurons. On the other hand, neural mass models (NMMs) such as the Wilson-Cowan model [67] provide effective theories of neural systems. The former, a more detailed class of models, is appropriate for representing single-cell recordings in animals or brain slices, but their state variables do not directly—at least without very large computational demands—capture the functional activity recorded with macroscopic level techniques such as Electroencephalography (EEG), Magnetoencephalography (MEG) or mesoscopic Local Field Potential (LFP) measurements. In contrast, NMMs are more useful for modeling brain activity at larger spatial and temporal scales, since they describe the mean activity of whole neural populations. While providing a lower level of detail, their parameters emerge from microscopically measurable quantities, such as dendritic time constants and mean excitatory/inhibitory postsynaptic potentials, and they are able to represent the physiology of the brain as observed by macroscale measurements.

An *HBM* is essentially a *physically-situated network* in which NMMs constitute the *nodes*. Depending on the data available or the scale of the model, network nodes can represent either single columns, cortical patches, or whole-brain areas (see the extended review by Breakspear [68] for a detailed discussion on the choices of dynamical equations). Accordingly, network edges or *links* are needed to describe appropriately the links between nodes. For example, to model whole-brain dynamics [67], coupling strength is often defined in proportion to the number of white matter tracts (structural connectivity) between brain areas using the well-known human connectome [69]. However, functional or effective connectivity can also be used to define these links [70–72].

As mentioned above, one of the advantages of HBMs is that they can make a connection with macroscopic measurements. For example, the activity of NMM nodes in the HBM can be used to simulate cortical dipole source activity field $J(x,t)$, where x denotes a cortical source location and t, time. Since the NMM network is embedded in a known physical matrix that describes its electrical characteristics, the dipole field can be mapped to *EEG* electrode space activity using the "lead field" forward map [64, 73, 74]. Similar methods can, in principle, be used to model *MEG* or *fMRI*. The effects of *tES* can be represented on the grounds of known or hypothesized interaction mechanisms. The *lambda-E* model [8, 27, 64, 75, 76], for example, posits that the main effect of tES is to modulate the polarization of pyramidal cells in a manner proportional to the electric field component parallel to the cells' main axis (from apex to soma). Similarly, TMS's effects are assumed to be mostly due to electric field magnitude and are known to cause neuron spiking from strong depolarization. All these effects are readily represented in an NMM and, in consequence, in a HBM. All that is required is to calculate the electric field on the realistic head model. The effects of *drugs* on neurons can also be represented if their physiological mechanisms are known [77, 78]. For example, in the case of antiepileptic drugs [79], some molecules decrease the excitability of pyramidal cells (e.g., voltage-gated sodium channel blockers such as carbamazepine, or voltage-gated calcium channel blocker such as Zonisamide) or modulate cellular connectivity (GABA-A enhancers such as Clobazam, or NMDA antagonists such as Felbamate). HBMs can also represent network *plasticity* and the plastic impact of tES [76]. Plastic phenomena can be adapted in these models by encoding known Hebbian mechanisms ("cells that fire together, wire together, cells that fire apart, wire apart") such as BCM or Oja's rules [80]. To first order, their implementation will include the change connectivity constants within the NMM nodes (local scale) as a function of the history of the activity of the model, across them (large network or structural scale), or both. Other parameters can be modified as well.

The *personalization* of a model starts by using individual MRI (anatomy) and DTI (connectivity) data (see Fig. 24.4). DTI and MRI are used to connect the NMMs, to have information about physiological connections, anatomy, and physical distance between brain regions, and to represent macroscale electrical phenomena. Bansal et al. [81] and Aerts et al. [82] review recent research on personalized whole-brain models. The former is related to the study of structure-function relationship in human brains, while the latter focuses on the impact of network lesions. The majority of the studies cited in these reviews only use the structural connectivity brain data derived from DTI to personalize whole-brain models. Moreover, most of the models in those studies are based on static model parameters, failing to reproduce some meaningful features on individual brain dynamics.

Crucially, since they can be used to simulate and predict measurements, in addition to the structural data, HBMs can ingest physiological measurements (e.g., EEG, SEEG, fMRI, and EN)—much as weather or climate models do. Physiological data are used to adjust the desired parameters of the model. The most currently used approaches fit the data in the form of Functional Connectivity (FC) profile between regions [73, 83], but others can be used. That is, parameters are adjusted so that

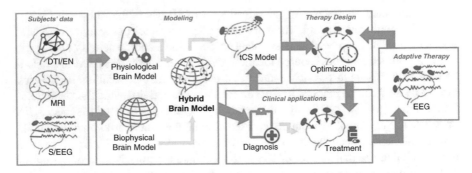

Fig. 24.4 Workflow for the creation of hybrid-model-driven tES optimization. The DTI and anatomical MRI data are combined to create a finite element biophysical model (FEM), which is then personalized using EEG and/or SEEG (S/EEG), EN, and other data to reflect both biophysical and physiologic characteristics—from excitation/inhibition balance to plastic potential (long-term effect physiological model). The personalized hybrid brain model can be used to generate EEG and to simulate the effects of brain stimulation. As a result, personalized diagnosis and treatment can be applied, such as optimized stimulation protocols. Since tES protocols are typically multisession, the EEG data collected over time (e.g., at patient's home, using telemedical solutions) can be used to refine models and adapt the stimulation protocols (target map, dosing)

model generated FC across cortical regions matches that inferred from dense EEG measurements (after cortical mapping, see [73] and [5], for example). More specifically, the EEG data can be processed to extract functional connectivity from the power envelope in a given frequency band [74, 75], which can then be matched with NMM activity at each parcel [73].

24.5   Tailoring and Adapting Interventions

As we have seen, today, tES montages are optimized on the assumption that the effects can be directly quantified from the knowledge of the electric field on the cortex. For example, a neurologist may want to reduce the excitability of a brain region under the assumption that this will lead to beneficial plastic network effects. In order to do so, it suffices to demand for the electric field to be adequately intense and properly oriented with respect to the cortical surface (pointing out, to be specific). However, such an approach ignores the complexity of nonlinear network interactions associated with brain physiology. *Specifying a target function* in such a manner is equivalent to making crucial assumptions about mechanisms and cascade effects at the system level. A more natural way of doing so would be to simply state "I want to disconnect this node from this network" in an epileptic patient, for example, or "I would like to increase gamma activity in these regions" (in AD, for example), and let a physiologically grounded algorithm take care of the analysis and solution. This is the vision of hybrid modeling: helping the clinician focus on the causes of the disease, presumably at the connectivity (micro or macro) level, and finding a computational grounded solution. Moreover, accurate modeling combined with regular patient monitoring, big data, and artificial intelligence approaches could pave the way for "adaptive therapeutics", where the individual patient data are used to refine tES parameters on a daily/weekly/monthly basis (see Fig. 24.4). Future implementations of hybrid models may allow the prediction of structural/functional brain changes induced by a given therapy, and, combined with the incoming patient data, "correct" the therapeutic trajectory accordingly.

From the large body of evidence that is accumulating regarding the effects of tES on brain activity, some possibilities of *future developments of this technique are emerging*. Since dynamic tES appears to mediate its effects mainly on endogenous rhythms, by matching the stimulation frequency with those endogenous rhythms, one possibility would be to characterize the function to be targeted in terms of associated neural oscillations. This would provide the temporal characteristics of the stimulation to be applied. To go further, mapping the functional network associated with the targeted function, and deriving corresponding multi-site tES montages through hybrid models, would provide the spatial characteristics of the stimulation protocol. By combining both types of information, tES could provide a spatiotemporal modulation of function-specific neuronal activity. That being said, what are the neurological disorders that could benefit the most from this "tES 3.0" strategy? First of all, conditions where the pattern of altered metabolic/functional activity is widespread—such as dementias in primis. In the case of Alzheimer's disease, multi-site tES could be optimized to tackle hypometabolic regions [84], areas affected by amyloid and tau deposition [85], as well as nodes of mostly affected brain functional networks (e.g., default mode network) [86]. Moreover, recent evidence points toward specific alterations of high-frequency activity within the gamma band, involving dysfunction of GABAergic parvalbumin (PV+) inhibitory interneurons. This specific neurophysiological substrate requires, among other aspects, the optimization of stimulation solutions able to entrain gamma activity, and potentially do so by leveraging cross-frequency coupling dynamics [87], or via precise modeling of the interaction between PV+ cell(s) and pyramidal cells (PV+ ↔ PV+ inhibition circuit, PV+ ↔ pyramidal cell circuit). A hybrid model accounting for such circuitry could suggest different simulation solutions based on the proportion of residual interneurons and pyramidal cells, which might differ across regions (due to protein deposit and atrophy) and disease state.

Differently, psychiatric conditions not involving neurodegeneration tend to present a more local pattern of alteration, such as in the case of subgenual and prefrontal lobe changes in depression and cerebellar-prefrontal changes in schizophrenia. However, even though alterations might be more focal, other disease-specific factors come into place and make novel tES solutions equally needed. For instance, differential alterations of prefrontal GABA-A and GABA-B circuitry have been documented in schizophrenia, suggesting future therapeutic interventions to focus more on modulation of GABA-B dynamics for optimal cognitive remediation [88]. While such neurotransmitter-level targeted modulation is more intuitive for drug-based interventions, hybrid tES models accounting for intracolumnar dynamics could eventually identify cell-class specific targets and the corresponding optimal therapies.

24.6 Conclusions

By using hybrid models to represent brain activity and the impact of tES, better optimization algorithms can be developed. This methodology is widely applicable beyond tES to other brain stimulation modalities. By forcing the field to quantify mechanisms and etiology in computational models, advanced algorithms can provide novel and powerful solutions. At the same time, technological advances provide more tolerable and flexible experimental protocols. Already today, hybrid, wireless tES/EEG systems allow for the recording of EEG signals and stimulation using the same system and the same electrodes. Both for basic and clinical research applications, tES studies typically involve multiple stimulation sessions, because the effects of tES are cumulative. For this reason, the field benefits from the existence of controlled and safe home deployment solutions, allowing subjects to participate in studies without the need to visit the research lab or hospital on multiple occasions. The same solutions, collecting EEG and allowing for remote protocol modifications, will eventually provide the means for adaptive interventions in telemedicine.

References

1. Price CJ, Moore CJ, Humphreys GW, Frackowiak RSJ, Friston KJ. The neural regions sustaining object recognition and naming. Proc R Soc Lond Ser B Biol Sci. 1996;263(1376):1501–7.
2. Fox MD, Halko MA, Eldaief MC, Pascual-Leone A. Measuring and manipulating brain connectivity with resting state functional connectivity magnetic resonance imaging (fcMRI) and transcranial magnetic stimulation (TMS). Neuroimage. 2012;62(4):2232–43.
3. Fox MD, Buckner RL, White MP, Greicius MD, Pascual-Leone A. Efficacy of transcranial magnetic stimulation targets for depression is related to intrinsic functional connectivity with the subgenual cingulate. Biol Psychiatry. 2012;72:595–603.
4. Fornito A, Zalesky A, Breakspear M. The connectomics of brain disorders. Nat Rev Neurosci. 2015;16(3):159–72.
5. RuffiniRuffini G, Wendling F, Sanchez-Todo R, Santarnecchi E. Targeting brain networks with multichannel transcranial current stimulation (tCS). Curr Opin in Biomed Eng. 2018;8:70–7.
6. Antal A, Alekseichuk I, Bikson M, Brockmöller J, Brunoni AR, Chen R, et al. Low intensity transcranial electric stimulation: safety, ethical, legal regulatory and application guidelines. Clin Neurophysiol. 2017;128(9):1774–809.
7. Nitsche MA, Paulus W. Excitability changes induced in the human motor cortex by weak transcranial direct current stimulation. J Physiol. 2000;527(Pt 3):633–9.
8. Ruffini G, Wendling F, Merlet I, Molaee-Ardekani B, Mekkonen A, Salvador R, et al. Transcranial current brain stimulation (tCS): models and technologies. IEEE Trans Neural Syst Rehabil Eng. 2013;21(3):333–45.
9. Kammer T, Beck S, Thielscher A, Laubis-Herrmann U, Topka H. Motor thresholds in humans: a transcranial magnetic stimulation study comparing different pulse waveforms, current directions and stimulator types. Clin Neurophysiol. 2001;112:250–8.
10. Peterchev AV, Rosa MA, Deng Z-D, Prudic J, Lisanby SH. ECT Stimulus Parameters: Rethinking Dosage. J ECT. 2010 Sep;26(3):159–74.
11. Peterchev AV, Wagner TA, Miranda PC, Nitsche MA, Paulus W, Lisanby SH, et al. Fundamentals of Transcranial Electric and Magnetic Stimulation Dose: Definition, Selection, and Reporting Practices. Brain Stimul. 2012 Oct;5(4):435–53.

12. Miranda PC, Mekonnen A, Salvador R, Ruffini G. The electric field in the cortex during transcranial current stimulation. Neuroimage. 2013;70:45–58.
13. Miranda PC, Mekonnen A, Salvador R, Ruffini G. The electric field in the cortex during transcranial current stimulation. Neuroimage. 2013;70:45–58.
14. Lefaucheur J-P, Antal A, Ayache SS, Benninger DH, Brunelin J, Cogiamanian F, et al. Evidence-based guidelines on the therapeutic use of transcranial direct current stimulation (tDCS). Clin Neurophysiol. 2017 Jan;128(1):56–92.
15. Bartolomei F, Lagarde S, Wendling F, McGonigal A, Jirsa V, Guye M, et al. Defining epileptogenic networks: contribution of SEEG and signal analysis. Epilepsia. 2017;58(7):1131–47.
16. Wendling F, Bartolomei F, Mina F, Huneau C, Benquet P. Interictal spikes, fast ripples and seizures in partial epilepsies--combining multi-level computational models with experimental data. Eur J Neurosci. 2012;36(2):2164–77.
17. Iosifescu DV. Electroencephalography-derived biomarkers of antidepressant response. Harv Rev Psychiatry. 2011;19(3):144–54.
18. Nyström C, Matousek M, Hällström T. Relationships between EEG and clinical characteristics in major depressive disorder. Acta Psychiatr Scand. 1986;73(4):390–4.
19. Baskaran A, Milev R, McIntyre RS. The neurobiology of the EEG biomarker as a predictor of treatment response in depression. Neuropharmacology. 2012;63(4):507–13.
20. Fitzgerald PJ, Watson BO. Gamma oscillations as a biomarker for major depression: an emerging topic. Transl Psychiatry. 2018;8(1):177.
21. Clancy K, Ding M, Bernat E, Schmidt NB, Li W. Restless 'rest': intrinsic sensory hyperactivity and disinhibition in post-traumatic stress disorder. Brain. 2017;140(7):2041–50.
22. Kirihara K, Rissling AJ, Swerdlow NR, Braff DL, Light GA. Hierarchical organization of gamma and theta oscillatory dynamics in schizophrenia. Biol Psychiatry. 2012;71(10):873–80.
23. Senkowski D, Gallinat J. Dysfunctional prefrontal gamma-band oscillations reflect working memory and other cognitive deficits in schizophrenia. Biol Psychiatry. 2015;77:1010–9.
24. van Diessen E, Senders J, Jansen FE, Boersma M, Bruining H. Increased power of resting-state gamma oscillations in autism spectrum disorder detected by routine electroencephalography. Eur Arch Psychiatry Clin Neurosci. 2015;265(6):537–40.
25. Sun L, Grützner C, Bölte S, Wibral M, Tozman T, Schlitt S, et al. Impaired gamma-band activity during perceptual organization in adults with autism spectrum disorders: evidence for dysfunctional network activity in frontal-posterior cortices. J Neurosci. 2012;32(28):9563–73.
26. Palop JJ, Mucke L. Network abnormalities and interneuron dysfunction in Alzheimer disease. Nat Rev Neurosci. 2016;17(12):777–92.
27. Ruffini G, Fox MD, Ripolles O, Miranda PC, Pascual-Leone A. Optimization of multifocal transcranial current stimulation for weighted cortical pattern targeting from realistic modeling of electric fields. Neuroimage. 2014;89:216–25.
28. Opitz A, Falchier A, Yan CG, Yeagle EM, Linn GS, Megevand P, et al. Spatiotemporal structure of intracranial electric fields induced by transcranial electric stimulation in humans and nonhuman primates. Sci Rep. 2016;6:31236.
29. Huang Y, Liu AA, Lafon B, Friedman D, Dayan M, Wang X, et al. Measurements and models of electric fields in the in vivo human brain during transcranial electric stimulation. eLife. 2017;6:e18834.
30. Göksu C, Hanson LG, Siebner HR, Ehses P, Scheffler K, Thielscher A. Human in-vivo brain magnetic resonance current density imaging (MRCDI). Neuroimage. 2018;171:26–39.
31. Kasinadhuni AK, Indahlastari A, Chauhan M, Schär M, Mareci TH, Sadleir RJ. Imaging of current flow in the human head during transcranial electrical therapy. Brain Stimul. 2017;10(4):764–72.
32. Rush S, Driscoll DA. EEG electrode sensitivity - an application of reciprocity. IEEE Trans Biomed Eng. 1969;16:15.
33. Johnson CR. Computational and numerical methods for bioelectric field problems. Crit Rev Biomed Eng. 1997;25:1–81.

34. Huang Y, Datta A, Bikson M, Parra LC. Realistic volumetric-approach to simulate transcranial electric stimulation—ROAST—a fully automated open-source pipeline. J Neural Eng. 2019;16(5):056006.
35. Saturnino GB, Puonti O, Nielsen JD, Antonenko D, Madsen KHH, Thielscher A. SimNIBS 2.1: a comprehensive pipeline for individualized electric field modelling for transcranial brain stimulation. bioRxiv. 2018;500314.
36. Opitz A, Paulus W, Will S, Antunes A, Thielscher A. Determinants of the electric field during transcranial direct current stimulation. Neuroimage. 2015;109:140–50.
37. Huang Y, Parra LC, Haufe S. The New York Head-a precise standardized volume conductor model for EEG source localization and tES targeting. NeuroImage [Internet]. 140. Available from: internal-pdf://100.120.191.80/NeuroImage_(_)2015p_.pdf http://www.ncbi.nlm.nih.gov/pubmed/26706450.
38. Windhoff M, Opitz A, Thielscher A. Electric field calculations in brain stimulation based on finite elements: an optimized processing pipeline for the generation and usage of accurate individual head models. Hum Brain Mapp. 2013;34:923–35.
39. Bikson M, Rahman A, Datta A. Computational models of transcranial direct current stimulation. Clin EEG Neurosci. 2012;43:176–83.
40. Saturnino GB, Antunes A, Thielscher A. On the importance of electrode parameters for shaping electric field patterns generated by tDCS. Neuroimage. 2015;120:25–35.
41. Wagner T, Eden U, Rushmore J, Russo CJ, Dipietro L, Fregni F, et al. Impact of brain tissue filtering on neurostimulation fields: a modeling study. Neuroimage. 2014;85(Pt 3):1048–57.
42. Gullmar D, Haueisen J, Reichenbach JR. Influence of anisotropic electrical conductivity in white matter tissue on the EEG/MEG forward and inverse solution. A high-resolution whole head simulation study. Neuroimage. 2010;51:145–63.
43. Opitz A, Windhoff M, Heidemann RM, Turner R, Thielscher A. How the brain tissue shapes the electric field induced by transcranial magnetic stimulation. Neuroimage. 2011;58:849–59.
44. Ruffini G, Fox MD, Ripolles O, Miranda PC, Pascual-Leone A. Optimization of multifocal transcranial current stimulation for weighted cortical pattern targeting from realistic modeling of electric fields. Neuroimage. 2014;89:216–25.
45. Kammer T, Vorwerg M, Herrnberger B. Anisotropy in the visual cortex investigated by neuro-navigated transcranial magnetic stimulation. Neuroimage. 2007;36:313–21.
46. Neuling T, Wagner S, Wolters CH, Zaehle T, Herrmann CS. Finite-element model predicts current density distribution for clinical applications of tDCS and tACS. Front Psych. 2012;3:83.
47. Miranda PC, Faria P, Hallett M. What does the ratio of injected current to electrode area tell us about current density in the brain during tDCS? Clin Neurophysiol. 2009;120:1183–7.
48. Salvador R, Wenger C, Miranda PC. Investigating the cortical regions involved in MEP modulation in tDCS. Front Cell Neurosci [Internet]. 2015;9. Available from: internal-pdf://80.246.106.242/FrontCellNeurosci9(_)2015pp.pdf http://www.frontiersin.org/Journal/Abstract.aspx?s=156&name=cellular_neuroscience&ART_DOI=10.3389/fncel.2015.00405.
49. Datta A, Bansal V, Diaz J, Patel J, Reato D, Bikson M. Gyri-precise head model of transcranial direct current stimulation: Improved spatial focality using a ring electrode versus conventional rectangular pad. Brain Stimul. 2009;2:201–7.
50. Datta A, Bikson M, Fregni F. Transcranial direct current stimulation in patients with skull defects and skull plates: high-resolution computational FEM study of factors altering cortical current flow. Neuroimage. 2010;52:1268–78.
51. Datta A, Baker JM, Bikson M, Fridriksson J. Individualized model predicts brain current flow during transcranial direct-current stimulation treatment in responsive stroke patient. Brain Stimul. 2011;4:6.
52. Dmochowski JP, Datta A, Bikson M, Su YZ, Parra LC. Optimized multi-electrode stimulation increases focality and intensity at target. J Neural Eng [Internet]. 2011;8. Available from: internal-pdf://0293331575/JNeuralEng8(4)2011p46011.pdf.
53. Jurcak V, Tsuzuki D, Dan I. 10/20, 10/10, and 10/5 systems revisited: their validity as relative head-surface-based positioning systems. Neuroimage. 2007;34:1600–11.
54. Laakso I, Tanaka S, Koyama S, De Santis V, Hirata A. Inter-subject variability in electric fields of motor cortical tDCS. Brain Stimul. 2015;8:906–13.

55. Fischer DB, Fried PJ, Ruffini G, Ripolles O, Salvador R, Banus J, et al. Multifocal tDCS targeting the resting state motor network increases cortical excitability beyond traditional tDCS targeting unilateral motor cortex. Neuroimage. 2017;157:34–44.
56. Radman T, Ramos RL, Brumberg JC, Bikson M. Role of cortical cell type and morphology in subthreshold and suprathreshold uniform electric field stimulation in vitro. Brain Stimul. 2009;2(215):28.
57. Reato D, Rahman A, Bikson M, Parra LC. Low-intensity electrical stimulation affects network dynamics by modulating population rate and spike timing. J Neurosci. 2010;30(45):15067–79.
58. Gerstner W, Kempter R, van Hemmen JL, Wagner H. A neuronal learning rule for sub-millisecond temporal coding. Nature. 1996;383(6595):76–81.
59. Modolo J, Thomas AW, Legros A. Possible mechanisms of synaptic plasticity modulation by extremely low-frequency magnetic fields. Electromagn Biol Med. 2013;32(2):137–44.
60. Schmidt SL, Iyengar AK, Foulser AA, Boyle MR, Fröhlich F. Endogenous cortical oscillations constrain neuromodulation by weak electric fields. Brain Stimul. 2014;7(6):878–89.
61. Fresnoza S, Christova M, Feil T, Gallasch E, Körner C, Zimmer U, et al. The effects of transcranial alternating current stimulation (tACS) at individual alpha peak frequency (iAPF) on motor cortex excitability in young and elderly adults. Exp Brain Res. 2018;236(10):2573–88.
62. Vossen A, Gross J, Thut G. Alpha power increase after transcranial alternating current stimulation at alpha frequency (α-tACS) reflects plastic changes rather than entrainment. Brain Stimul. 2015;8(3):499–508.
63. Reato D, Rahman A, Bikson M, Parra LC. Effects of weak transcranial alternating current stimulation on brain activity—a review of known mechanisms from animal studies. Front Hum Neurosci [Internet]. 2013 [cited 2019 Sep 13];7. Available from: http://journal.frontiersin.org/article/10.3389/fnhum.2013.00687/abstract.
64. Merlet I, Birot G, Salvador R, Molaee-Ardekani B, Mckonnen A, Soria-Frish A, et al. From oscillatory transcranial current stimulation to scalp eeg changes: a biophysical and physiological modeling study. PLoS One [Internet]. 2013.; Available from: http://www.scopus.com/inward/record.url?eid=2-s2.0-84874530177&partnerID=MN8TOARS.
65. Coombes S. Waves, bumps, and patterns in neural field theories. Biol Cybern. 2005;93(2):91–108.
66. Hodgkin AL, Huxley AF. A quantitative description of membrane current and its application to conduction and excitation in nerve. Bull Math Biol. 1990;52(1–2):25–71.
67. Wilson HR, Cowan JD. Excitatory and Inhibitory interactions in localized populations of model neurons. Biophys J. 1972;12(1):1–24.
68. Breakspear M. Dynamic models of large-scale brain activity. Nat Neurosci. 2017;20(3):340–52.
69. Hagmann P, Kurant M, Gigandet X, Thiran P, Wedeen VJ, Meuli R, et al. Mapping human whole-brain structural networks with diffusion MRI. PLoS One. 2007;2(7):e597.
70. Bassett DS, Bullmore ET. Human brain networks in health and disease. Curr Opin Neurol. 2009;22(4):340–7.
71. Feldt S, Bonifazi P, Cossart R. Dissecting functional connectivity of neuronal microcircuits: experimental and theoretical insights. Trends Neurosci. 2011;34(5):225–36.
72. Bassett DS, Sporns O. Network neuroscience. Nat Neurosci. 2017;20(3):353–64.
73. Sanchez-Todo R, Salvador R, Santarnecchi E, Wendling F, Deco G, Ruffini G. Personalization of hybrid brain models from neuroimaging and electrophysiology data. BioRxiv. 2018.
74. Ruffini G. Application of the reciprocity theorem to EEG inversion and optimization of EEG-driven transcranial current stimulation (tCS, including tDCS, tACS, tRNS). arXiv. 2015;29(2013):1–11.
75. Molaee-Ardekani B, Márquez-Ruiz J, Merlet I, Leal-Campanario R, Gruart A, Sánchez-Campusano R, et al. Effects of transcranial Direct Current Stimulation (tDCS) on cortical activity: a computational modeling study. Brain Stimul. 2013;6:25–39.
76. Lefaucheur J-P, Wendling F. Mechanisms of action of tDCS: a brief and practical overview. /data/revues/09877053/unassign/S0987705319301790/ [Internet]. 2019 24 [cited 2019 Oct 1]; Available from: https://www.em-consulte.com/en/article/1306771.

77. Liang Z, Duan X, Su C, Voss L, Sleigh J, Li X. A pharmacokinetics-neural mass model (PK-NMM) for the simulation of EEG activity during propofol anesthesia. PLoS One. 2015;10(12):1–21.
78. Kurbatova P, Wendling F, Kaminska A, Rosati A, Nabbout R, Guerrini R, et al. Dynamic changes of depolarizing GABA in a computational model of epileptogenic brain: insight for Dravet syndrome. Exp Neurol. 2016;283(Pt A):57–72.
79. Goldenberg MM. Overview of drugs used for epilepsy and seizures. P T. 2010;35(7):392–415.
80. Dayan P, Abbott LF. Theoretical neuroscience: computational and mathematical modeling of neural systems. Cambridge: The MIT Press; 2005.
81. Bansal K, Nakuci J, Muldoon SF. Personalized brain network models for assessing structure-function relationships. Curr Opin Neurobiol. 2018;52:42–7.
82. Aerts H, Fias W, Caeyenberghs K, Marinazzo D. Brain networks under attack: robustness properties and the impact of lesions. Brain. 2016;139(Pt 12):3063–83.
83. Cabral J, Luckhoo H, Woolrich M, Joensson M, Mohseni H, Baker A, et al. Exploring mechanisms of spontaneous functional connectivity in MEG: how delayed network interactions lead to structured amplitude envelopes of band-pass filtered oscillations. Neuroimage. 2014;90:423–35.
84. Marchitelli R, Aiello M, Cachia A, Quarantelli M, Cavaliere C, Postiglione A, et al. Simultaneous resting-state FDG-PET/fMRI in Alzheimer disease: relationship between glucose metabolism and intrinsic activity. Neuroimage. 2018;176:246–58.
85. Villemagne VL, Doré V, Burnham SC, Masters CL, Rowe CC. Imaging tau and amyloid-β proteinopathies in Alzheimer disease and other conditions. Nat Rev Neurol. 2018;14(4):225–36.
86. Sepulcre J, Sabuncu MR, Li Q, Fakhri GE, Sperling R, Johnson KA. Tau and amyloid β proteins distinctively associate to functional network changes in the aging brain. Alzheimers Dement. 2017;13(11):1261–9.
87. Canolty RT, Edwards E, Dalal SS, Soltani M, Nagarajan SS, Kirsch HE, et al. High gamma power is phase-locked to theta oscillations in human neocortex. Science. 2006;313(5793):1626–8.
88. Farzan F, Barr MS, Levinson AJ, Chen R, Wong W, Fitzgerald PB, et al. Evidence for gamma inhibition deficits in the dorsolateral prefrontal cortex of patients with schizophrenia. Brain. 2010;133(5):1505–14.

Printed in the United States
by Baker & Taylor Publisher Services